Biomedical Visualization

Volume 5

Series Editor

Paul M. Rea, Anatomy Facility, School of Medicine, Dentistry and Nursing, College of Medical, Veterinary and Life Sciences, University of Glasgow, Glasgow, UK

The Biomedical Visualization book series invites contributions related to visualization and imaging in the biomedical sciences and related fields such as medicine, dentistry, veterinary surgery, informatics, and the allied health professions.

This can encompass work in image analysis, workflow methodologies, photogrammetry in science, animations, digital reconstructions and applications, big data and visualizations, educational methodologies, usability and evaluations, augmented and virtual reality, and 3D and 4D technologies, including 3D printing, as well as informatics, e-tutorials, MOOCs, HCI and public engagement. It can be from macroscopic to microscopic but show how we can view data and information related to the biomedical field in a much more accessible, innovative and engaging way using technology.

This series is intended for researchers, clinicians, students, and teaching staff in biomedical and medical schools who use and develop visualization and imaging techniques in medical education, patient care, and biomedical and medical research.

Jenny Clancy • Matthieu Poyade
Editors

Medical Visualization and Applications of Technology – Volume 2

Springer

Editors
Jenny Clancy
School of Medicine, Dentistry and Nursing
University of Glasgow
Glasgow, UK

Matthieu Poyade
School of Innovation and Technology
Glasgow School of Art
Glasgow, UK

ISSN 2731-6130 ISSN 2731-6149 (electronic)
Biomedical Visualization
ISBN 978-3-031-63462-8 ISBN 978-3-031-63463-5 (eBook)
https://doi.org/10.1007/978-3-031-63463-5

Cover Illustration: Catherine MacRobbie.

This Springer imprint is published by the registered company Springer Nature Switzerland AG
The registered company address is: Gewerbestrasse 11, 6330 Cham, Switzerland

Preface

This book features the innovative research projects of graduates of the MSc Medical Visualisation and Human Anatomy programme. This unique postgraduate taught programme is offered jointly by University of Glasgow and The Glasgow School of Art and is accredited by the Institute of Medical Illustrators. This collaborative approach allows students to study anatomy at the Anatomy Facility at the University of Glasgow while also learning how to perform digital reconstruction of human anatomy, at the School of Innovation and Technology, The Glasgow School of Art. Students also learn how to design and develop engaging and interactive digital user-experiences in the field of life sciences. By the end of the programme students have obtained the skills to create realistic and anatomically accurate 3D digital representations of the human body and can incorporate these into online or mobile applications, animations and/or Extended Reality for use in medical education, simulation and training.

The 10 chapters included in this book detail the range of techniques, tools and methodologies used to create a variety of applications. Chapters 1–6 are based on the use of Extended Reality to enhance education and training of health professionals or to facilitate public engagement. These Extended Reality projects include the use of Augmented Reality to train paramedics in ECG interpretation in collaboration with the Scottish Ambulance Service (Chap. 1) and to enhance paediatric surgery in collaboration with the Royal Hospital for Children (Chap. 4). The potential of Virtual Reality was investigated in surgical planning or training in Chaps. 2, 5 and 6. In addition, a novel virtual reality app presenting a 10m long interactive muscle cell was developed to facilitate public engagement (Chap. 3).

The potential of online interactive 3D animation was investigated as a potential method to educate parents/carers about vertebral fractures in juvenile osteoporosis (Chap. 7) and to enhance education of doctors in Indonesia in cerebral angiogram interpretation (Chap. 8). Lastly, gamification approaches were utilised to improve public understanding of schistosome infection (Chap. 9) and to provide a revision tool for students learning about cranial nerves (Chap. 10).

The diversity of the methods used and applications produced showcase the range of potential uses for these technologies in medical education, simulation and training. Furthermore, these chapters also include evaluations of the applications, adding to the growing evidence supporting the incorporation of digital technologies into medical education and training.

Glasgow, UK Jenny Clancy
Glasgow, UK Matthieu Poyade

Contents

Editors and Contributors

About the Series Editor

Paul M. Rea Paul M. Rea is Professor of Digital and Anatomical Education at University of Glasgow. He is Director of Innovation, Engagement and Enterprise within the School of Medicine, Dentistry and Nursing. He is also a Senate Assessor for Student Conduct, Council Member on Senate and coordinates the day-to-day running of the Body Donor Programme and is a Licenced Teacher of Anatomy, licenced by the Scottish Government.

He is qualified with a medical degree (MBChB), an MSc (by research) in craniofacial anatomy/surgery, a PhD in neuroscience, Diploma in Forensic Medical Science (DipFMS), and an MEd with Merit (Learning and Teaching in Higher Education). He is a Senior Fellow of the Higher Education Academy, Fellow of the Institute of Medical Illustrators (FIMI) and a registered medical illustrator with the Academy for Healthcare Science.

Paul has published widely and presented at many national and international meetings, including invited talks. He is the Series Editor for Biomedical Visualisation's 21 published volumes and is the founding editor for this book series. This has resulted in over 155K downloads across these volumes, with contributions from over 430 different authors, across 133 institutions from 24 countries across the globe. These volumes are read in 75 countries and have over 765 citations and 472 social media mentions. He is Associate Editor for the European Journal of Anatomy and has reviewed for 25 different journals/publishers. He is a Public Engagement and Outreach lead coordinating collaborative projects with the Glasgow Science Centre, NHS and Royal College of Physicians and Surgeons of Glasgow. Paul is also a STEM ambassador and has visited numerous schools to undertake outreach work.

His research involves a long-standing strategic partnership with the School of Simulation and Visualisation, The Glasgow School of Art. This has led to multi-million pound investment in creating world leading 3D digital datasets to be used in undergraduate and postgraduate teaching to enhance learning and assessment. This successful collaboration resulted in the creation of the world's first taught MSc Medical Visualisation and Human Anatomy combining anatomy and digital technologies for which he was the Founding Director having previously managed the degree for 12 years since its inception. The

Institute of Medical Illustrators also accredits it. It has created college-wide, industry, multi-institutional and NHS research linked projects for students.

About the Editors

Jenny Clancy is a lecturer in anatomy at the University of Glasgow and is the postgraduate lead for anatomy. She is also the programme director of the Medical Visualisation and Human Anatomy MSc, delivered jointly with The Glasgow School of Art and accredited by the Institute of Medical Illustrators (IMI). Jenny is a council member of the British Association of Clinical Anatomists and is assistant editor for the journal Clinical Anatomy.

Jenny obtained a degree in Anatomy (BSc Hons, first class) from University of Glasgow and an MSc in Human Identification from University of Dundee before moving to University of Leeds where she obtained a PhD in Neuroscience. Jenny is also a Fellow of the Higher Education Academy.

She is interested in the use of 3D digital models to teach complex areas of anatomy, particularly neuroanatomy and embryology. She has presented her work at numerous national and international conferences and has been widely published. Jenny has also been invited to speak at several conferences on the pedagogical evidence underpinning the incorporation of extended reality in life sciences and medical curricula, including delivering a workshop at AMEE 2023.

Matthieu Poyade is the programme leader of the MSc Medical Visualisation and Human Anatomy jointly offered with University of Glasgow, and a lecturer in Volumetric Visualisation, and Human Computer Interaction and Extended Reality. He is a member of the European Association for Extended Reality (EuroXR) and has been an executive member and secretary for several years.

He completed his PhD in Human Computer Interaction at the University of Malaga, Spain. His PhD thesis investigated the development of fine motor skills using haptic force feedback devices for industrial maintenance tasks.

Before joining the School of Innovation and Technology at the Glasgow School of Art, he was working as Research Associate at the University of Malaga, Spain, in a major EU-funded project, ManuVAR, which investigates the development of a methodological and technological framework including AR/VR, to support the product lifecycle of European industries.

His activities at the School of Innovation and Technology include several research projects in the field of Human Machine Interaction, Virtual Reality, Visualisation and Training applied to manufacturing and life sciences. He has been involved in several projects funded by the European Social Fund, Social Innovation Fund at the Scottish Government, Art and Humanities Research Council, Medical Research Council, Advanced Forming Research Centre, European Space Agency, National Health System Education Scotland.

He has presented his work in several journals and international conferences. Some of his developments have been demo'd in technological exhibition showcases such as Top Coder Open 2014 in San Francisco and Consumer Electronic Show CES2015 in Las Vegas.

Contributors

Daisy Abbott School of Innovation and Technology, Glasgow, UK

Emma Bailey School of Medicine, Dentistry and Nursing, College of Medical, Veterinary and Life Sciences, University of Glasgow, Glasgow, UK

Hannah Bialic Wellcome Centre for Integrative Parasitology, School of Infection & Immunity, College of Medical, Veterinary and Life Sciences, University of Glasgow, Glasgow, UK

Georgena Buesnel School of Innovation and Technology, The Glasgow School of Art, Glasgow, UK

School of Medicine, Dentistry and Nursing, College of Medical, Veterinary and Life Sciences, University of Glasgow, Glasgow, UK

Ibrahim Daniel Buksh School of Innovation and Technology, The Glasgow School of Art, Glasgow, UK

Matt Burke Medtronic, St Paul, MN, USA

Jenny Clancy School of Medicine, Dentistry and Nursing, University of Glasgow, Glasgow, UK

Junlong Dai Division of Liver Surgery, Department of General Surgery, West China Hospital, Sichuan University, Chengdu, Sichuan, China

School of Medicine, Dentistry and Nursing, College of Medical, Veterinary and Life Sciences, University of Glasgow, Glasgow, UK

School of Innovation and Technology, Glasgow, UK

Craig Daly School of Cardiovascular and Metabolic Health, University of Glasgow, Glasgow, UK

Fraser Dougan School of Innovation and Technology, The Glasgow School of Art, Glasgow, UK

Peter Faulds Motherwell, UK

Rowan Fitzpatrick School of Innovation and Technology, Glasgow, UK

School of Medicine, Dentistry and Nursing, College of Medical, Veterinary and Life Sciences, University of Glasgow, Glasgow, UK

David Fitzpatrick Auchterarder, UK

Nicole Gourlay School of Medicine, Dentistry and Nursing, College of Medical, Dentistry and Nursing, University of Glasgow, Glasgow, UK

School of Innovation and Technology, The Glasgow School of Art, Glasgow, UK

Julien Guevar College of Veterinary Medicine, University of Bern, Bern, Switzerland

Madeleine Guillery School of Medicine, Dentistry and Nursing, University of Glasgow, Glasgow, UK

School of Innovation and Technology, The Glasgow School of Art, Glasgow, UK

Fathul Huda Faculty of Medicine, Universitas Padjadjaran, Bandung, Indonesia

Michael Jacovides University of Glasgow, Glasgow, UK

Royal Hospital for Children, Glasgow, UK

Mirja Koponen School of Medicine, Dentistry and Nursing, College of Medical, Dentistry and Nursing, University of Glasgow, Glasgow, UK

School of Innovation and Technology, Glasgow School of Art, Glasgow, UK

Karen Lacey School of Innovation & Technology, The Glasgow School of Art, Glasgow, UK

School of Medicine, Dentistry and Nursing, College of Medical, Veterinary and Life Sciences, University of Glasgow, Glasgow, UK

Scott Lowenstein HealthPartners Regions Hospital, St. Paul, MN, USA

Department of Surgery, University of Minnesota, Minneapolis, MN, USA

Ryan McGonagle School of Innovation and Technology, The Glasgow School of Art, Glasgow, UK

School of Medicine, Dentistry and Nursing, College of Medical, Veterinary and Life Sciences, University of Glasgow, Glasgow, UK

Tara M. Mulyawan School of Medicine, Dentistry and Nursing, University of Glasgow, Glasgow, UK

School of Simulation and Visualisation, The Glasgow School of Art, Glasgow, UK

Liam Pearce School of Medicine, Dentistry and Nursing, College of Medical, Dentistry and Nursing, University of Glasgow, Glasgow, UK

School of Simulation and Visualisation, The Glasgow School of Art, Glasgow, UK

Matthieu Poyade School of Innovation and Technology, Glasgow School of Art, Glasgow, UK

Rodrigo Gutierrez Quintana School of Biodiversity, One Health and Veterinary Medicine, University of Glasgow, Glasgow, UK

Paul M. Rea School of Medicine, Dentistry and Nursing, College of Medical, Veterinary and Life Sciences, University of Glasgow, Glasgow, UK

Uti Nilam Sari PT. Teknologi Informasi Medimedi, Depok, Indonesia

Giuliana Torpiano Royal Hospital for Children, Glasgow, UK

University of Glasgow, Glasgow, UK

Sze Choong Wong Human Nutrition, School of Medicine, Dentistry and Life Sciences, University of Glasgow, Glasgow, UK

Department of Paediatric Endocrinology, Royal Hospital for Children, Glasgow, UK

Part I

Extended Reality

1 ECG-in-AR: Enhancing Learner Comprehension of Cardiac Electrophysiology Using an Augmented Reality Mobile Application

Rowan Fitzpatrick, Matthieu Poyade, Paul M. Rea, David Fitzpatrick, and Peter Faulds

Abstract

An electrocardiograph (ECG) consists of an assessment of cardiac electrophysiology and a complex diagnostic of heart health. During emergency situations, a high degree of importance is assigned to ECG interpretation. As first responders, ambulance personnel need a strong understanding of the ECG to assess a patient's needs quickly and accurately. However, the cardiac electrophysiology of an ECG is an intangible and complex system with clinical indicators commonly deemed difficult to comprehend. Interpretation remains an ongoing challenge for new and experienced paramedics and hence novel ways to support interpretation are needed. An interactive Augmented Reality mobile application which conveys a 3D anatomical heart model alongside varying clinical ECG presentations to enhance user knowledge of cardiac electrophysiology was developed. The usability and effectiveness of the application was tested on a cohort of newly qualified paramedics (NQP's) in the Scottish Ambulance Service, using the System Usability Scale (SUS), and comparing initial and post-intervention knowledge of ECG interpretation. Ten NQP's agreed to participate. Knowledge significantly increased on an average of 22% from pre- ($M = 4.8 \pm 1.62$) to post-test ($M = 7.0 \pm 1.49$) scoring. The application received an average usability score of 82.8, 24.8 points higher than the SUS standardised reference benchmark of 68. Improving interpretation of ECG may improve paramedics' diagnostic accuracy and therefore positively impact on patient outcome. Our experimental findings suggest the current efficacy of the application in facilitating user knowledge and support recommendations for future research, though further testing is needed to confirm the current trends and validate the application in a medical context.

R. Fitzpatrick (✉)
School of Innovation and Technology, Glasgow, UK

School of Medicine, Dentistry and Nursing, College of Medical, Veterinary and Life Sciences, University of Glasgow, Glasgow, UK

M. Poyade
School of Innovation and Technology, Glasgow, UK
e-mail: M.Poyade@gsa.ac.uk

P. M. Rea
School of Medicine, Dentistry and Nursing, College of Medical, Veterinary and Life Sciences, University of Glasgow, Glasgow, UK
e-mail: Paul.Rea@glasgow.ac.uk

D. Fitzpatrick
Scottish Ambulance Service, NHS, Auchterarder, UK
e-mail: David.fitzpatrick4@nhs.scot

P. Faulds
Scottish Ambulance Service, NHS, Motherwell, UK
e-mail: AlexanderPeter.Faulds@nhs.scot

J. Clancy, M. Poyade (eds.), *Medical Visualization and Applications of Technology – Volume 2*, Biomedical Visualization 5, https://doi.org/10.1007/978-3-031-63463-5_1

Keywords

Cardiac electrophysiology · Electrocardiograph · Paramedicine · Augmented reality · 3D · Mobile learning

1.1 Introduction

Cardiovascular disease (CVD) is the worldwide leading cause of death annually with 18.6 million deaths in 2019 (Roth et al. 2020). Moreover, CVD costs the EU economy an estimated €210 billion yearly with 53% (€111 billion) attributed to health care costs according to most recent reports (Wilkins et al. 2017). Prehospital ECG (PHECG) patterns are analysed to identify any cardiac abnormalities and possible myocardial infarctions (MI) (Quinn et al. 2014). As the first to examine patients during emergency situations, ambulance clinicians need a strong understanding of ECG rhythms in order to assess a patient's needs quickly and accurately. The cardiac electrophysiology of an ECG, however, is complex with clinical indicators commonly deemed difficult to comprehend (Sigg et al. 2010; Breen et al. 2019). It has been theorised that PHECG interpretation of critical ECG abnormalities such as myocardial infarctions could expedite treatment at definitive care facilities and improve outcomes for the patient population (Quinn et al. 2014). It can thus be inferred that improved education regarding ECG rhythmology could lead to improved diagnostics and patient care outcomes in paramedic first response.

Utilisation of supplemental learning techniques within healthcare fields has risen in recent years due to advancements in extended reality (XR) technologies (Birt et al. 2017; Parsons and MacCallum 2021; Turan et al. 2021; Birtill et al. 2023). Augmented reality (AR), a technology that allows overlaying digital models onto the real-world view (Birtill et al. 2023), in particular, has offered unique perspectives in medical training (Parsons and MacCallum 2021). Specifically in paramedic education, the use of AR to enhance student achievement and self-efficacy has been shown (Birt et al. 2017; Turan et al. 2021). Despite these positive outlooks, few interventions have been practically realised and many still call for future research on the subject. Therefore, the *ECG-in-AR* application was developed to reaffirm paramedic knowledge of cardiac electrophysiology (CEP) and ECG pathology.

The aim of this research was to develop an interactive AR mobile/tablet application visualising a 3D anatomical heart alongside varying clinical ECG presentations to enhance knowledge of cardiac electrophysiology (CEP) in ambulance technicians/paramedics. The usability and educational validity whilst engaging with the app was evaluated in collaboration with the Scottish Ambulance Service (SAS).

1.2 Background Context

1.2.1 Cardiac Electrophysiology and the 12-Lead ECG

Cardiac electrophysiology is the conduction system regulating the electrical pathways of the heart to control heart rate, rhythm, and contraction (Klabunde 2017). The initiation of this system, i.e., the triggering of a heartbeat, begins on the sub-cellular level in which ions traverse across cell membranes impacting levels of voltage across the plasma membrane. The rapid change in voltage affects depolarisation and repolarisation across cardiac cells stimulating an action potential, or nerve impulse, thus generating an electrical excitation to contract surrounding heart muscle (Sigg et al. 2010; Klabunde 2017). In healthy systems, the impulse begins in the sinoatrial (SA) node and follows a coordinated pathway through the heart (Sigg et al. 2010). Knowledge of this cardiac activation and its associated anatomical landmarks is essential for clinically translating ECGs.

An electrocardiogram is a graphical mapping of the electrical activity occurring throughout the heart (Klabunde 2017). ECG functions through the specific placement of 12 electrodes on the body to track activation across the heart from different lead views. The electrical activity is subsequently visualised by a series of waves marked as

P, Q, R, S, and T. Normality of each wave is determined by a set of criteria regarding the wave's appearance (Atienza et al. 2012; Klabunde 2017). If a wave or PQRST complex is deemed irregular, an arrhythmia may be diagnosed (Atienza et al. 2012). The location (and shape) of the irregularity may additionally provide insight to where in the heart something is wrong; for example, P-waves represent atrial diastole, QRS complexes represent the transition from atrial to ventricular systole, and T-waves represent ventricular diastole (Atienza et al. 2012). Accurate interpretation of ECG readings is integral in the diagnosis and treatment of myocardial infarction (MI) and many other life-threatening disorders. Here, ambulance clinicians will look specifically for changes to the ST segment of an ECG which will generally show elevation in myocardial infarction. Therefore, a comprehensive understanding of ECG interpretation is crucial for ambulance clinicians.

An extensive amount of knowledge is expected to be learned in ECG training. Kopeć et al. (2015) assessed ECG interpretation skills of 536 medical students on 18 ECG strips. Competency in ECG analysis was 7% higher in students who reported self-learning techniques; however, no difference in competency was found between students who attended versus those who did not attend ECG lectures. Kopeć et al. (2015) concluded that the overall ability for interpreting ECG was good but low when recognising signs of emergency thus indicating inadequacies in understanding, and, therefore, presented an opportunity to refine and improve their education methodology. Russo et al. (2021) implemented a survey of education satisfaction on cardiology fellows. Of 334 responses, 40% recorded not receiving formal lessons on CEP but 71% received lessons on clinical arrhythmias, i.e. ECG interpretation. This indicates an approach of teaching that focuses on identifying problems rather than comprehending them. A systematic review conducted by Cook et al. (2020) examined 78 studies related to ECG interpretation in both medical students and professionals. Key findings included deficiencies in ECG interpretation across all experience levels: 42% accuracy for medical students, 56% for residents, 69% for physicians, and 75% for cardiologists. Due to these and many more findings, the Accreditation Council for Graduate Medical Education has called for a significant change in teaching methodology in both 2007 and 2015 (Swing 2007; Balady et al. 2015), and only recently has a proposal for alternative training been formalised (Mendes et al. 2022). Specifically, regarding literature on ECG comprehension in ambulance technicians, little has been explored. Alrumayh et al. (2022) evaluated 84 paramedics of varying levels of experience to identify categories of MI on ECGs alone. ST-segment elevated myocardial infarctions (STEMIs) were correctly identified by only 41% of participants, and the proportion of participants who answered additional rhythms correctly (bundle branch blocks, pericarditis, ventricular hypertrophy, etc.) never exceeded 33%. A systematic review by Funder et al. (2020) identified 9 relevant studies investigating paramedic ability to interpret ECG data; however, not all were acknowledged to be of sufficient quality. Their findings concluded that paramedics who were supplied additional educational or learning tools usually achieved greater recognition of clinical ECGs. Despite the need, implementing a common standard curriculum for ECG education across all medical education schools is logistically unlikely.

Supplemental support for pairing anatomical and electrical knowledge in CEP via 3D visualisations, software, and applications has been advocated by clinicians and educators alike (Mendes et al. 2022). Aptly stated by Southworth et al. (2020), interactive education applications allow the user to visualise, participate, or experience the content in a controlled yet customisable manner. Additionally, necessity of a virtual approach has been brought to the forefront of education considering the recent COVID-19 pandemic (Han et al. 2021). Warriner et al. (2017) tested medical students ($n = 112$) with an interactive web-based model of the cardiovascular system. Students reported an overall positive experience and subsequently improved 33% knowledge score in a 6-question assessment derived from their standard curriculum. Mobile applications specifically have risen to the forefront in medical education support due to accessibility, popularity, and range of capabilities (Ventola 2014; Lumsden et al. 2015; Mohapatra et al. 2015). Coelho et al. (2018) developed a mobile application featuring an interactable 3D model of the heart simulated from real-time ECG data. User testing of this application included 17 biomechanical engineering students with prior rudimentary knowledge of CEP. Students were directed to rate the app by ranking several statements on a scale of 1[highly disagree]-5[highly agree]. Key statements of 'improves ECG interpretation' and 'easy to realize ECG with heart beating' ranked highly in 100% and 70% of students, respectively. These results indicate an applicability of supplemental CEP mobile learning in novice students; however, testing by paramedic students should be conducted for increased validity. Overall, there is substantial evidence and support for integrated virtual learning in CEP and other medical education regardless of modality.

1.2.2 Technology Enhanced Paramedic Education

Utilisation of supplemental learning techniques within healthcare fields has risen in recent years due to advancements in extended reality (XR) technologies (Birt et al. 2017; Logeswaran et al. 2021; Parsons and MacCallum 2021; Turan et al. 2021; Birtill et al. 2023). XR technology blends virtual with physical environment and includes three primary forms: virtual reality (VR), mixed reality (MR), and augmented reality (AR) (Logeswaran et al. 2021). VR entirely encapsulates the user's visual, and sometimes auditory, perception into a virtual environment, MR seamlessly integrates virtual and physical interactions together, and AR encompasses overlaying digital data onto the real world—thus 'augmenting' the environment (Logeswaran et al. 2021). These techniques allow learners a variety of ways to realistically incorporate and practise tasks in a professional environment (Parsons and MacCallum 2021). AR, in particular, has offered unique perspectives in medical trainings (Logeswaran et al. 2021; Parsons and MacCallum 2021). Comparable to other XR modalities, AR utilises hardware such as headsets, smart glasses, or widely accessible mobile devices to visualise augmented data within the real world. Conversely, AR has been argued as a safer method of XR visualisation as it can be less likely than VR and MR to compromise the user's proprioception in the real-world (Mohapatra et al. 2015; Southworth et al. 2020; Parsons and MacCallum 2021).

Few reviews and investigations have been conducted on the efficacy of AR specifically in ambulance technician education. Birtill et al. (2023) conducted a scoping review of emergent XR technology in overall paramedic education yielding only 11 relevant records. From this and their content, Birtill et al. (2023) concluded that the benefit of XR is not yet clear and that more research should be allocated to its usage in paramedicine and similar healthcare disciplines. Birt et al. (2017) investigated the value of XR in paramedic distance learning. Of 137 distance-learning paramedic students, 55 were supplied with 3D printed tools along with an AR mobile application concerning laryngoscopy and foreign body removal. Upon in-person testing of the learned skills, those supplied with the simulated education tools achieved significantly greater scores than those who were not. Lastly, Turan et al. (2021) investigated the efficacy of an AR versus traditional ECG education in first-year paramedic students. Thirty students were supplied with a traditional book and 31 were provided with an AR book that allowed them to view 3D animations and videos on a mobile device. Following completion of the learning term, the post-test academic achievement and self-efficacy scores of the AR group were significantly higher than the paramedic students in the traditional group. Furthermore, in a post-intervention interview, it was stated that

> *... paramedic education should definitely be supported by these devices*

Overall, these reviews and investigations provide a positive outlook for the benefits of integrating XR into paramedic education programmes, and all support the development of an XR based cardiac electrophysiology learning tool.

1.3 Materials and Methodology

1.3.1 Materials

The hardware, software, and datasets utilised in the design and development of this application are displayed alongside their purposes in Tables 1.1 and 1.2. The hardware materials used in the creation of this application included an HP Victus laptop computer for the primary design and development, and a Samsung Galaxy A52s mobile device for the download and testing of the application. The primary software utilised was selected due to availability and licensing provided by the Glasgow School of Art.

1.3.2 Methodology

1.3.2.1 Concept

The initial aim of this application was for it to be utilised as a supplementary learning aid for trainee ambulance clinicians during ECG training of STEMI recognition; however, it was extended to encompass certified ambulance technicians and paramedics who wish to refresh or enhance their existing knowledge of cardiac anatomy, electrophysiology, ECGs (both normal and pathological), and STEMI pathology recognition.

1.3.2.2 Storyboard

The preliminary storyboard design for this application and of scenes with annotated functionalities was created to guide workflow. A MoSCoW priority matrix was also used to organise the key features of the application as 'must have', 'should have', 'could have', and 'will not have' (Table 1.3). The priority of features was determined through consultations with ambulance clinicians and limited by time constraints.

1.3.2.3 Asset Creation

1.3.2.3.1 Segmentation

To ensure anatomical accuracy, the source model of the heart was segmented from the sample *CTACardio* DICOM dataset (Table 1.2) from 3D Slicer. Prior to segmentation, the scan's window level contrast was adjusted for clearer threshold differentiation between structures and a new region of interest was defined for cropping. Isometric spacing at a scale 1.10x was inputted for cropping the volume. A Laplacian sharpening filter was applied to denoise and refine edges. Within the segment editor the paint tool was used to fill portions of the following anatomical regions: left ventricle, left atrium, right ventricle, right atrium, superior vena cava, aorta, pulmonary artery, and 'other'. The grow-from-seed tool was used to expand the painted portions into each anatomical structure based on threshold similarity. Then, margin smoothing was applied at 3 mm, and the segments were refined with the paint and eraser tool. After being exported as a label-map, the 3D model of the heart was created and a final Laplacian smoothing filter was applied.

A singular model of the whole heart was also segmented. The first segmentation was duplicated, and the segments of the heart regions were deleted, leaving only the external space as 'other'. The segment 'other' was grown by 1.5 mm and smoothed by 3 mm. A new segment named 'wholeheart' was added and the threshold tool expanded to maximum and minimum limit was used to fill outside all visible segments. The resultant 3D model after Laplacian filtering can be seen in Fig. 1.1b. Finally, models were saved and exported as OBJ files.

1.3.2.3.2 Modelling

Following segmentation, the heart model was imported into 3DS Max for initial retopology of vertices reducing the polygon count to 19,667. This model was then imported into ZBrush for refinement. After being sculpted for anatomical accuracy using smooth and morph brushes, the

Table 1.1 Software materials used in the design and development of this application

Software	Publisher	Purpose
Slicer 3D	Slicer 3D https://www.slicer.org/	Segmentation and 3D visualisation of anatomical structures
3Ds Max	Autodesk, Inc. https://www.autodesk.co.uk/products/3ds-max/overview	3D modelling, retopology, UV mapping, and animation
Zbrush	Pixologic https://pixologic.com/	3D model refinement and texturing
Unity 3D	Unity Technologies https://unity.com/	Application development
Visual Studio Code	Microsoft Corp. https://code.visualstudio.com/	C# Scripting
Adobe Substance 3D Painter	Adobe, Inc. https://www.adobe.com/uk/products/substance3d-painter/	Model texturing and mapping
Adobe Illustrator	Adobe, Inc. https://www.adobe.com/uk/products/illustrator/	2D illustration design

(continued)

Table 1.1 (continued)

Software	Publisher	Purpose
Microsoft Office Word	Microsoft Corp. https://www.microsoft.com/en-gb/microsoft-365/p/word/	Formal write-up
Microsoft Office Excel	Microsoft Corp https://www.microsoft.com/en-gb/microsoft-365/p/excel/	Data compilation and organisation
Mendeley Reference Manager	Mendeley Ltd. https://www.mendeley.com/	Reference organisation and bibliography creation
PSPP	GNU Project https://www.gnu.org/software/pspp/	Statistical analysis of results

heart model was again retopologied in ZBrush to approximately 50,000 polygons (Fig. 1.2).

Once sculpted to anatomical accuracy, the model was imported back into 3DS Max to begin modelling the coronary arteries. The right coronary, left anterior descending, and circumflex arteries were modelled using the snap tool to adjust splines onto the model of the heart. Once a general pathway was outlined, an *edit poly* and *turbosmooth* were attached to allow the spines to take on a cylindrical structure and the terminal points of the splines were then tapered to appear similar to that of an artery (Fig. 1.3). The modelled arteries were enlarged compared to anatomically accurate specimens to emphasise their structures and locations during the educational scenes in the application.

The electrical conduction system animation was developed in 3DS Max by attaching the 2D illustration of the heart's conduction system to a plane of the same dimensions. The ECG segment was modelled with a spline and the electricity activation current was modelled with spheres and cylinders. The animation was organised by matching the waves to their corresponding activations on the pathway (Fig. 1.4). The pink and purple circles represent the growing wave of electrical current travelling across the electrical branches in yellow.

The pre-made model of the ribs was downloaded later on in the development of the application from Sketchfab (https://sketchfab.com/3d-models/ribcage). The file was imported into 3DS Max and retopologied. Cylinders were modelled and placed to represent electrode placements for an ECG examination (Fig. 1.5).

Table 1.2 Datasets used in the design and development of this application

Data	Publisher	Purpose
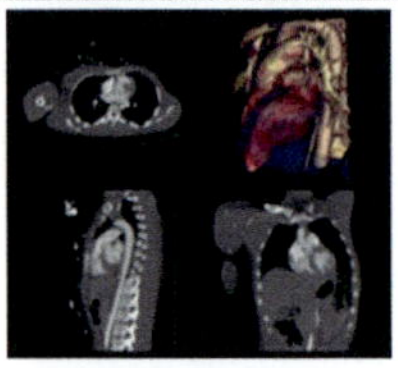 CTACardio	Slicer 3D https://www.slicer.org/	Dataset used for segmentation of the heart
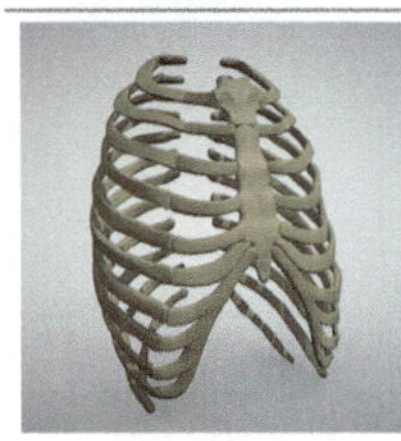 Ribcage	Sketchfab https://sketchfab.com/3d-models/ribcage	3D ribcage model used in the home scene to help visualise lead placements
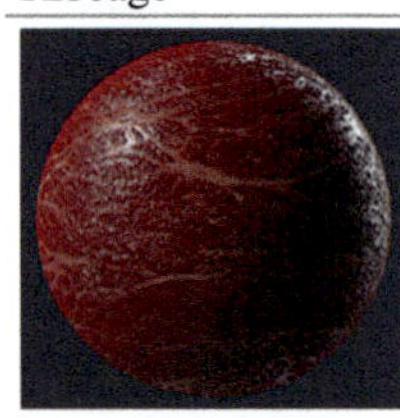 Organic Flesh	Adobe, Inc. https://www.adobe.com/uk/products/substance3d-painter/	Preset texture used for texturing the surface of the heart
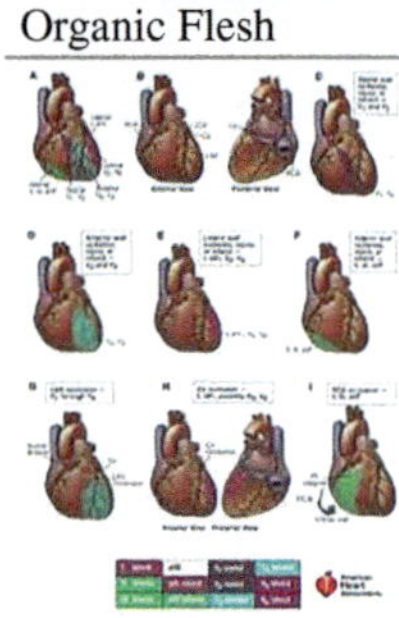 STEMI Location	American Heart Association https://www.ahajournals.org/	Reference image used for localising affected myocardium of specific STEMIs
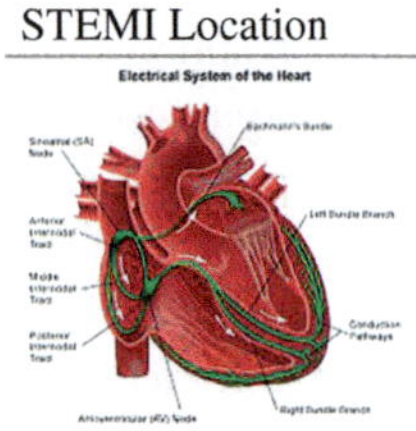 Electrical Conduction System	Stanford Medicine https://www.stanfordchildrens.org/en/topic/default?id=anatomy-and-function-of-the-electrical-system	Reference image for illustrating and animating the electrical conduction pathway of the heart

1.3.2.3.3 Texturing

To texture the 3D heart model, it first underwent UVW unwrapping in 3DS Max. Seams were selected manually along the natural form of the model, then peeled and scaled to create the texture maps seen in Fig. 1.6.

The UVW unwrapped model of the heart was exported as an OBJ file and imported into Adobe Substance Painter to begin colouring and texturing. The export statistics of the structures include the polygon count of the whole model totalling 51,168. The model and texture map of the heart were imported into Adobe Substance 3D Painter without the coronary arteries. The model was painted in various layers using paint fill and black masks while following the natural colourisation of a human heart. A final texture was added from the preset *Organic Flesh*. The colour and texture were then baked into the maps of the heart before it was prepared for export. A personalised output template was created for texture outputting. Albedo, emissive, normal, ambient occlusion, metallic, and height maps were all saved as PNGs and later attached to their corresponding material spaces in Unity.

1.3.2.3.4 2D Content

The colour palette for this application was selected according to colour theory and aimed to be colour blind friendly (Monigatti 2022). The primary colour for this application (#136162) and its lighter shade (#73F0A3) were selected as an altered shade of blue. According to colour psychology, blue is representative of serenity, knowledge, and professionalism (Yu et al. 2021). It is also commonly associated with the medical field (Yu et al. 2021) making it appropriate for this medical education application. The secondary colour for the application (#FFD700) was

Table 1.3 MoSCoW prioritisation of sections key to the application design and development

Must have	Should have	Could have	Will not have
AR affected myocardium STEMI learning Electrical conduction learning	Coronary artery learning Animation Quiz	ECG lead view learning	Additional dysrhythmias Internal cardiac cross-section

a

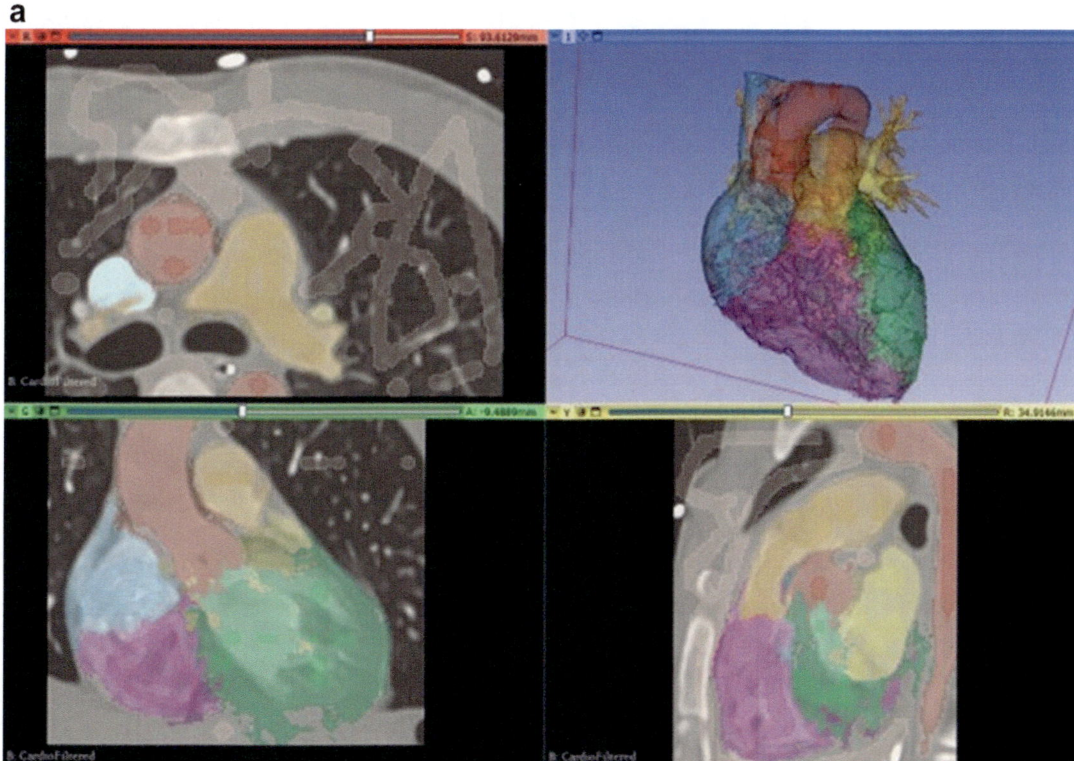

Fig. 1.1 Initial 3D Slicer segmentation preview of heart structures where each colour represents a different structure (**a**), and segmentation of the heart as a whole structure (**b**)

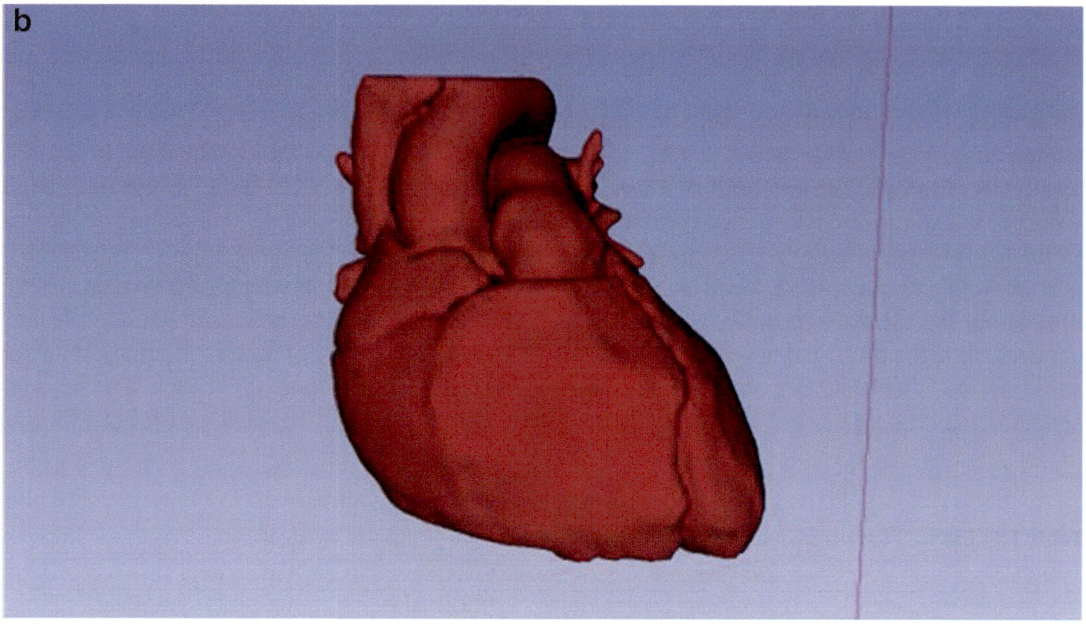

Fig. 1.1 (continued)

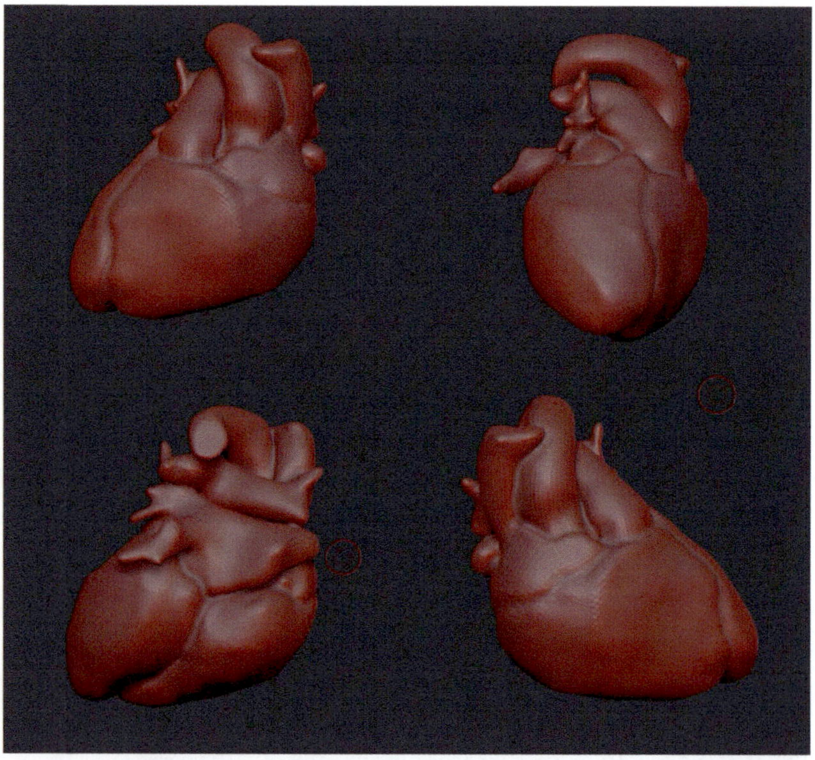

Fig. 1.2 3D model of the heart after being sculpted for greater anatomical accuracy and retopologied a second time in ZBrush

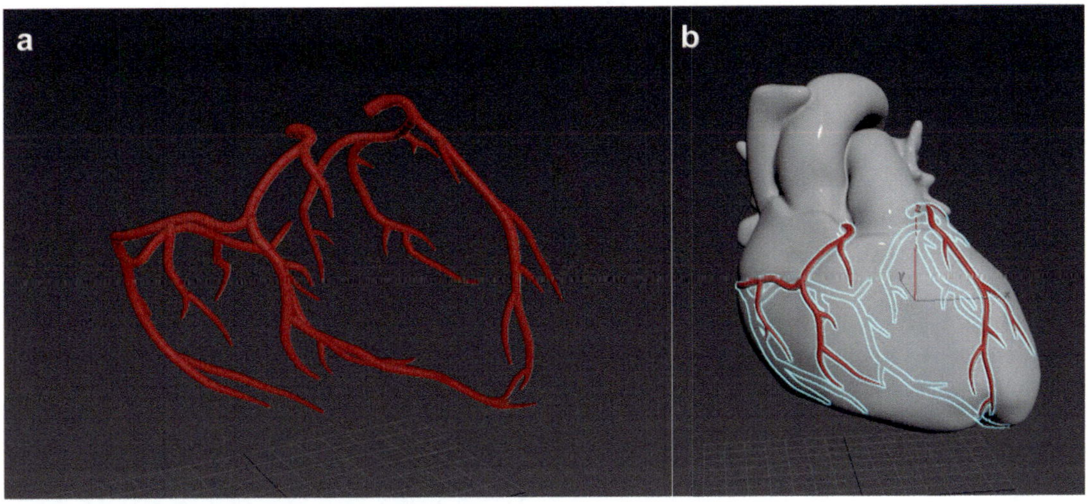

Fig. 1.3 Final model of the coronary arteries with (a) and without (b) the heart

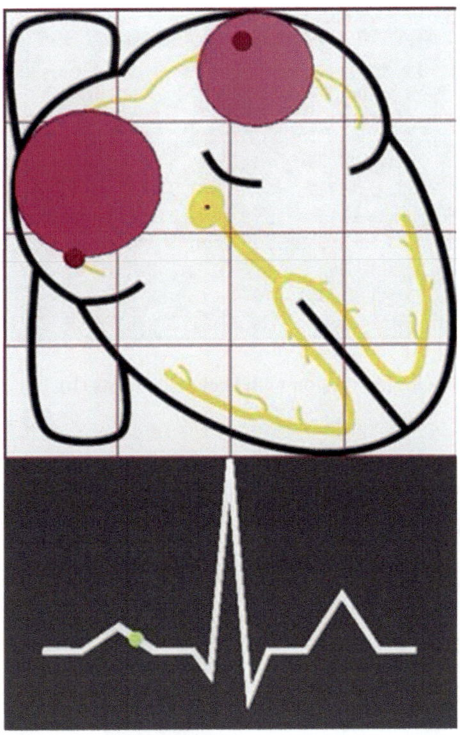

Fig. 1.4 Screenshot of the electrical conduction system animation in 3DS Max

derived from yellow which has been deemed representative of happiness and is commonly associated with electricity (Yu et al. 2021). The accent colour for this application encompasses the undertones of the heart model and is the standard RGB for blood (#880808) (Figs. 1.7 and 1.8).

2D illustrations such as the UI buttons, the electrical pathway of the heart (Fig. 1.9), and the application logo (Fig. 1.10) were created in Adobe Illustrator. The electrical pathway of the heart (Fig. 1.9) was designed in reference to reviewed anatomical images. It includes the SA node, Bachmann's branches through the atria, the AV node, atrioventricular branch, bundle branches, and Purkinje fibres.

The logo for the application also acts as the reference image for the augmented reality overlay (Fig. 1.10). The design is the title of the application over a minimalistic outline of a human heart with coronary arteries on a blue field. The font of the title aims to represent the sharp spikes of an ECG recording. In the initial concept design, the AR reference image was meant to be an image of an ECG recording; however, these were unable to be used due to constraints in the software's ability to recognise symmetrical, graph-like patterns. Hence, the logo was substituted.

1.3.2.4 Application Development

The application was developed using Unity 3D with imported assets and was scripted using Visual Studio Code. For the development of an augmented reality capability on an android device, the AR Foundation and AR Core plugins were used. The flow of development was organised by specific scenes and their necessary functionalities (Fig. 1.11). Prototype scenes were used to test functionality, review UI, and debug scripts before importing assets.

The design of the application allows the user to quit at any time and switch between scenes in no set order. This was achieved by attaching scripts (Fig. 1.12) to correlating UI buttons. Upon selecting a new scene, a pop-up panel with directions on how to use the scene is generated. The user can revisit these directions by selecting the information button on the bottom toolbar.

The majority of interactions were able to be implemented using UI buttons. For example, the OnClick event of each button in the learn scene sets a variety of GameObjects to active or inactive. Additionally, in scenes such as the STEMI learning, selecting a specific button can change the appearance of the heart model triggering a material change with the OnClick event.

More complex functionalities such as touch interactions had been achieved through scripting.

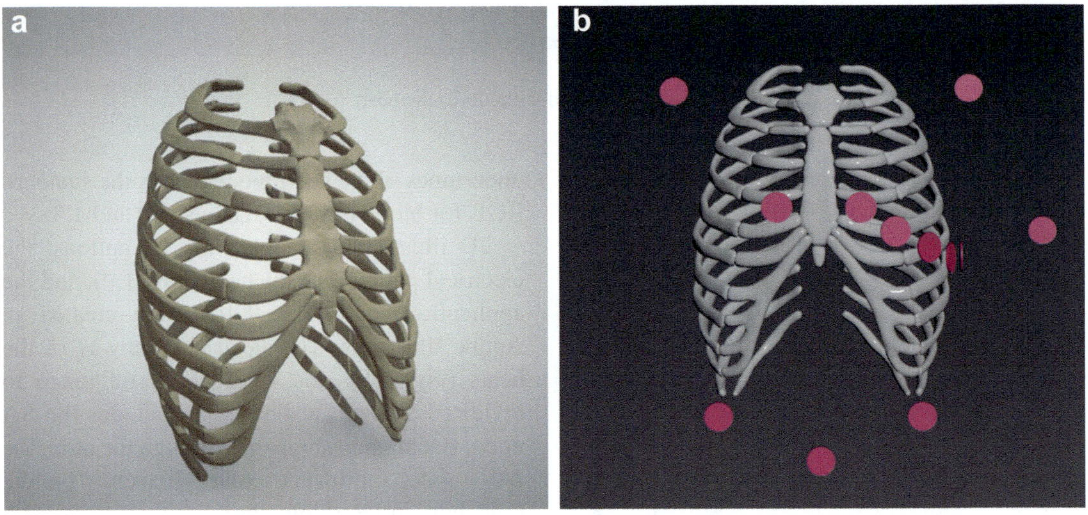

Fig. 1.5 Sketchfab downloaded model of the ribcage (**a**) and retopologied version with lead placements (**b**)

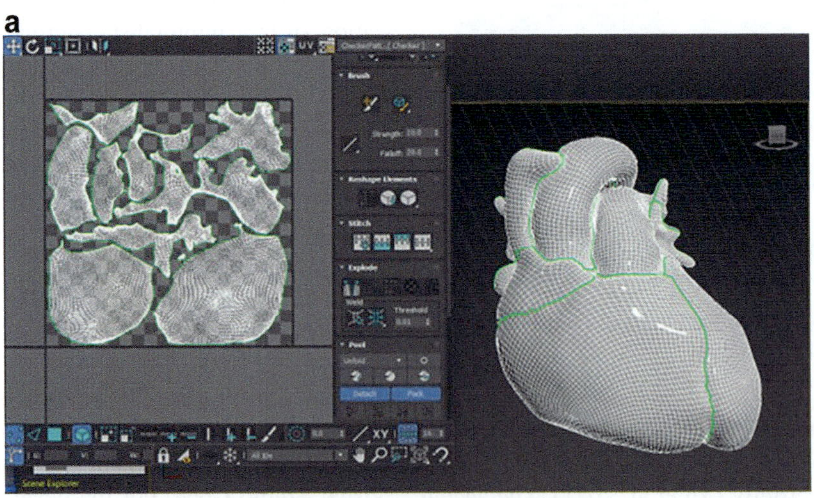

Fig. 1.6 UVW unwrap texture map and model seams in 3DS Max (**a**) and final painted 3D heart model with corresponding texture map in Adobe Substance 3D Painter (**b**)

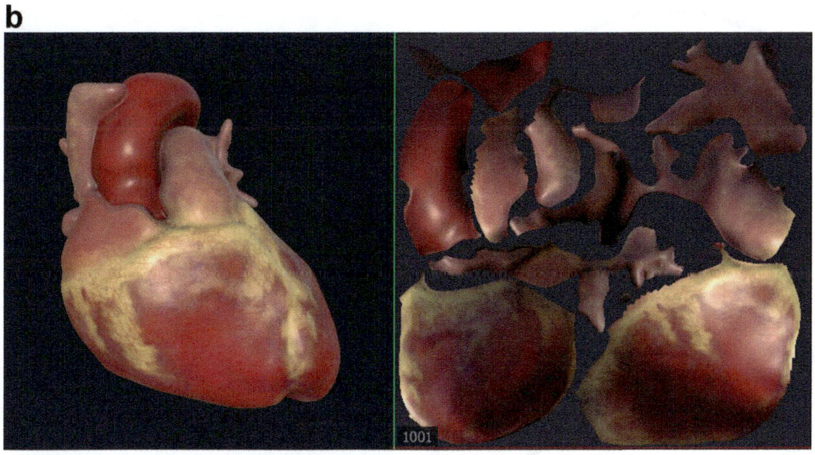

Fig. 1.6 (continued)

Fig. 1.7 The colour palette used in the application in RGB

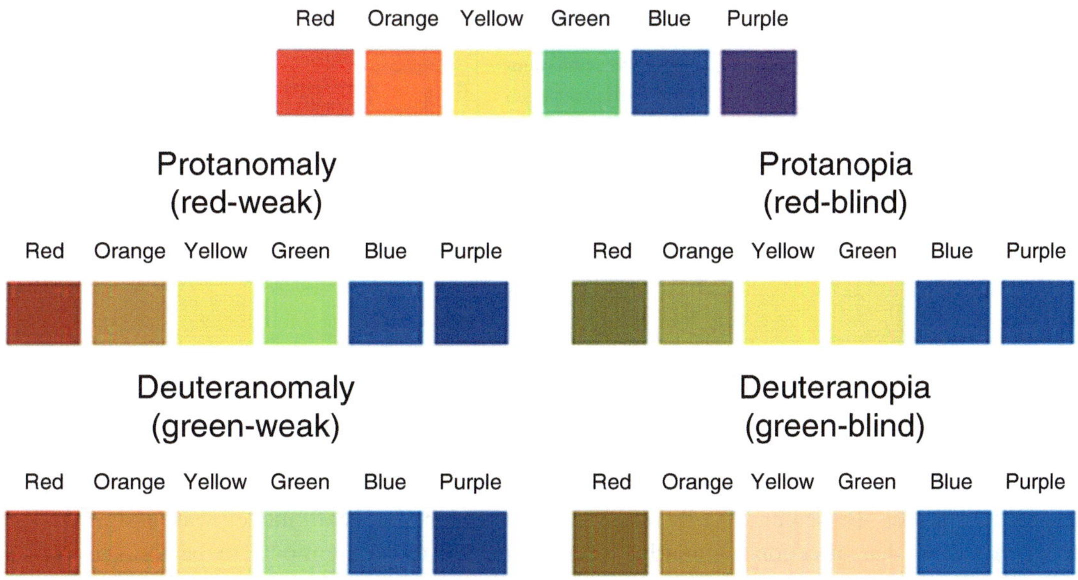

Fig. 1.8 Traditional colour rainbow compared with several variants of colour blindness

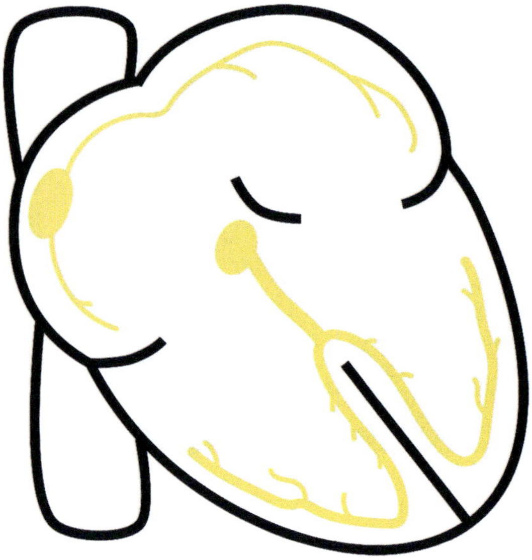

Fig. 1.9 Electrical conduction pathway illustration of the heart

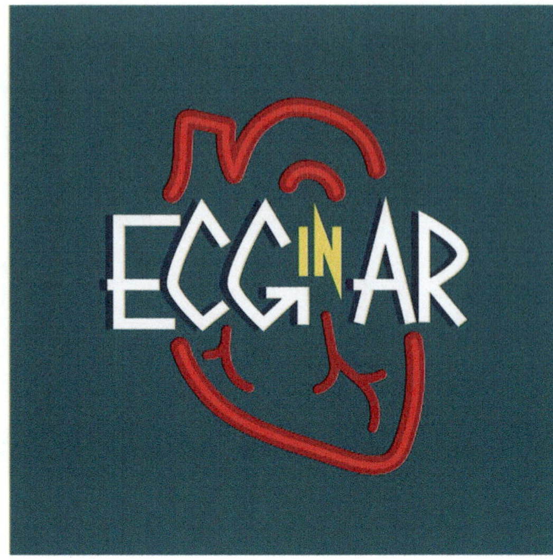

Fig. 1.10 Application logo and the reference image for AR overlay

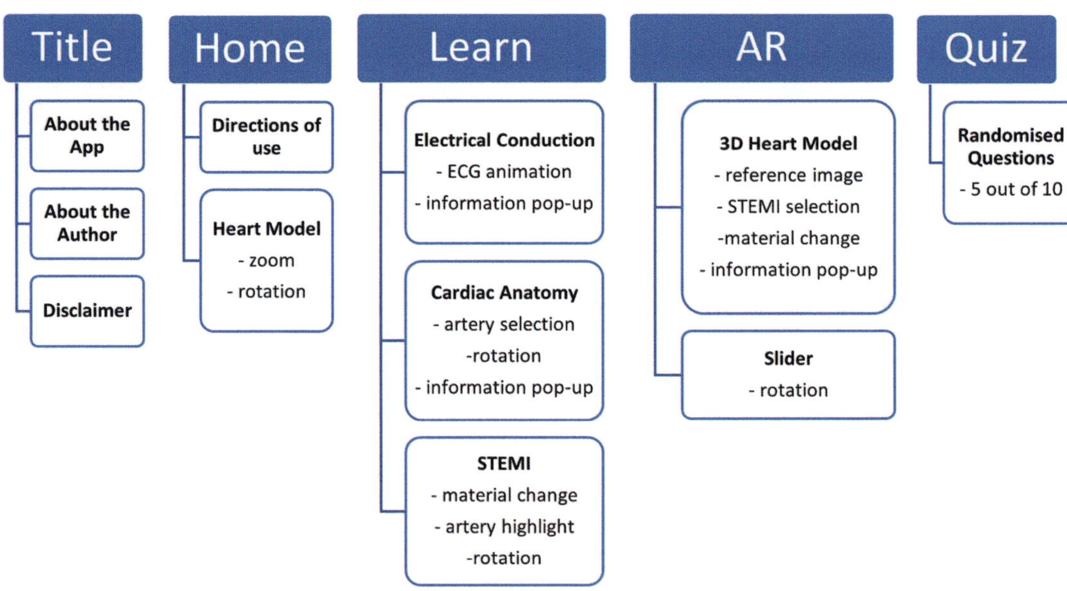

Fig. 1.11 Scene development functionality map

On the mobile device, if the user uses a one-finger drag across the screen, it will rotate the heart model in that direction. Similarly, if the user uses a two-finger pinch on the screen, it will zoom the heart model in and out. Both of these touch interactions were created on the same script (Fig. 1.13). The script was attached to the scene camera and included a public GameObject to which the heart model was assigned. This enabled the heart model to be the only object affected by the rotate and zoom function.

Augmented reality was implemented using the AR Core plugin within the AR Foundation package of Unity3D. This permitted the

a

```
public class SceneChange: MonoBehaviour
{
    // change to new scene
    public void MovetoScene(int sceneID)
    {
        SceneManager.LoadScene(sceneID);
    }
}
```

b

```
public class QuitManager : MonoBehaviour
{
    // close the app
    public void OnApplicationQuit()
    {
        Debug.Log("app quit");
        Application.Quit();
    }
}
```

Fig. 1.12 Scene change (**a**) and quit (**b**) functions of the application

```
void Update()
{
    if (Input.touchSupported)
    {
        //Rotate model
        if (Input.touchCount == 1)
        {
            Touch tZero = Input.GetTouch(0);
            //Debug.Log(tZero.deltaPosition);
            focusObj.transform.Rotate(tZero.deltaPosition.y /speed,tZero.deltaPosition.x /speed * (-1.0f),0.0f, Space.World);
        }

        // Pinch to zoom
        if (Input.touchCount == 2)
        {
            // get current touch positions
            Touch tZero = Input.GetTouch(0);
            Touch tOne = Input.GetTouch(1);

            // get touch position from the previous frame
            Vector2 tZeroPrevious = tZero.position - tZero.deltaPosition;
            Vector2 tOnePrevious = tOne.position - tOne.deltaPosition;

            float oldTouchDistance = Vector2.Distance (tZeroPrevious, tOnePrevious);
            float currentTouchDistance = Vector2.Distance (tZero.position, tOne.position);

            // get offset value
            float deltaDistance = oldTouchDistance - currentTouchDistance;
            Zoom (deltaDistance, TouchZoomSpeed);
        }
```

Fig. 1.13 Touch inputs of the PinchZoom script

development to be functional on an android device. Within the augmented reality scene, functionalities previously employed via buttons were required to be completed through scripting. This is because the AR heart model prefab was not present within the hierarchy and was only called into the running scene when triggered by the reference image. Therefore, any script was first required to be attached to an empty GameObject in the hierachy called *HeartManager*. The script was then written to reference the *ARObjOverlayImage* script and find the clone of the heart model prefab by name. An example of this can be seen in the script for the slider rotation in Fig. 1.14.

Similarly, for the material change per STEMI type in the AR scene, an array of the materials was created and attached to the *HeartManager* (Fig. 1.15). The STEMI buttons then triggered their correlating material change function class. For example, the lateral STEMI matches with material #3 (Fig. 1.15).

The quiz scene functions were achieved using two scripts. The *QuestionManager* script utilises UI toggles which are set as either a 'correct' or 'incorrect' answer depending on the question. Upon selecting an answer and clicking the confirm button, a pop-up correlating to whether the correct answer was selected or not is triggered (Fig. 1.16a). The *QuizManager* script randomises

```
void Start()
{
    // find slider and call the clone of my AR prefab from ARObjectOverlay script
    rotateSlider = GameObject.Find("RotateSlider").GetComponent<Slider>();

    arScript = GetComponent<ARObjOverlayImage>();
}
```

Fig. 1.14 Start function of the RotateSlider script calling the ARObjectOverlayImage script

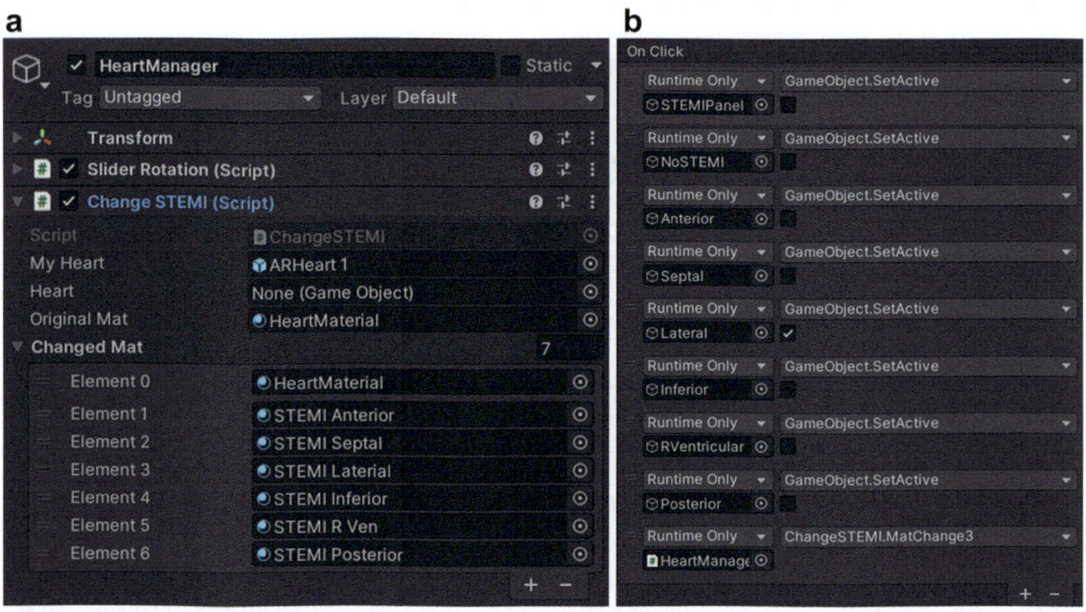

Fig. 1.15 ChangeSTEMI script with material array attached to the empty game object HeartManager (**a**) and example on-click function template for STEMI buttons (**b**)

```
public void OnConfirmClick()
{
    if(transform.GetComponent<ToggleGroup>().ActiveToggles().FirstOrDefault() != null)
    {
        if(transform.GetComponent<ToggleGroup>().ActiveToggles().FirstOrDefault().gameObject == correctAnswer)
        {
            //correct answer
            instructions.SetActive(false);
            positiveResponse.SetActive(true);

            //update score
            transform.parent.GetComponent<QuizManager>().scoreNb += 1;
        }
        else
        {
            //wrong answer
            instructions.SetActive(false);
            negativeResponse.SetActive(true);
        }
```

Fig. 1.16 Correct and Incorrect response functionality from QuestionManager script (**a**) and randomisation of questions functionality from QuizManager script (**b**)

```
public void OnNextClick()
{
    maxQuestions = maxQuestions -1;

    if(maxQuestions > 0)
    {
        myQList[itemNb].SetActive(false);
        myQList.RemoveAt(itemNb);

        itemNb = Random.Range (0, myQList.Count-1);
        myQList[itemNb].SetActive(true);
    }
    else
    {
        //remove the used question
        myQList[itemNb].SetActive(false);
        myQList.RemoveAt(itemNb);

        scoreObj.SetActive(true);
        //update score text
        scoreObj.GetComponent<TextMeshProUGUI>().text += " " + scoreNb.ToString();
    }
```

Fig. 1.16 (continued)

the questions from a pre-made list and removes the used question from that list, so it is not repeated during the session (Fig. 1.16b). The question answers are recorded and then shown as a score out of five after finishing the quiz.

1.4 ECG-in-AR Application

The opening title can be seen in Fig. 1.17 including panels about the application, about the author and collaborators, and a disclaimer. A video recording of the full application can be viewed at https://www.youtube.com/watch?v=NjQg7iKSieE.

1.4.1 Home Scene

When selecting the 'BEGIN' button on the title scene, the user is transported to the home scene. The aim of the home scene is to inform the user about the primary uses of the app and to install base knowledge of 12-lead locations in relation to the human heart. The scene first displays a pop-up panel containing information about the buttons on the bottom toolbar panel (Fig. 1.18). Closing this panel reveals the 3D model of the heart within a transparent ribcage. This model is able to be zoomed in/out and rotated by the user for better perspective. The model is surrounded by 12-lead ECG placements which glow in specified colours when their corresponding buttons are selected. The colours of these buttons are meant to mirror their matching contiguous leads.

1.4.2 Learning Scenes

The learn scene is triggered when the magnifying glass button is selected on the bottom toolbar. A pop-up panel informing the user of the learning buttons is displayed first (Fig. 1.19). The aim of the learn scenes is to educate the user on how the ECG and coronary arteries correlate and how they are affected during STEMIs.

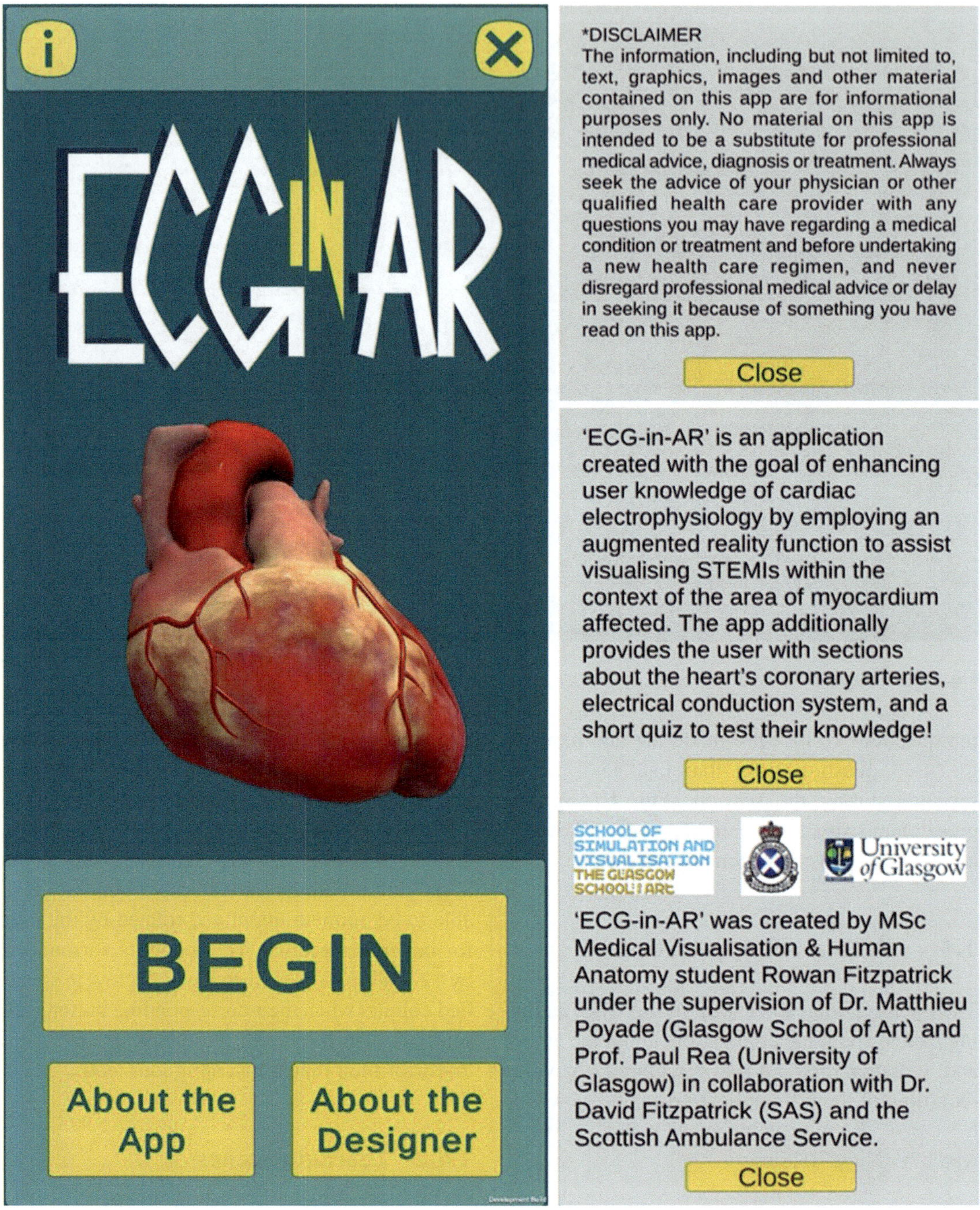

Fig. 1.17 Opening title scene and pop-up panels

1.4.2.1 Electrical Pathway

The electrical pathway (ECG and conduction pathway) section of the learn scene aims to educate the user specifically about how electricity travels through the heart and is recorded as waves. The scene includes a 2D illustration of the heart's conduction pathway with a 3D animation playing on loop (Fig. 1.20). The animation plays over both the electrical activation through the pathway and the matching flow through a normal

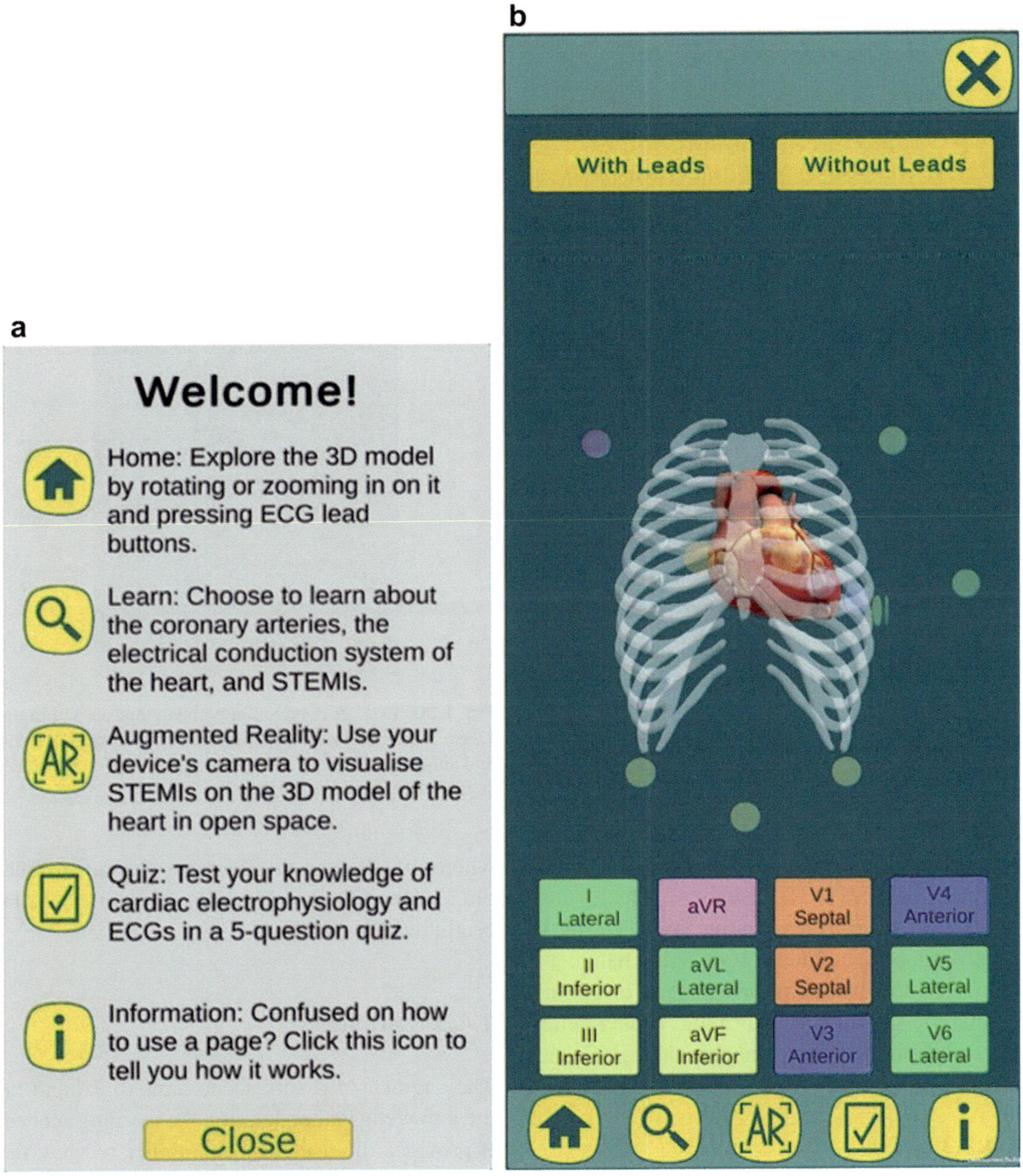

Fig. 1.18 Home scene pop-up panel with directions about each button (**a**) and the home heart/lead exploration (**b**)

ECG rhythm. This allows the user to visualise where in the heart each waves' activation is occurring. Additionally, a set of buttons provides information about each significant segment of the ECG rhythm (P-wave, QRS segment, J-point, T-wave).

1.4.2.2 Coronary Arteries

The coronary artery learning page aims to educate the user about the main arteries of the heart and their branches as well as what leads are affected by occlusion. The scene contains a rotatable 3D model of the heart with coronary

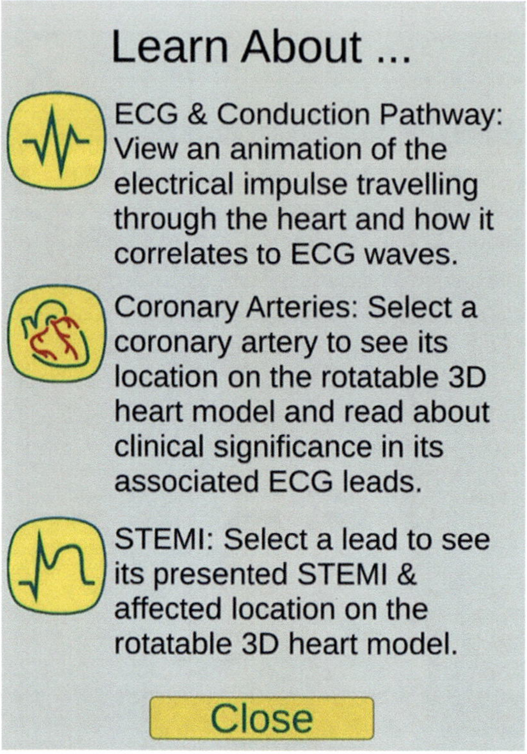

Fig. 1.19 Learn scene pop-up panel with directions about each button

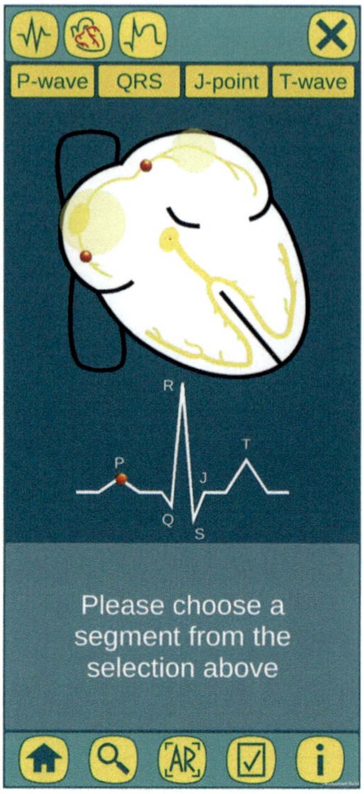

Fig. 1.20 ECG & conduction pathway option within the Learn scene. Includes an animation of electrical activity and information about selected segments (P-wave, QRS segment, J-point, T-wave)

arteries being displayed a transparent white colour (Fig. 1.21). The user can select which artery they wish to learn about by selecting its according button. The button will change the colour of the matching artery to a bright red colour and summon an information panel detailing its origin, branches, and clinical significance (Fig. 1.21).

1.4.2.3 STEMI

When entering the STEMI page, a pop-up panel is shown to first inform the user about what a STEMI is. The aim of this learning page is to inform the user of STEMIs as they relate to ECG contiguous leads. The scene includes a rotatable 3D model of the heart and 12-lead ECG set of labelled buttons. These buttons represent themselves as contiguous leads and upon selection highlight the occluded artery and affected myocardial area. For example, selecting either V3 or V4 purple buttons will display an anterior STEMI where the affected myocardium changes to purple and the left anterior descending artery turns bright red (Fig. 1.22).

1.4.3 AR Scene

The augmented reality scene aims to expand on the knowledge gained during the learning scenes. It provides the user with the ability to view the affected myocardium of particular STEMIs while rendered in space. An information pop-up tells the user how to use the AR function and provides a link to where the reference image can be freely downloaded.

Aiming the camera at the reference image will cause the 3D heart model to appear without any STEMI presentation. The user can select the STEMI they want to visualise from a drop-down menu which will both highlight the affected area of the heart and summon a panel detailing which

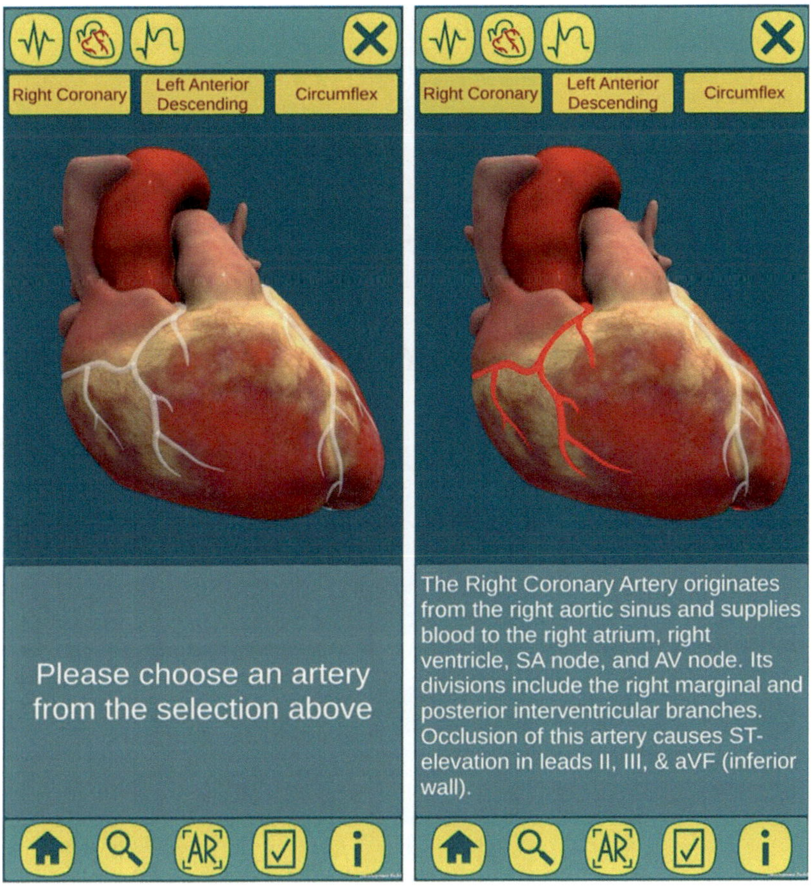

Fig. 1.21 Coronary Artery option within Learn scene. Includes a rotatable heart model and information about selected arteries

artery is occluded and which lead(s) will present ST-elevation. Then the user can either use the slider to rotate the model or physically move the android device to view different angles of the heart. Examples of these capabilities can be seen in Fig. 1.23.

1.4.4 Quiz Scene

The quiz scene is for the user to test their knowledge of ECG leads, coronary arteries, and STEMIs (Fig. 1.24). The quiz itself is comprised of five multiple-choice questions randomly generated from a pool of ten. The questions were provided by educators within the Scottish Ambulance Service after viewing the application prototype to reflect their training curriculum and the information offered by the learn scenes. The user is able to complete the quiz at any point while using the application and any number of times by refreshing the scene.

1.5 Analysis

The following section overviews the methods of analysis and subsequent results. The validity of the application was determined as knowledge acquisition and if it was effective at enhancing learner knowledge of CEP. The usability of the application was determined via a standardised system usability assessment completed by participants.

1.5.1 Methods

1.5.1.1 Participants

Ten newly qualified paramedics (degree level SCQF 9) completing their clinical induction

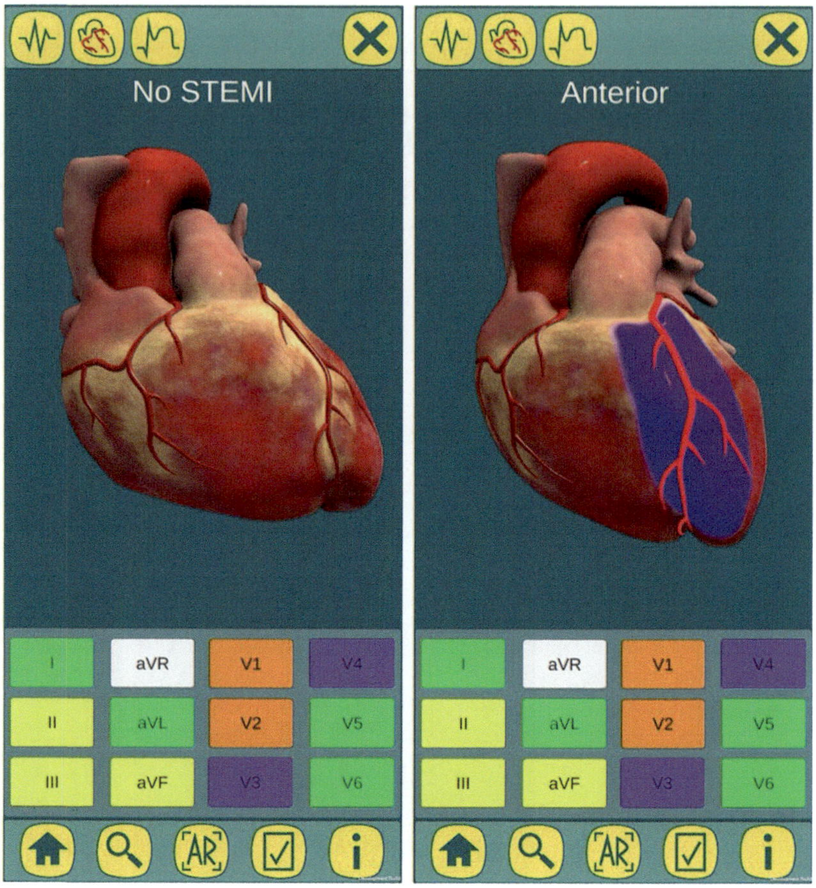

Fig. 1.22 STEMI option within the Learn scene. Includes a rotatable heart and visualisation of STEMIs from contiguous leads

module with the SAS were recruited. Participants were provided with an information sheet to inform them of the details about the study. Those who wished to participate were then given consent forms to be signed by themselves and the researcher on the day of testing. Demographic information was not collected from participants as they were all at the same qualification level and in the same training course. Any further demographic data was extraneous to the current investigation.

Ethics approval for this research was provided by the Glasgow School Art ethics committee and by the Scottish Ambulance Service research and development committee.

1.5.1.2 Equipment

The equipment utilised during testing included two Samsung Galaxy A52s mobile phones installed with the *ECG-in-AR* application and a printed A3 size poster. The poster included the logos of each collaborating body, the name of the author and supervisors, and the *ECG-in-AR* application logo (Fig. 1.25).

1.5.1.3 Procedure

Prior to using the application, participants completed a pre-test which comprised ten multiple-choice questions to assess their initial knowledge of cardiac electrophysiology. The participants were then given a mobile device with which they were asked to explore freely the *ECG-in-AR* application. As pre-test questions were the same as the questions included in the Quiz Scene of the application, participants were directed not to enter the Quiz Scene when given access to the application, to avoid any bias. Testing lasted approximately 10–15 min per participant.

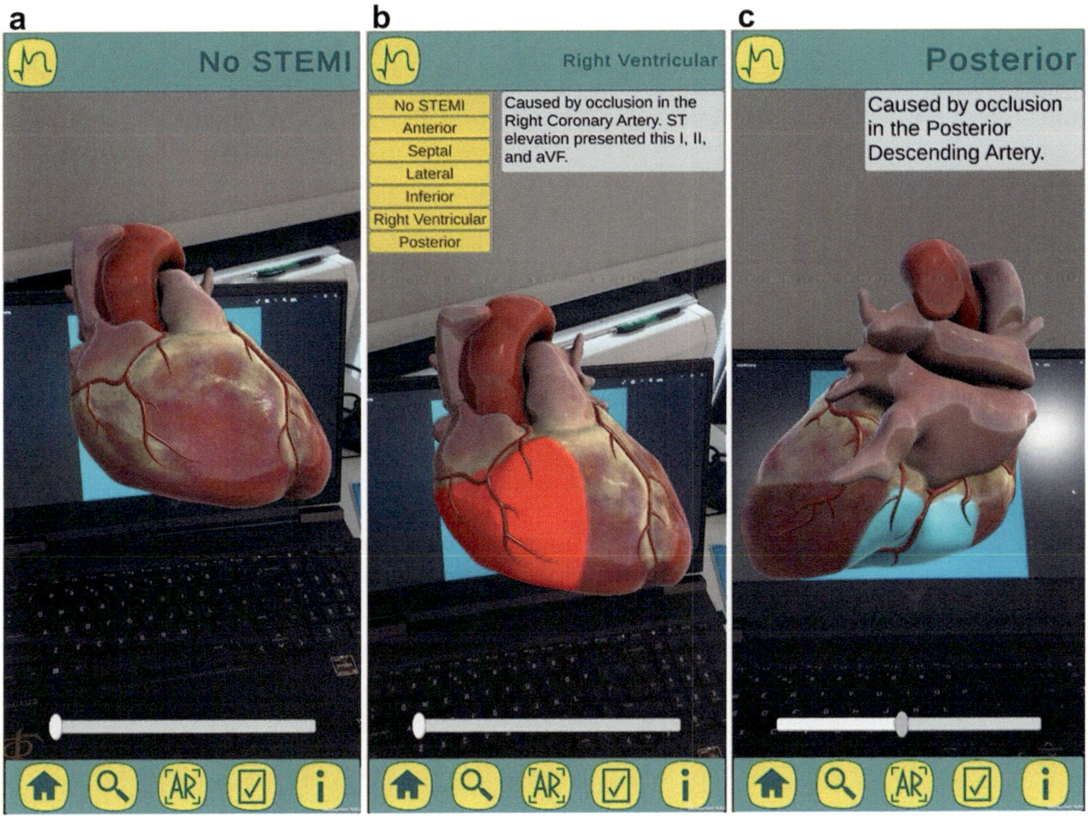

Fig. 1.23 AR scene with heart model, slider for rotation, and drop-down selection of STEMIs with correlating information. No STEMI (**a**), right ventricular (**b**), and posterior (**c**)

The researcher remained in the testing facility with participants to answer any questions and assist when necessary. Participants were allowed an unlimited time to explore the application and given the following directions:

(a) Press every button
(b) Read all information in full
(c) Scan the poster during the AR Scene (taped to the wall of the testing facility)
(d) Do *not* enter the Quiz Scene.

Once finished using the application, participants returned the mobile device and were immediately given the post-test and a usability questionnaire (Brooke 1996) to complete. The post-test was comprised of the same questions and answers as the pre-test but reordered. These tests were used to establish educational efficacy of the application.

1.5.1.4 Data Analysis

The normality of the data was first assessed by determining the skewness of the pre- and post-test scores. Data were not normally distributed; therefore, a Wilcoxon signed-rank test was used to compare pre- and post-test scores. Significance was determined by a p-value <0.05 (Laerd Statistics 2020).

The usability questionnaire was acquired from Brooke (1996) System Usability Scale (SUS). The questionnaire included ten statements for the user to rate. Responses were rated along the following Likert scale: 1 = strongly disagree, 2 = disagree, 3 = neutral, 4 = agree, and 5 = strongly agree. The possible SUS scoring range is 0–100; however, this does not represent a percentage. The SUS score was calculated by first scoring each question response and following the steps below:

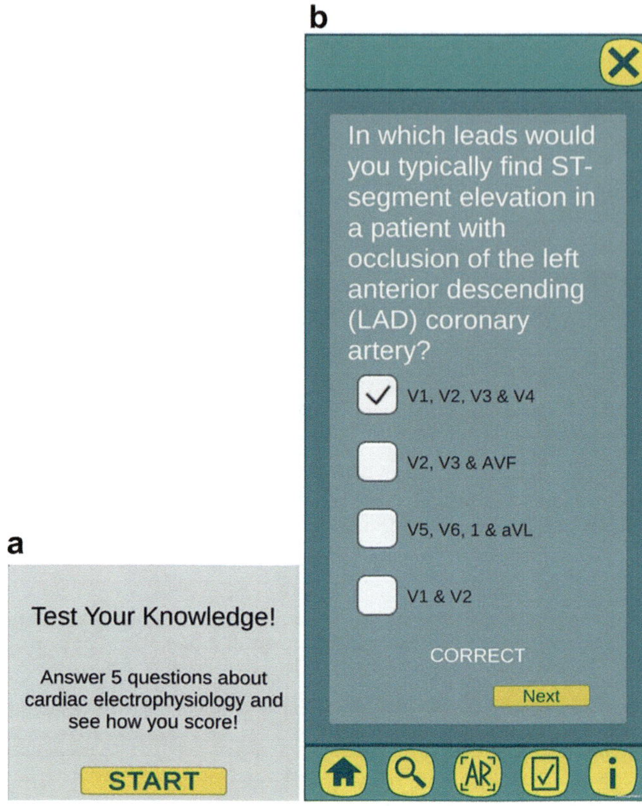

Fig. 1.24 Quiz scene pop-up panel with directions (**a**) and example question layout (**b**)

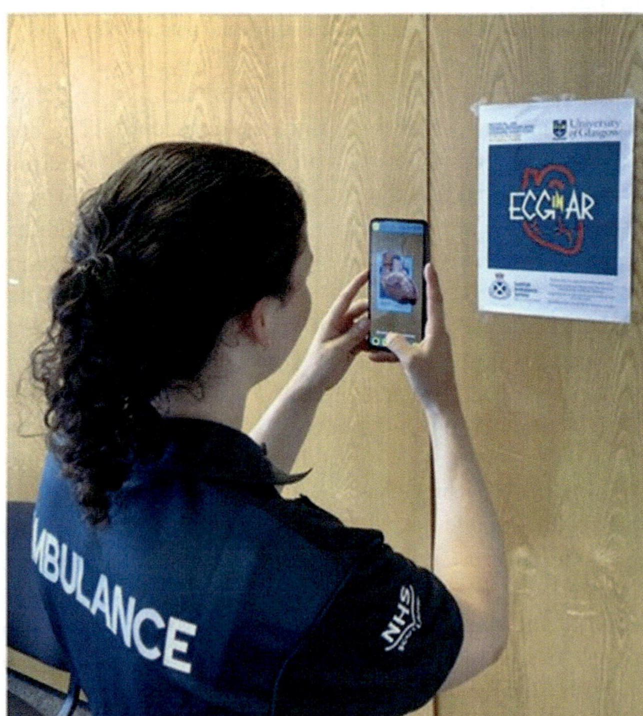

Fig. 1.25 Experimental testing set-up at SAS facility

1. Odd numbered question = [scale position]—1
2. Even numbered question = 5—[scale position]
3. SU score = [sum of the question scores] * 2.5

The collected data was transferred to Microsoft Excel for organisation and graphical analysis. Any statistical analysis was conducted via PSPP from the collated data.

1.5.2 Results

1.5.2.1 Validity

The statistical analysis suggested a significant increase in knowledge post-test scores with a mean score of *4.8 ± 1.62*) pre-test compared to po *7.0 ± 1.49* post-test (p = 0.024) (Figs. 1.26 and 1.27).

1.5.2.2 Usability

The application received a usability score of 82.8 (Fig. 1.28) which is 24.8 points higher than the SUS standardised reference benchmark of 68 (Sauro 2011).

Regarding knowledge acquisition, results of the Wilcoxon signed-rank test showed that the observed difference between both measurements was significant ($z = -2.26, p = 0.024$). Therefore, it can be assumed that the significant increase in participant knowledge was due to using the application and not due to an external influence (Meek et al. 2007). The 22% improvement from pre- to post-test scores indicates the efficacy of this application in facilitating user knowledge acquisition. Nine of the ten questions received post-test scores greater than or equal to that of their pre-test scores. Conversely, Question 10, which received the highest number of correct answers in the pre-test, was the only question to decrease in the number of correct responses from pre- to post-test. This could be due to participants second-guessing their answers during the pre-test and not wishing to duplicate those responses; however, the reason for this outlier cannot be confirmed without further testing.

Responses from the usability questionnaire were highly satisfactory from a developmental perspective. The SUS testing scored 82.8 receiving an A grade and *excellent* denomination. A score greater than 80.3 receives an A letter grade

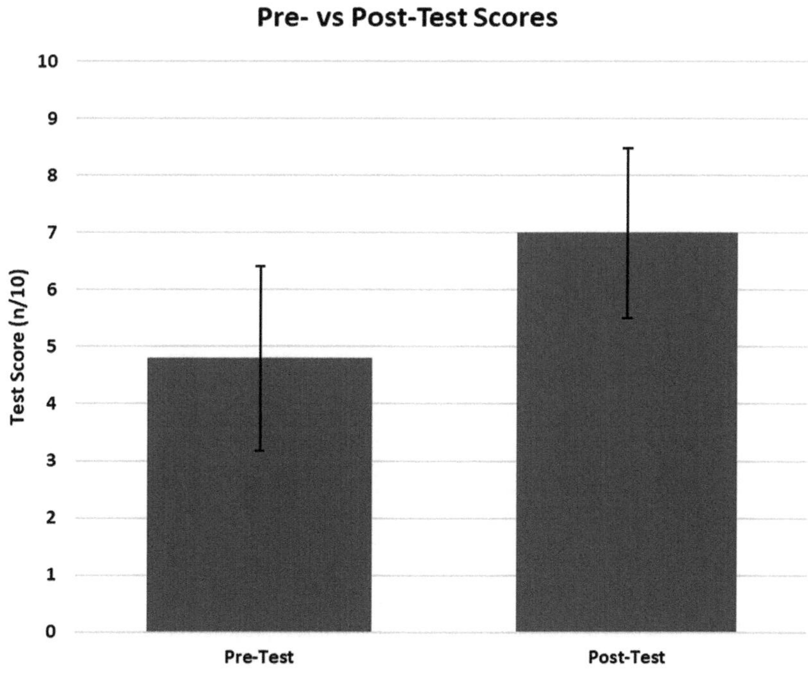

Fig. 1.26 Pre-test and post-test scores presented as mean ± standard deviation (Pre: 4.8 ± 1.62; Post: 7.0 ± 1.49)

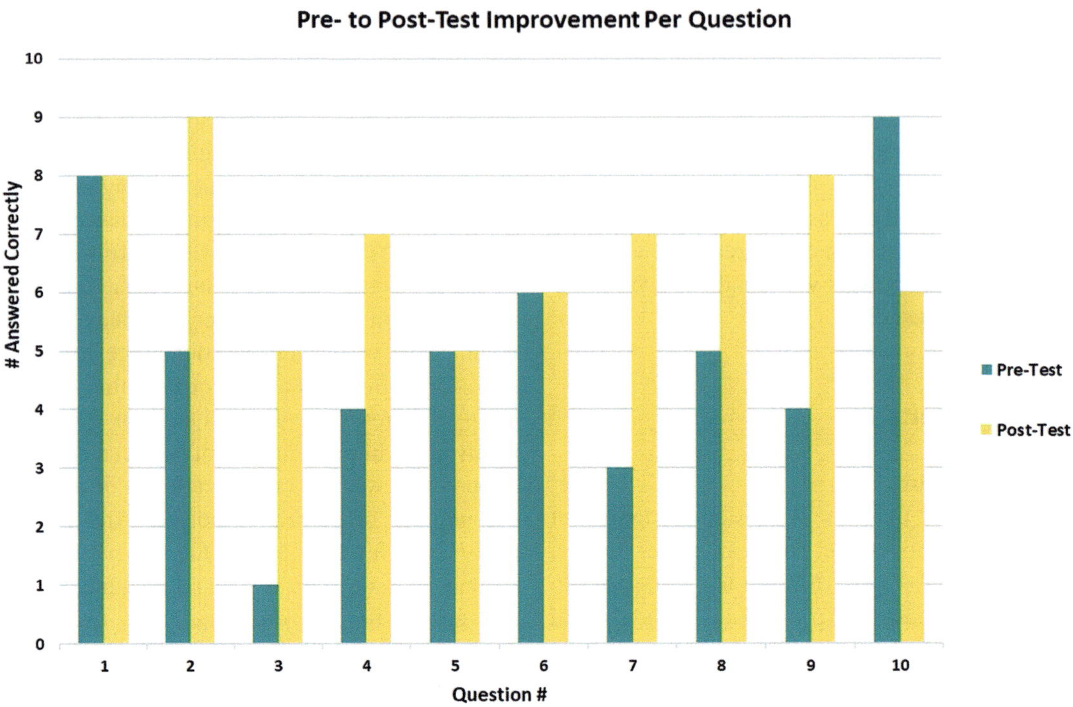

Fig. 1.27 The number of participants who answered each question correctly showing the difference per question between pre- and post-test

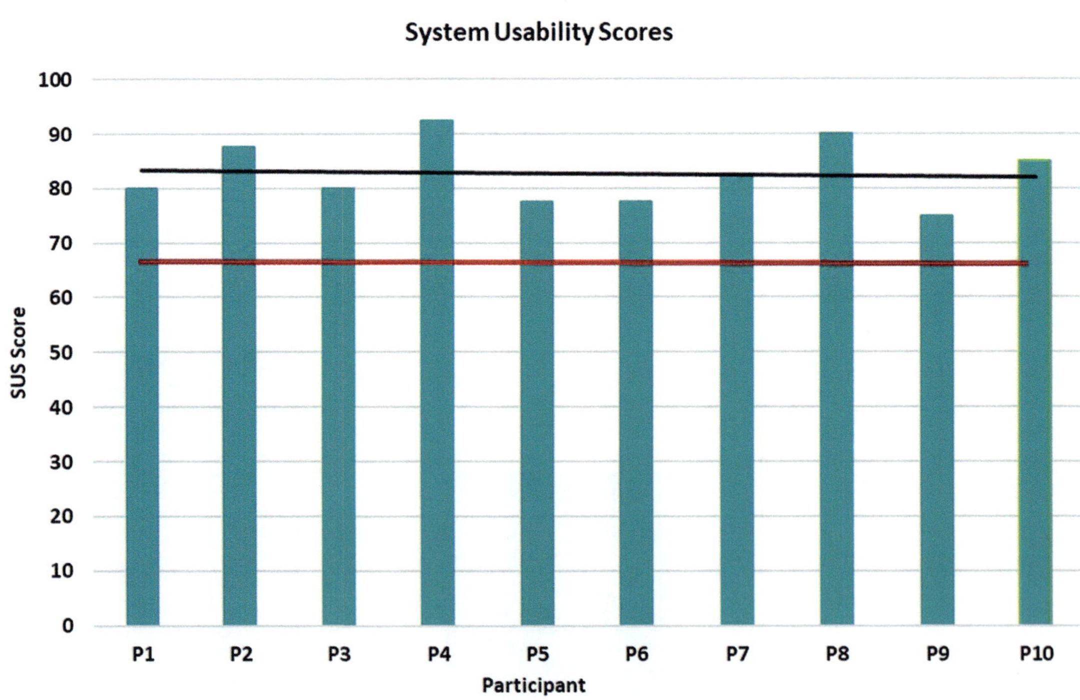

Fig. 1.28 SUS scores per participant where the red line represents the standardised reference score (SUS = 68.0), and the black line represents the mean score of this application (M = 82.8)

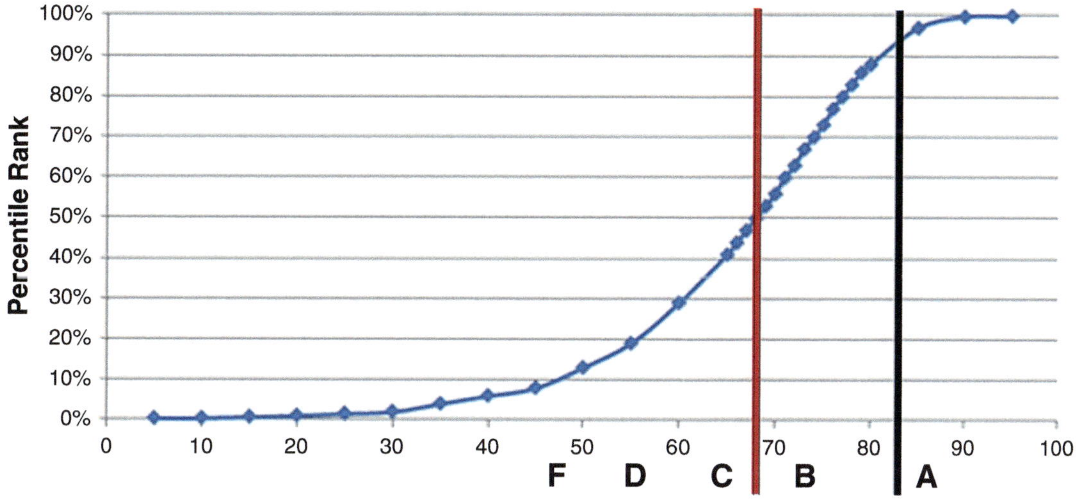

Fig. 1.29 SUS score percentile ranks as letter grades (Sauro 2011). The red line represents the standardised reference score (SUS = 68.0), and the black line represents the mean score of this application (M = 82.8)

and 'excellent' adjective result placing the application in the top 10% of scores (Fig. 1.29) (Bangor et al. 2009; Sauro 2011).

This placed the application 24.8 points above the standardised SUS benchmark and within the top 10% of scores indicating its promise as a user-friendly application. This is in line with similar AR learning applications about the spinal cord (Fernandes et al. 2020) and molecular geometry (Nazar et al. 2020) which scored 69 and 92.7, respectively. Anecdotally, no correlation was identified between pre-/post-test scores and SUS ratings. Future research should include additional text boxes to allow users to input their individual and specific feedback about the application.

In all, the outcomes of user testing were positively indicated. The efficacy of the application, *ECG-in-AR*, at enhancing user knowledge of cardiac electrophysiology was validated through pre- and post-test questionnaires. The usability of the application was shown to be excellent according to high SUS scores and user feedback. Overall results suggest the promise of this application if introduced on a wider scale. Future investigations should be conducted to further validate the current findings.

1.6 Discussion

1.6.1 Design and Development

The design and development of *ECG-in-AR* was successful but not without challenge. As seen in the initial storyboard for the application (Fig. 1.1), several changes were implemented to achieve the final application. Many of these changes were in respect to recommendations made by supervisors and consults with SAS educators. Moreover, the final application includes all major aspects included in the MoSCoW prioritisation.

Retrospectively, the segmentation process could have been more definitive in its goal of segmenting the heart. Though 3D Slicer was not difficult to use, it did require several trial-and-error attempts to properly segment the heart. The first segmentations included segmenting each individual region of the heart, yet none progressed passed this stage as they were deemed secondary to the educational goals of the application. Only the segmentation of the whole heart was exported for modelling. Future developments of the application might include a section on heart anatomy in which these segmentations could be utilised.

The 3D modelling and texturing phase was successful in all goals. The primary difficulty of this process was the UVW unwrapping which required several trials of drawing and relaxing seams on the model. In hindsight, the only alteration would be to increase the number of polygons in the final heart retopology. This would allow the model to be higher quality and provide more depth to textures. Additionally, modelling the arteries separate to the heart meant that painting the model required some guesswork when texturing the area surrounding where the arteries were meant to be placed. The painting and texturing of the heart from anatomical references was the developers most satisfactory accomplishment.

The Unity development and scripting provided the greatest challenge. The UI was the first aspect created of the application with accompanying button functions. The majority of scripts were able to be implemented without difficulties and only the scripts associated to the AR scene represented a certain degree of challenge. Figuring out how to add functionality to the AR rendered heart was the most time-consuming as the model was not in the scene hierarchy. Numerous attempts were written to include the heart model before incorporating the *HeartManager* gameobject and linking it to the *ARObjOverlayImage* script.

Lastly, the interactions in the Home Scene were added after completing the application as the scene seemed plain and without purpose. The concept of the lead placements on the ribcage was influenced by the initial storyboard's camera analogy scene. Due to being a last-minute addition, the ribcage was downloaded as a model from SketchFab rather than being segmented and modelled from scratch.

Overall, the creation process and final application realised the expectations of the researcher and was only negatively impacted by time constraints.

1.6.2 Evaluation

1.6.2.1 Limitations and Future Recommendations

The primary limiting factor during this project was time. Though all major aspects listed in the MoSCoW matrix (Table 4) were able to be included in the final development, additional features imagined by the research during the development were not incorporated to maintain the strict schedule for development and analysis. The recommendations for future development are the inclusion of voice-over audio components for users with hearing impairment, internal cross-section views of the heart for more in depth cardiac anatomy training, AR version of the lead views present in the Home Scene, 3D animated heartbeat to assist in correlating the ECG rhythm in real time, and a video animation of how arteries become occluded to restrict blood flow to the surrounding myocardium for greater comprehension of the pathological mechanism behind STEMIs. Expansion of the application may also include education on additional ECG presented dysrhythmias beyond STEMI.

Regarding the experimental design of this project, several recommendations can be made. Firstly, the small sample size recruited for this experiment ($n = 10$) should be increased for greater reliability and more extensive statistical testing. The population demographic could also be expanded upon in both experience level and specialisation as this study only tested on newly qualified paramedic students not ambulance technicians and clinicians with years of experience. Moreover, students learning cardiac electrophysiology within other health fields such as medicine, nursing, or exercise physiology could be tested. Expanding the testing population in either of these demographic directions would help to determine the efficacy of the application as an educational tool. Similarly, expanding the questionnaire question pool and allowing for individual feedback on the application would be beneficial. Additionally, a comparison study of conventional learning methods (e.g., textbook, 2D education, etc.) versus the application as supplementary learning may be advised to evaluate efficacy further. Also, knowledge retention following usage of the application could be examined via longitudinal investigations.

1.6.3 Conclusion

Overall, the *ECG-in-AR* application shows potential for becoming a widely utilised educational application within ambulance personnel. The application was effective at improving paramedic knowledge of CEP and STEMI presentations. This could lead to more accurate and rapid diagnoses in the future and improve patient care outcomes. Our experimental findings suggest the current efficacy of the application in facilitating user knowledge and support recommendations for future research, though further testing is needed to confirm the current trends and validate the application in a medical context.

References

Alrumayh AA et al (2022) Paramedic ability in interpreting electrocardiogram with ST-segment elevation myocardial infarction (STEMI) in Saudi Arabia. J Multidiscip Healthc 15:1657–1665. https://doi.org/10.2147/JMDH.S371877

Atienza F, Martins RP, Jalife J (2012) Translational research in atrial fibrillation. Circ Arrhythm Electrophysiol 5(6):1207–1215. https://doi.org/10.1161/CIRCEP.111.970335

Balady G et al (2015) COCATS 4 task force 3: training in electrocardiography, ambulatory electrocardiography, and exercise testing. J Am Coll Cardiol 65(17):1763–1777

Bangor A, Kortum P, Miller J (2009) Determining what individual SUS scores mean: adding an adjective rating scale. J Usability Stud 4(3):114–123

Birt J, Moore E, Cowling M (2017) Improving paramedic distance education through mobile mixed reality simulation. Australas J Educ Technol 33(6). https://doi.org/10.14742/ajet.3596

Birtill M et al (2023) The use of immersive simulation in paramedicine education: a scoping review. Interact Learn Environ 31(4):2428–2443. https://doi.org/10.1080/10494820.2021.1889607

Breen C, Bond R, Finlay D (2019) A clinical decision support tool to assist with the interpretation of the 12-lead electrocardiogram. Health Informatics J 25(1):51–61. https://doi.org/10.1177/1460458216683534

Brooke J (1996) SUS: a quick and dirty usability scale, Usability evaluation in industry, vol 189, pp 189–194

Coelho RC, Rangel Lourenço NCG, de Godoy CMG (2018) A mobile device tool to assist the ECG interpretation based on a realistic 3D virtual heart simulation. Simulation 94(6):465–476. https://doi.org/10.1177/0037549717733038

Cook DA, Oh S-Y, Pusic MV (2020) Accuracy of physicians' electrocardiogram interpretations. JAMA Intern Med 180(11):1461. https://doi.org/10.1001/jamainternmed.2020.3989

Fernandes J, Teles A, Teixeira S (2020) An augmented reality-based mobile application facilitates the learning about the spinal cord. Educ Sci 10(12):376. https://doi.org/10.3390/educsci10120376

Funder JL, Ross L, Ryan S (2020) How effective are paramedics at interpreting ecgs in order to recognize STEMI? A systematic review. Aust J Paramedicine 17:1–9

Han JK et al (2021) Virtual transformation and the use of social media: cardiac electrophysiology education in the post-COVID-19 era. Curr Treat Options Cardiovasc Med 23(11):70. https://doi.org/10.1007/s11936-021-00948-9

Klabunde RE (2017) Cardiac electrophysiology: normal and ischemic ionic currents and the ECG. Adv Physiol Educ 41(1):29–37. https://doi.org/10.1152/advan.00105.2016

Kopeć G et al (2015) Competency in ECG interpretation among medical students. Med Sci Monit 21:3386–3394. https://doi.org/10.12659/MSM.895129

Laerd Statistics (2020) *Lund Research Ltd*. Available at: https://statistics.laerd.com/features-selecting-tests.php. Accessed 11 Aug 2023

Logeswaran A et al (2021) The role of extended reality technology in healthcare education: towards a learner-centred approach. Future Healthc J 8(1):e79–e84. https://doi.org/10.7861/fhj.2020-0112

Lumsden CJ et al (2015) Using mobile devices for teaching and learning in clinical medicine. Arch Dis Child Educ Pract Ed 100(5):244–251. https://doi.org/10.1136/archdischild-2014-306620

Meek GE, Ozgur C, Dunning K (2007) Comparison of the t vs. Wilcoxon signed-rank test for Likert scale data and small samples. J Mod Appl Stat Methods 6(1):91–106. https://doi.org/10.22237/jmasm/1177992540

Mendes LA et al (2022) Competency-based alternative training pathway in cardiovascular disease and clinical cardiac electrophysiology. J Am Coll Cardiol 79(25):2540–2542. https://doi.org/10.1016/j.jacc.2022.04.022

Mohapatra D et al (2015) The scope of mobile devices in health care and medical education. Int J Adv Med Health Res 2(1):3. https://doi.org/10.4103/2349-4220.159113

Monigatti L (2022) Why your data visualizations should be colorblind-friendly. https://towardsdatascience.com/is-your-color-palette-stopping-you-from-reaching-your-goals-bf3b32d2ac49

Nazar M et al (2020) Development of augmented reality application for learning the concept of molecular geometry. J Phys Conf Ser 1460(1):012083. https://doi.org/10.1088/1742-6596/1460/1/012083

Parsons D, MacCallum K (2021) Current perspectives on augmented reality in medical education: applications, affordances and limitations. Adv Med Educ Pract 12:77–91. https://doi.org/10.2147/AMEP.S249891

Quinn T et al (2014) Effects of prehospital 12-lead ECG on processes of care and mortality in acute coronary syndrome: a linked cohort study from the myocardial Ischaemia National Audit Project. Heart 100(12):944–950. https://doi.org/10.1136/heartjnl-2013-304599

Roth GA et al (2020) Global burden of cardiovascular diseases and risk factors, 1990–2019. J Am Coll Cardiol 76(25):2982–3021. https://doi.org/10.1016/j.jacc.2020.11.010

Russo V et al (2021) Cardiac electrophysiology and pacing educational and training needs among early-career cardiologists: a national survey of the young Committee of the Italian Association of Arrhythmology and cardiac pacing. J Cardiovasc Med (Hagerstown) 22(10):744–750. https://doi.org/10.2459/JCM.0000000000001169

Sauro J (2011) Measuring usability with the system usability scale (SUS), measuring U. Available at https://measuringu.com/sus/. Accessed 11 Aug 2023

Sigg D et al (2010) In: Sigg DC et al (eds) Cardiac electrophysiology methods and models. Springer US, Boston, MA. https://doi.org/10.1007/978-1-4419-6658-2

Southworth MK, Silva JR, Silva JNA (2020) Use of extended realities in cardiology. Trends Cardiovasc Med 30(3):143–148. https://doi.org/10.1016/j.tcm.2019.04.005

Swing SR (2007) The ACGME outcome project: retrospective and prospective. Medical teacher 29(7): 648–654. https://doi.org/10.1080/01421590701392903

Turan Z, Gürol A, Uslu S (2021) A mixed-methods study exploring the effect of augmented learning for paramedic students in ECG training. Innov Educ Teach Int 58(2):230–241. https://doi.org/10.1080/14703297.2020.1752282

Ventola CL (2014) Mobile devices and apps for health care professionals: uses and benefits. P & T 39(5):356–364

Warriner DR et al (2017) Computer model for the cardiovascular system: development of an e-learning tool for teaching of medical students. BMC Med Educ 17(1):220. https://doi.org/10.1186/s12909-017-1058-1

Wilkins E et al (2017) European cardiovascular disease statistics 2017. European Heart Network, Brussels

Yu L et al (2021) Colour associations and consumer product-colour purchase decisions. Color Res Appl 46(5):1119–1127. https://doi.org/10.1002/col.22659

2 Virtual Reality Surgical Simulation Model to Train Microsurgical Digit Revascularization and Replantation

Madeleine Guillery, Matthieu Poyade, Jenny Clancy, Matt Burke, and Scott Lowenstein

Abstract

Virtual Reality has become a common tool in surgical simulation and training. Its application in microsurgery presents opportunities for immersive learning and skill refinement, as these non-biological simulators can significantly aid in teaching intricate microsurgical techniques.

This chapter presents a case for using VR in microsurgical training, spotlighting its application in managing ring avulsion injuries and facilitating adept replantation procedures. Ring avulsion injuries frequently necessitate microsurgical measures for effective replantation. Tracing back to the traditional Halsted residency model of "see one, do one, teach one," this chapter explores the shift towards a competency-based training approach. Simulation, in this context, has emerged as a pivotal tool, enabling safe and repetitive training for surgical residents. A description of the development and evaluative analysis of a VR-based simulator designed for mastering microsurgical digit revascularization and replantation is offered. The virtual reality simulator was tested using Oculus Quest 2 by seven participants to assess the face and content validity of the surgical simulator. The participants were surgeons, doctors, and other medical professionals, and experts in surgical simulation training. Feedback was gathered using a Likert-Scale, and suggestions were implemented in an updated version. This innovative tool, which offers a 3D immersive surgical environment, not only serves as a comprehensive guide through the stages of digit replantation but also demonstrates VR's potential in microsurgical education and refresher training in under-served hospitals. Through the proposed VR's immersive experience, even medical professionals in lesser-equipped hospitals can gain access to

M. Guillery (✉)
School of Medicine, Dentistry and Nursing, University of Glasgow, Glasgow, UK

School of Innovation and Technology, The Glasgow School of Art, The Hub, Pacific Quay, Glasgow, UK

M. Poyade
School of Innovation and Technology, The Glasgow School of Art, The Hub, Pacific Quay, Glasgow, UK
e-mail: M.Poyade@gsa.ac.uk

J. Clancy
School of Medicine, Dentistry and Nursing, University of Glasgow, Glasgow, UK
e-mail: Jenny.Clancy@glasgow.ac.uk

M. Burke
Medtronic, St Paul, MN, USA

S. Lowenstein
HealthPartners Regions Hospital, 640 Jackson Street, St. Paul, MN, USA

Department of Surgery, University of Minnesota, Minneapolis, MN, USA
e-mail: Scott.N.Loewenstein@healthpartners.com

J. Clancy, M. Poyade (eds.), *Medical Visualization and Applications of Technology – Volume 2*, Biomedical Visualization 5, https://doi.org/10.1007/978-3-031-63463-5_2

standardized training on finger revascularization and replantation.

Keywords

Virtual reality (VR) · Microsurgical training · Ring avulsion injuries · Replantation · Surgical simulation

2.1 Introduction

Ring avulsion injuries are unique injuries with treatment options ranging from amputation to replantation. Data from 2014 shows approximately 45,000 patients in the USA sustained injuries resulting in finger amputation (Giladi et al. 2014). These injuries are 90% of the US amputations costing the American healthcare system billions of dollars annually (Cho et al. 2019). Over the same time period, hand trauma care has been centralized to high-volume trauma care centers (Cho et al. 2018).

The advancement of microsurgery has greatly impacted digit revascularization and replantation as it has made for better visualizations of arterial anastomosis, nerve grafts, or autografts, as well as venous anastomoses. To aid in training, synthetic models like rubber gloves, surgical gauze, and sewing needles have been developed to aid in microsurgical training simulations. However, a survey of members of the American Society for Surgery of the Hand (ASSH) showed that only 63% of microsurgeons feel confident in performing microsurgery. With the advent of Virtual Reality (VR) simulators in surgical training, new opportunities are emerging to aid microsurgery training (Abi-Rafeh et al. 2019).

Finding ways to provide exposure to rare injuries to low-volume hospital staff is important to ensure they are confident in their knowledge of these injuries when they present to their emergency rooms. For this reason, providing accessible and cost-effective solutions can potentially help surgeons familiarize themselves with different digit revascularization cases.

The study's aim was to develop and examine the efficacy of VR simulation in presenting 3D models of digit revascularization injuries and providing an interactive environment to aid in understanding replantation candidates. These aims were achieved through the completion of the following objectives:

1. Create anatomically accurate 3D models of various stages of digit replantation and animations further showcasing the anatomy of the injury.
2. Build and develop an interactive virtual reality environment that allows the viewer to interact with models using their hands.
3. Determine the feasibility of the application through a study focused on content validity and usability.
4. Formulate conclusions and future considerations.

2.2 Background Context

Hand surgery is an umbrella term that refers to a variety of operations, all of which are performed on the hand. Hand injuries are some of the most common injuries that present to emergency rooms in the USA. A large portion of these are occupational laceration injuries that affect mostly young individuals (Kohan et al. 2022). The other common procedures performed on the hand include skin grafts, skin flaps, closed reduction fixation, tendon repair, nerve repair, fasciotomy, surgical drainage or debridement, joint replacement, and replantation ("Overview of Hand Surgery," 2021). (e.g., Fig. 2.1).

Although not every hand injury requires microsurgery, an essential component in orthopedic surgery and plastic surgery, replantation is one of these injuries that do require it. Microsurgical interventions in a simplified form can be described as the "Three M's"; microscopy, micro-instruments, and micro-sutures.

Ring avulsion injuries have been defined as the following: a forcible separation or detachment: such as a tearing away of a body part accidentally or surgically (www.merriam-webster.com, n.d.). As explained by Yoon (2021), replantation is the reattachment of a completely ampu-

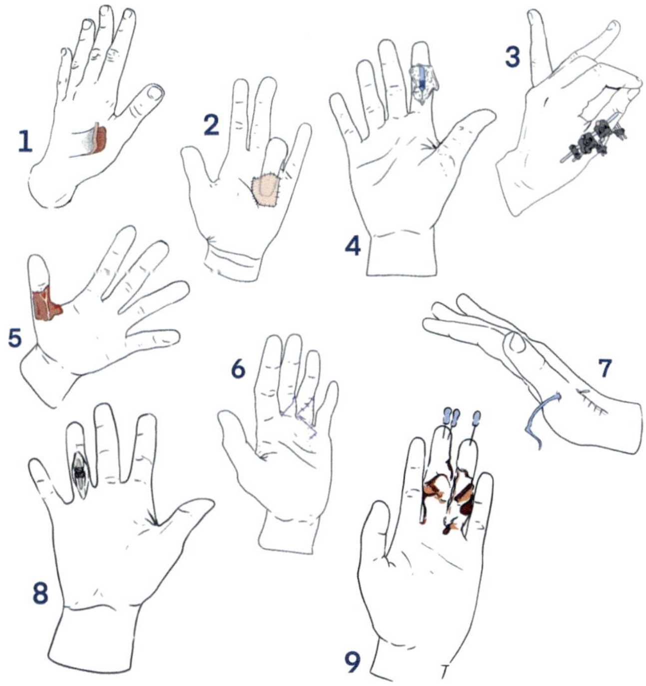

Fig. 2.1 Hand Injury Examples 1: Skin graft, 2: Skin flap, 3: Closed reduction fixation, 4: Tendon repair, 5: Fasciotomy, 7: Surgical drainage, 8: Joint replacement, 9: Replantation (Guillery 2023a, b)

tated finger, and revascularization is the reattachment of a partially amputated finger. The Urbaniak Classification System (Urbaniak et al. 1981) classifies these injuries into three classes: Class I: Circulation adequate; Class II: Circulation inadequate; and class III: Complete degloving or complete amputation (Urbaniak et al. 1981) shown in Fig. 2.2.

This classification system was referenced in many cases that reported ring avulsion injuries (Jones and Gujral (2016), Barbato and Salsac (2020), Struckmann et al. (2020), Jewett et al. (2021)). While class I and class II injuries can be treated with surgical intervention, these remain highly challenging. Replantation of a digit requires success in microsurgical anastomosis of arteries, veins, and nerves as well as a complete repair of any bone and or tendon injuries (Breahna et al. 2016). The mechanism of injury, the surgeon's years in practice, as well as the venous repairs all impact the success rate of digit replantation (Cho et al. 2019). Class III injuries can also be treated with surgical intervention as the advancement of microsurgery has improved the outcomes of replants after such critical injury (Cullen et al. 2022).

This classification system is a means to provide surgeons with a tool to assess the condition of the functional prognosis. Communication with the patient is an important first step in identifying if replantation is an option, as the patient must agree to this (Barbato and Salsac 2020).

Treatment options for ring avulsion injuries are constantly adapted as technology advances. However, surgeons continue to face challenges in determining whether amputation or replantation has better functional outcomes for the patient (Davis Sears and Chung 2011). The three treatment options are revised amputation, failed replantation, and successful replantation (Cho et al. 2018). Revised amputation is more often considered for class II and III injuries where more severe damages to the arteries, nerves, and bone are encountered. Replantation of digits is more common in the case of class I & II injuries and has been a controversial treatment option because of the cost of the procedure for the patient and the local healthcare system, as well as varied functional outcomes for the patient (Sebastin and Chung 2013).

Recent reviews of the existing patient data on functional outcomes of ring avulsion injuries

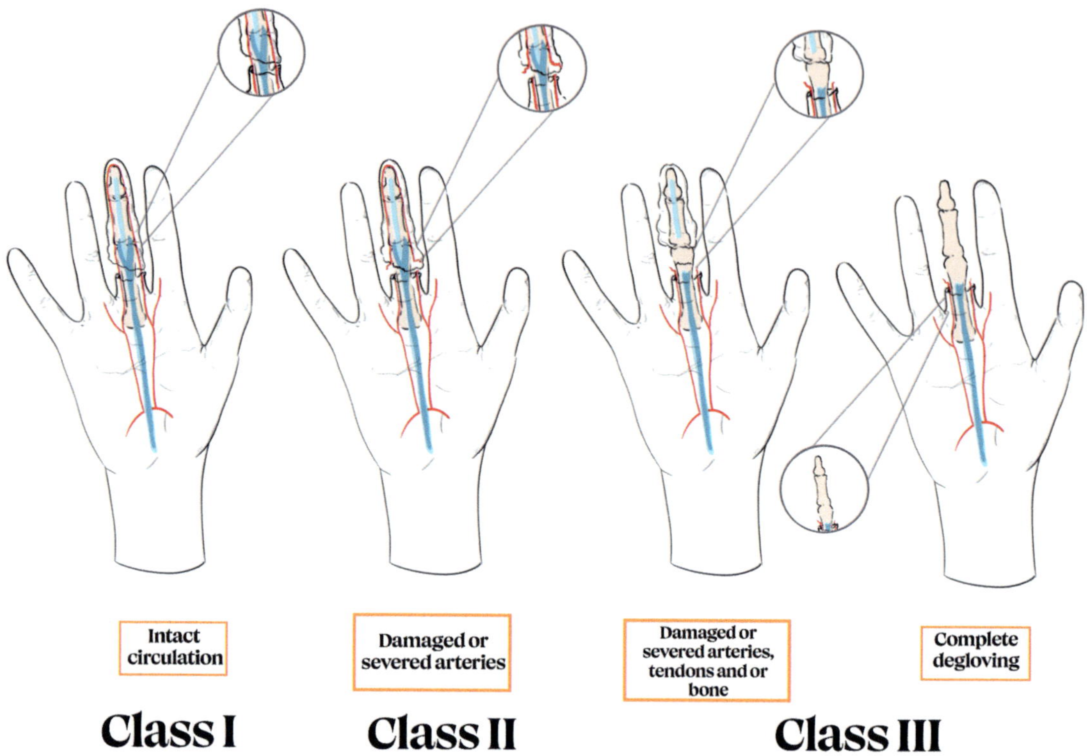

Fig. 2.2 Urbaniak Classification System illustration (Guillery 2023a, b)

show that the advancement of microsurgical revascularization skills has greatly impacted the surgeon's ability to achieve good functional outcomes post-operatively (Davis Sears and Chung 2011; Chiu et al. 2019). Patients who have undergone a successful replantation report minimized pain, better functional outcomes, improved long-term quality of life, and enhanced patient satisfaction. There are high success rates for Class I and II finger injury replants (Brown et al. 2017). Replantation process of a class III injury is possible because of the severity and complexity is difficult, optimal outcomes for microsurgical replantation warm and cold ischemia time is now under 6 h (Konczalik et al. 2019).

In the USA, digit replantation attempt rates have been declining over the last few decades, this is attributed to rising health costs, scarcity, and maldistribution of hand surgeons with microsurgical skills, low reimbursement rates for digit replantation, and unavailability of on-call hand surgeons (Fufa et al. 2013, Hustedt et al. 2016, Brown et al. 2017, Mahmoudi and Chung 2017). In an optimization study on national digit replantation trends in the USA, results showed that only half of the hand surgeons certified in microsurgery performed digit replantation. Additionally, the surgeons who performed digit replantation performed fewer than 5 cases per year (Cho et al. 2018). This highlights how the limited availability of microvascular services and the uneven distribution of case volume per hospital increase the need for patient transfers. Cases that present to a small rural hospital will be transferred to a large teaching hospital by helicopter or ambulance; however, the data shows that nearly half of these patients that are transferred were deemed ineligible for replantation. Responding ER doctors not being informed on what characteristics make a good candidate and what are indications for failed replantation's (Cho et al. 2018).

A study published in The Journal of Hand Surgery by Hustedt et al. (2016) reviewed all digit replants documented in the National

Inpatient Sample between 1998 and 2012. There were 101,693 amputations identified, and 15,822 cases were replants. Their findings showed that the success rate of replants dropped from 74.5% success rate between 2004 and 2006 to 64.7% between 2010 and 2012. Overall, these studies found high-volume centers to have a 2.5 times greater likelihood of obtaining a successful replantation compared to a low-volume center (Hustedt et al. 2016). In a research study on the patterns and epidemiology of digit replantation in the USA, Long et al. (2019) stated hospitals that are level 1 trauma centers located in metropolitan areas and teaching hospitals have higher rates of replantation compared to hospitals that do not fit into those categories. Long et al. (2019) also highlighted those patients who lived in zip codes with a higher median income had higher rates of replantation.

2.2.1 Simulation in Microsurgery Training

Simulation has been identified as a critical component of microsurgery training (Abi-Rafeh et al. 2019). These can include living and nonliving models/specimens, such as rat vessels, chicken thighs, and plastic and latex tubes (Winter and Petropolis 2021). Simulators are typically categorized into two groups: high and low fidelity (Odobescu et al. 2018). Low-fidelity models are designed to train the user on microscope setup, suture training, and handling the instruments; these are more often the nonliving models. High-fidelity training methods are typically using living simulation models. They are designed to train the user on technical aspects such as tissue dissection, technique, and suture placement, improving operative skills, which in turn improves patient safety (Winter and Petropolis 2021). Nonetheless, the current microsurgical simulation models have been reported to be limited in accessibility as well as having a lack of fidelity (Winter and Petropolis 2021).

In the USA, residents can get microsurgery training from various specialties. Although it has been reported, there are inconsistencies to residency training resources and practices depending on the specialty (Elliott et al. 2012). A survey conducted among hand surgeons (N = 131) between 2008 and 2010 revealed a variation in microsurgical experience, with 10 respondents who had not been exposed to replantation, 30 had not been exposed to free flap surgery, and 73 of the respondents did not have additional dedicated time for research during their fellowship. Free flap surgical techniques are very common when performing replantation procedures (Kakar et al. 2012). Kakar et al. (2012) study also highlighted that among those surgeons in the USA who completed a hand surgery fellowship, 74% (97) were trained in orthopedics, 16% (21) were trained in plastic surgery, and 10% (13) in general surgery. It has been suggested that the average perceived competence level dropped to 60% when performing replantation and 30% when performing free flap surgery (Kakar et al. 2012). Found that orthopedic surgery produces more microsurgeons than specialties like plastic or general surgery. However, orthopedically trained microsurgeons report lower confidence in microsurgical procedures than those trained in plastic surgery (Kakar et al. 2012). The ASSH survey revealed that only 53% of orthopedically trained surgeons performed replantation surgery, compared to 70% of plastic surgeons.

Virtual reality (VR) is a computer graphics technology that allows for real-time interactions with 3D models, combined with an immersive technology that physically places the user in immersion within the digital world (Cipresso et al. 2018; Yeung et al. 2021). M. Meehan et al. (2003) and D. A. Bowman and McMahan (2007) explain that immersion refers to the objective level of sensory fidelity a VR system provides, and that presence refers to a user's subjective psychological response to a VR system.

The benefits of VR-induced immersion, motion tracking, and its ability to provide a means for the user to view tangible, physically realistic 3D objects in a computer-generated environment have been well documented. It has been suggested that the key components to creating realistic and useful VR simulators for surgical training rely on a combination of advanced interaction paradigms, tissue deformation, collision detection, and high-resolution graphics (Abi-Rafeh et al. 2019). In study on the feasibility which using a VR device under the medical prototyping platform Mevis Lab, Egger et al.(2016), found that reviewing the 3D models in a virtual space supports training for improving the recognition of lesions from various angles.

According to the knowledge of the authors, the available literature on VR applied to microsurgery is limited. Abi-Rafeh, J. et al. (2019) found five VR simulators that are dedicated to microsurgery training, two of which consisted of knot-tying simulations. The other three provided haptic feedback while the user was doing simulated surgical tasks featuring threading models with collision detection systems as well as a suturing system training for grasping, suture placement, needle insertion, and knot tying. Given the limited availability of VR applications and tools for training, this study set out to develop and examine VR simulation's efficacy in presenting 3D models of digit revascularization injuries.

2.3 Methods

2.3.1 Materials

2.3.1.1 Software
See Table 2.1.

2.3.1.2 Hardware
See Table 2.2.

2.3.1.3 Source Data
See Table 2.3.

Building upon the previous analysis of the literature, there is a need for additional VR simulators related to microsurgery training to further understand the role VR can play in microsurgical training. To measure this, additional focused resources and research efforts are required. To address this need, the development and evaluation of the VR tool for reinforcing knowledge for digit revascularization and replantation was pursued.

The aim of the study was to examine the efficacy of VR simulation in presenting 3D models of digit revascularization injuries and providing an interactive environment to aid in understanding replantation candidates.

2.3.2 Workflow

The design and development of the application followed the workflow presented in Fig. 2.3. The activities throughout the workflow used the technologies presented in Fig. 2.4.

2.3.3 Concept

The concept consisted of an interactive VR environment aimed at familiarizing microsurgeons with ring avulsion cases. These injuries vary in severity levels, enabling microsurgeons to gain a better understanding of which cases warrant replantation attempts. Serving as a pilot experience, the project aims to offer a valuable means of visualizing digit revascularization cases at different stages and levels of severity, providing microsurgeons with a resource to analyze, visualize, and enhance comprehension of the anatomical aspects related to ring avulsion injuries.

The MoSCoW technique was used to inform the planning of the design and development by classifying requirements into priority categories ("Must have, should have, Could have, and Won't have") technique (Hudaib et al. 2018) to analyze the functional and user requirements (Fig. 2.5). This well-established prioritization technique was helpful for planning and identifying the critical components of the application.

2.3.4 Storyboard

A storyboard (Fig. 2.6) was designed to showcase some 3D model examples and three main scenes. The first scene illustrates the "landing page" with information about the application, how-to instructions as well as a visual of a ring avulsion injury modeled in 3D spinning in front

Table 2.1 The software used in this study is shown in the table

Software	Publisher	Use
Unity 3D	Unity Technologies https://unity.com/	Application development engine
Blender	Blender https://www.blender.org/	Animation and rendering of 3D objects
3Ds Max	Autodesk Inc. https://www.autodesk.co.uk/	UV unwrapping and retopologies
ZBrush	Pixologic Zbrush https://pixologic.com/zblanding/?v=2#	Make many of the models
Wacom	Wacom https://www.wacom.com/en-gb	3D modeling and texturing
Adobe Substance Painter	Adobe inc. https://www.adobe.com/uk/products/substance3d-painter.html	Materials made for all 3D objects in Adobe Substance Painter
Visual Studio Code	Microsoft https://code.visualstudio.com/	Code manager for the project
3D Slicer	3D Slicer https://www.slicer.org/	Segmentations of the bone models
Procreate	Savage Interactive https://procreate.com/	Storyboard, mood board, All 2D illustrations

(continued)

Table 2.1 (continued)

Software	Publisher	Use
Adobe Color	Adobe Inc. https://color.adobe.com/create/color-wheel	Creation of color pallet
Adobe Substance Sampler	Adobe Inc. https://www.adobe.com/uk/products/substance3d-sampler.html	Texture bases for Adobe Substance Painter
Microsoft Word	Microsoft https://www.microsoft.com	Primary writing application
Canva	Canva Pty Ltd https://www.canva.com/	Made Figs. 2.1, 2.2, 2.12

(continued)

Table 2.1 (continued)

Software	Publisher	Use
Kiri Engine	Kiri Innovation https://www.kiriengine.app/	App used for photogrammetry scans of hand
Miro	RealtimeBoard, Inc. https://miro.com/templates/moscow-matrix/	Used to make Figs. 2.6, 2.7, 2.8
Hardware	**Company**	**Use**
MacBook Pro	Apple Inc. www.apple.com	Blender, Zbrush, Substance Painter, 3D slicer, Microsoft Word
Oculus Quest2	Meta Quest https://www.oculus.com/	Final application development
Windows Desktop PC	Microsoft Windows https://www.microsoft.com/en-gb/windows?r=1	3Ds Max Use & Unity 3D

(continued)

Table 2.1 (continued)

Software	Publisher	Use
IPhone XS	Apple Inc. www.apple.com	Used the Kiri Engine App

Table 2.2 The hardware used in this study is shown in the table

Hardware	Company	Use
MacBook Pro	Apple Inc. www.apple.com	Blender, Zbrush, Substance Painter, 3D slicer, Microsoft Word
oculus Oculus Quest2	Meta Quest https://www.oculus.com/	Final application development
Windows 11 Windows Desktop PC	Microsoft Windows https://www.microsoft.com/en-gb/windows?r=1	3Ds Max Use & Unity 3D
IPhone XS	Apple Inc. www.apple.com	Used the Kiri Engine App

Table 2.3 The source data used in this study is shown in the table

Data	Source	Use
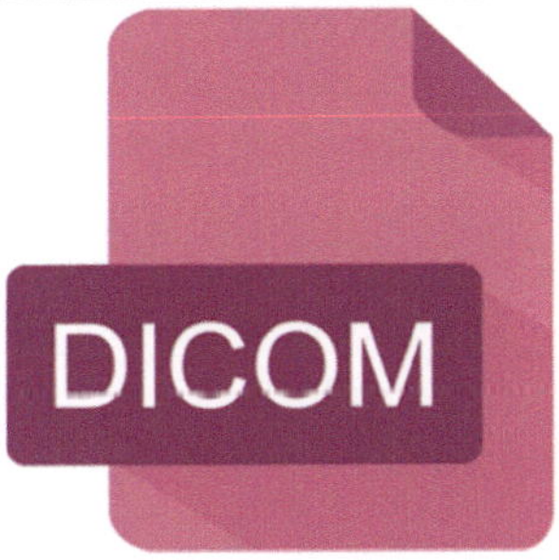 CT & MRI data of avulsion injuries of the fingers and hand	Dr. Megan Mills and Taylor Conkey from the Department of Radiology at the University of Utah	Dataset used for segmentation of the hand bones as well as the full hand
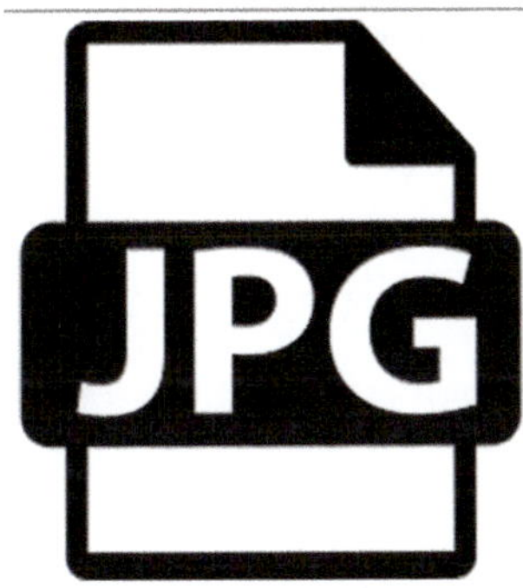 Figures from "Avoiding Ring Avulsion Injuries with Silicone Rings: A Biomechanical Study"	Dr. Callie A. Jewett	Image data used as a reference when modeling ring avulsions
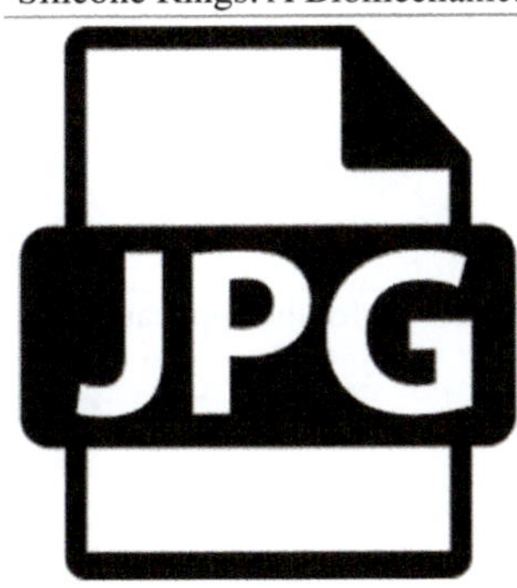 Figures from "Ring Injuries of the Finger: Long-Term Follow-up"	Dr. John D. Lubahn	Image data was used as a reference to avulsion injury 2 and the vein graft model
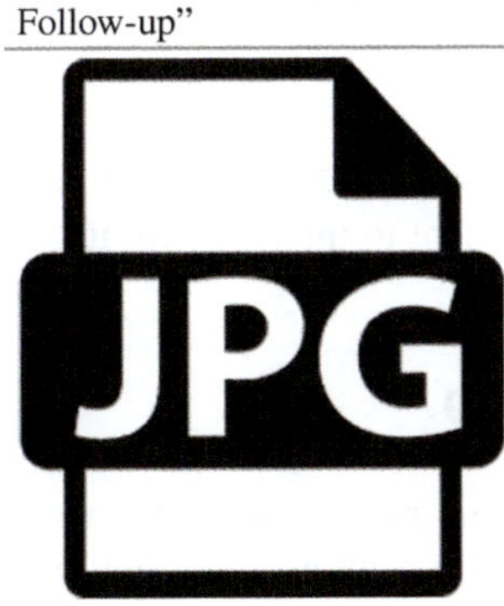 Image and video data from Dr. Scott Loewensein	Dr. Scott Loewensein	Image data was used as supporting data when building replantation models. The data provided highlighted the replantation procedure from start to finish

(continued)

Table 2.3 (continued)

Data	Source	Use
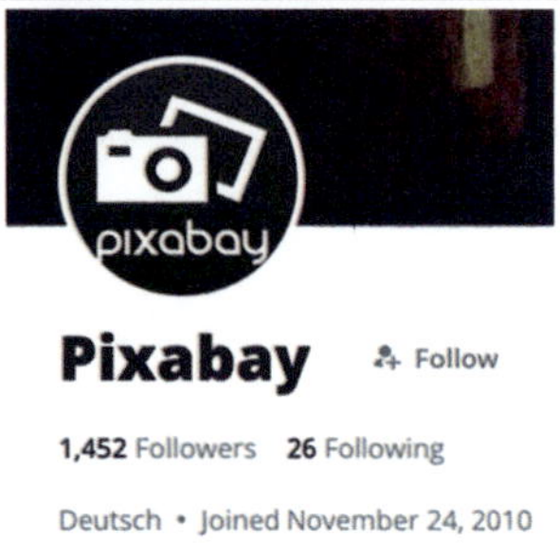 High-Pitch Click	https://pixabay.com/	Button click sound
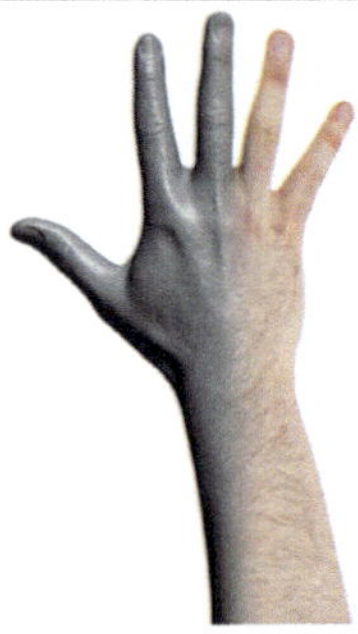 Hand Model	https://www.digitalrealitylab.com/sample-model/	Used photogrammetry model for avulsion model 1 used in the first scene
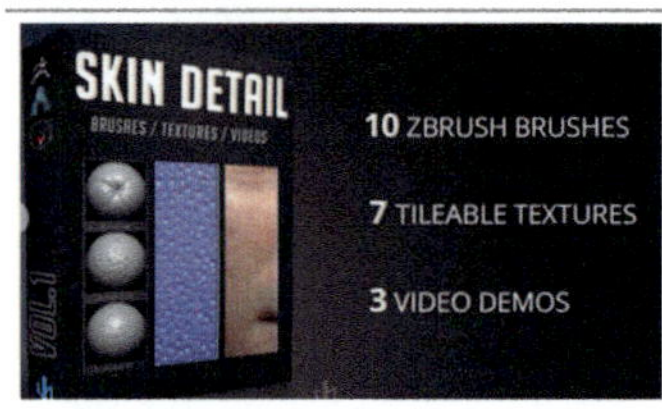 JH Skin Pack	http://www.artofjhill.com	Brushes for skin textures used in Zbrush on models
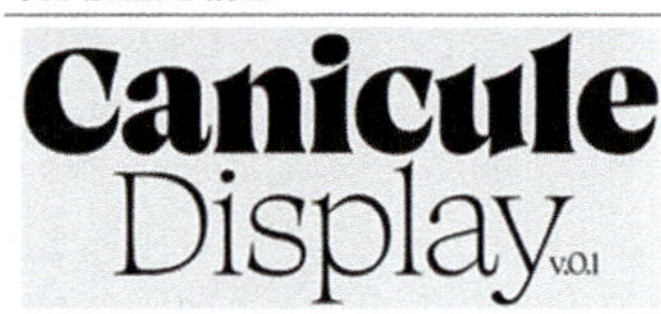 Canicule Typeface	https://www.behance.net/gallery/151899333/Canicule-Typeface-(Free-Trial)	Font used for the application

of the viewer. The final three scenes showcase the main part of the application. This is where the user will be presented with a larger-than-life 3D model of a hand with a finger avulsion injury. Each model will include the superficial components of the injuries and all relevant anatomical structures.

The storyboard below shows the 3D models of the bones of the finger, tendons, and arteries. The user will be prompted with questions about each model and encouragement to interact with it.

2.3.5 3D Modeling

The 3D models for this project were primarily built in Zbrush by using a photo reference. For anatomical accuracy, hand bones were segmented and exported into an .OBJ file and used a photo-

Fig. 2.3 Workflow Chart

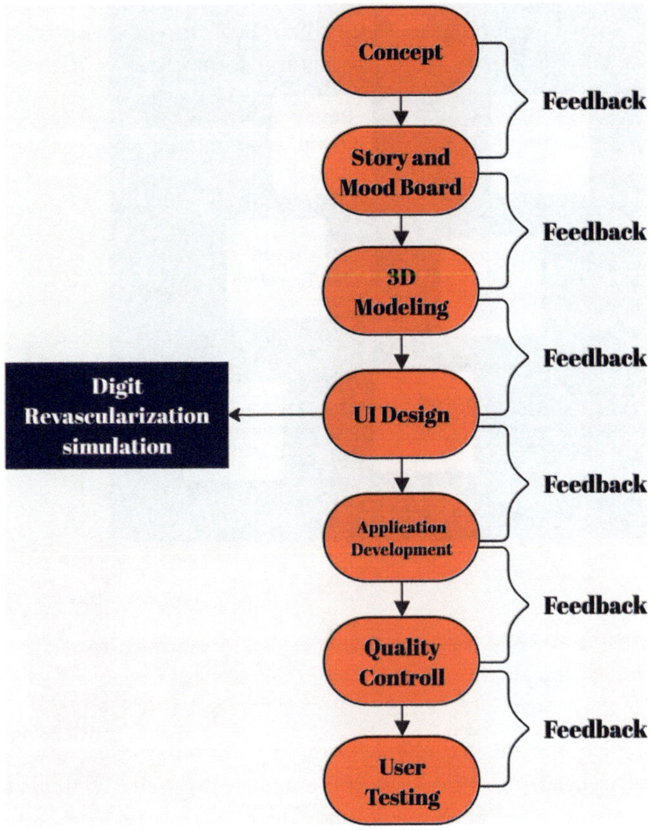

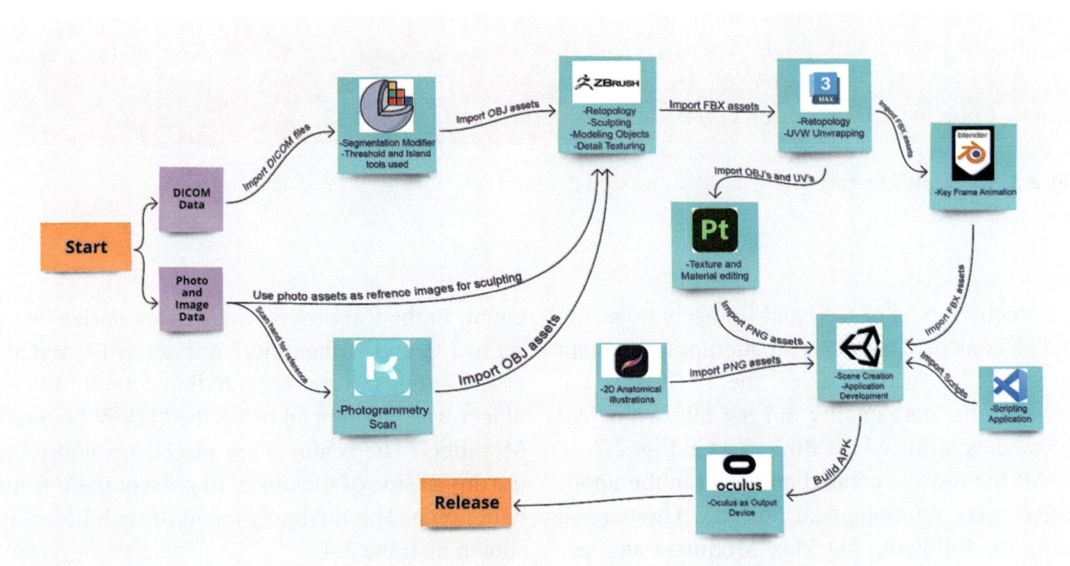

Fig. 2.4 This flow chart illustrates the application workflow used during the project. It depicts the association between the data, technology, and the process

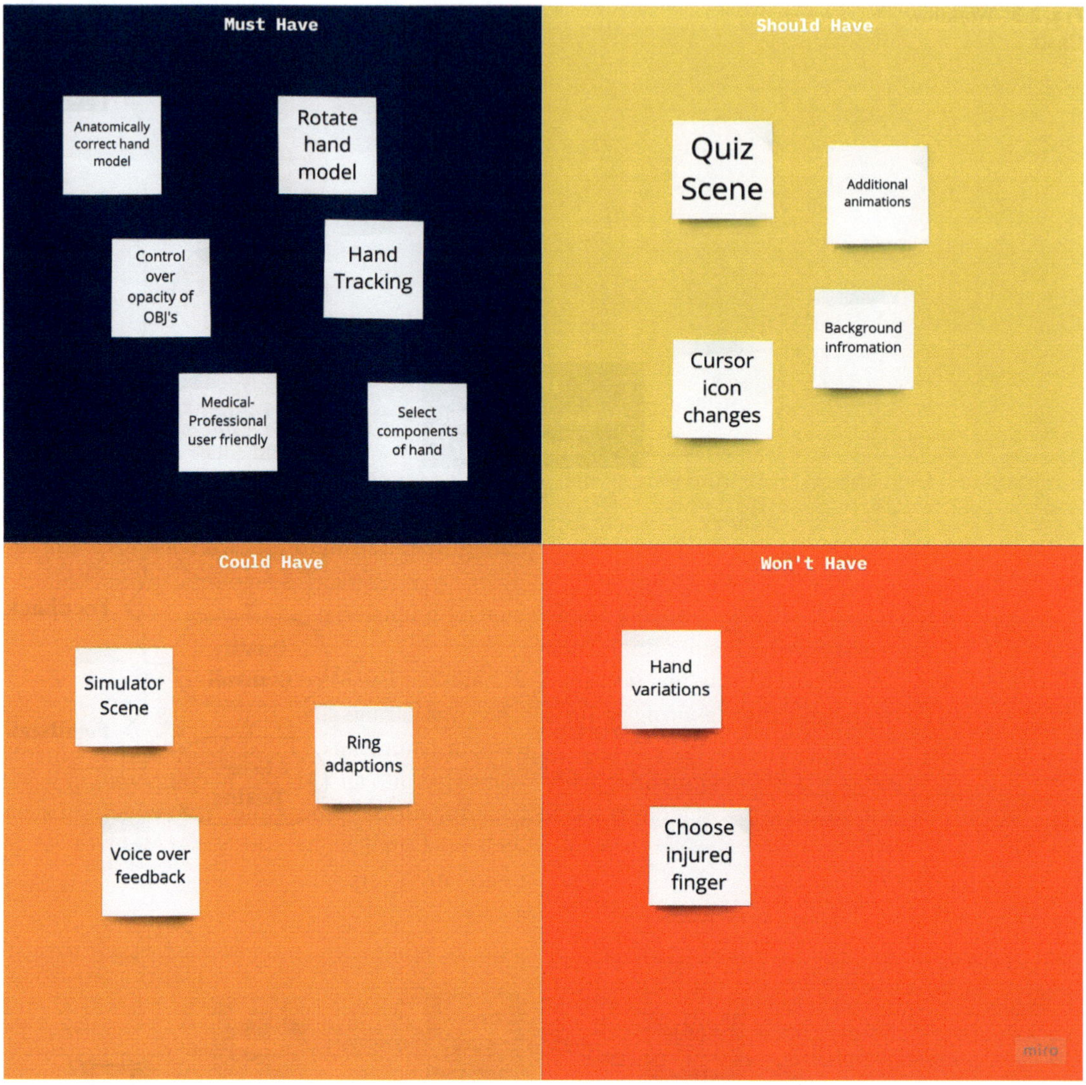

Fig. 2.5 MoSCoW chart

grammetry model of the hand for accurate sizing and placement. There was an attempt to segment more hand structures from the DICOM data; however, the data quality did not allow this. All the models followed the flow chart in Fig. 2.7.

All the models created and used in the application were retopologized and UV Unwrapped using the following 3D Max Modifiers and settings. The "Retopologize" Modifier was applied on each object with the settings set to "ReForm" and "Face Count" set to the intended polygon count. In the ReForm Settings, "Regularize" was set to 1.0, and "Adaptivity" was set to 1.0 and all other settings were kept at the default. Every object was unwrapped using the "UVW Unwrap Modifier." The seams were placed manually on the dorsal side of the object to prevent them from being seen. The final poly count of each object is shown in Table 2.4.

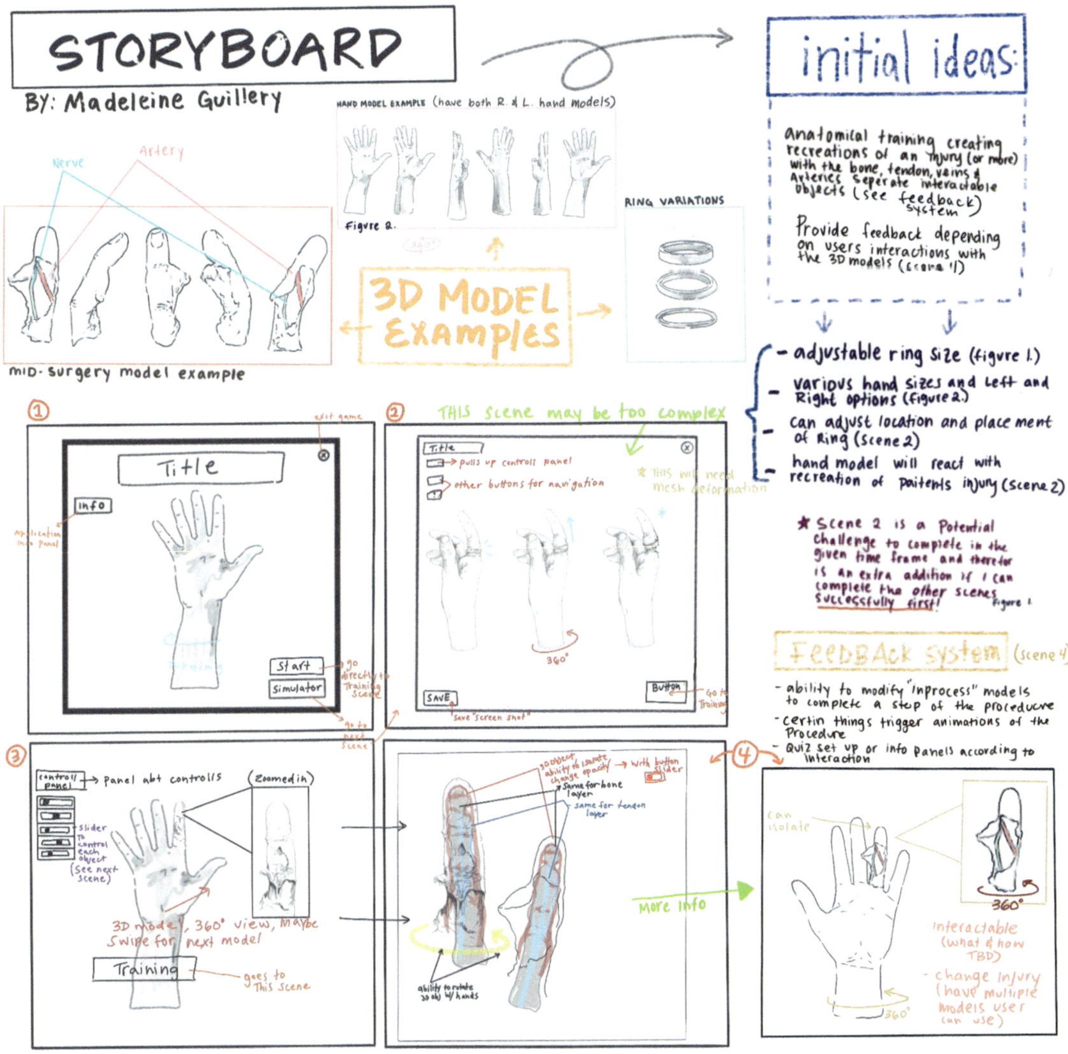

Fig. 2.6 Storyboard

2.3.6 Hand Model for Welcome Scene

A right-hand photogrammetry scan named "Hand Scan Sample" was downloaded from Digital Reality Lab initially as a backup, and imaging taken of a right hand of a volunteer for real life representation (Fig. 2.7. A ring avulsion injury was sculpted on this hand in ZBrush using the "Move" brush, "Smooth" brush, and "Deco" brush. This model was then textured in Substance Painter. It was then used in the Welcome Scene when users first entered the application.

A standard ring was built in Blender using the primitive shape "Torus." The hand model was used to reference size and ensure a proper fit of the ring to the finger. The ring model was then textured in Substance Painter, using a preset texture, "Metal Polished." Using the "Hard Brush" to paint the material onto the ring.

The application Kiri Engine was used to create a photogrammetry replica of a hand. After completing the photogrammetry scan, the model was exported as an OBJ file and imported into Zbrush. However, most of the fingers had webbing issues, so they were individually cut between

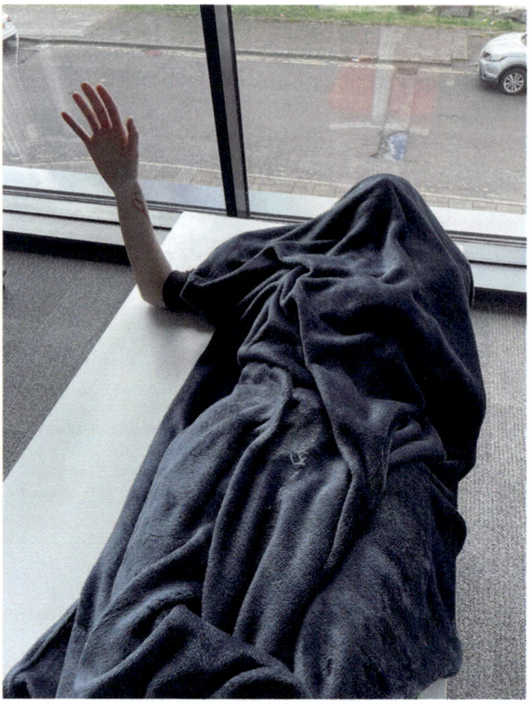

Fig. 2.7 Generic Hand Model

Table 2.4 Every object's final poly count

Object	Poly count
Ring avulsion model	11,700
The ring	792
The right hand	98,386
The bones	60,000
Veins	809
Arteries	5000
Nerves	5200
Cruciform part of the fibrous sheath	6700
Synovial tendon sheath	3100
Muscles	10,000
The common flexor tendon sheath	3070
The articular capsules of the interphalangeal joints	2109
Injury one	8900
Injury two	4997
Injury three	7500
Injury four	10,000
Injury five	2800

every single finger using the "Select Rect" brush. After that, the geometry was revised in Zbrush by applying the "Close holes" modifier in the "Modify Geometry" modifier to ensure that each finger was correctly separated. The poly count at this stage was 16,316.

After the separation of the fingers, Zremesher was used to re-mesh the hand to prepare it for more detailed modeling. The details of the fingernails, creases of the inner palm as well as skin details were added using the clay build-up brush, move brush, and smoothing brush. JHill's skin pack was used at the end for fine details of the skin, such as small pores and bumpy skin texture. After this, the fingernails were made by using the "Mask" brush in ZBrush to mask the area where the fingernails would be. Then using the move brush, the surrounding geometry was pulled out to create the ridges where the skin meets the fingernails. Finally, the mask applied was inverted, resulting in masking everything but the fingernails. This is when the "Move" brush was used to pull on the fingernails to create a ridge slightly going over the fingertip. At this stage, the hand model had 331,183 polygons and was exported from ZBrush as an FBX and imported into 3DS Max.

The model was then imported into Substance Painter, where the texture was baked. Following this using a mixture of layers of base colors, fill layers as well as part of the "Skin Human Simple" Starter Asset Texture to create the texture for the hand. All the layers listed in Fig. 2.8 were turned into a material asset named "skin" that was able to be saved in Substance Painter to apply to the injured finger objects to ensure the skin matched the hand (Fig. 2.9).

To start building this model, both the high poly right-hand object and the bone objects were imported into ZBrush. The two objects were aligned by resetting the transform on each object. Once they were aligned, the Standard pen tool was used with Zsub to carve out the palmer side of the hand. This method was used to push back the mesh until the bones were visible. The remaining structures were built from appended objects.

The 3D models of the bones were first extracted from a DICOM dataset using 3D Slicer. The models were created using the segmentation editor function in 3D Slicer. Using the threshold modifier in the segmentation editor produced a

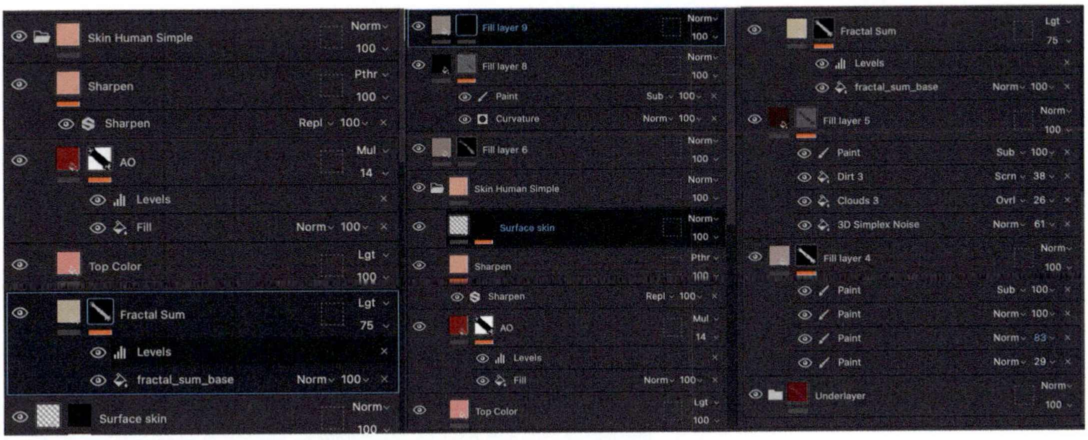

Fig. 2.8 "Skin" prefab settings in Substance Painter

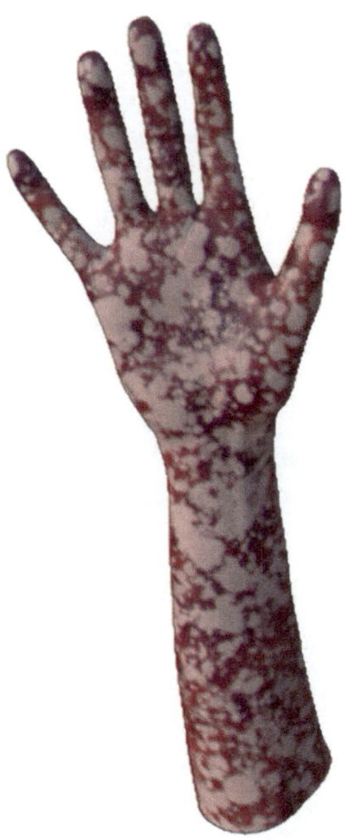

Fig. 2.9 Painting process in Substance Painter

good-quality model of the hands of the bones. However, there were small islands of voxels that were removed using the "remove small islands" function in the "Islands" modifier. Using the mouse, all the islands were selected that were not part of the bones; the thumb and wrist were not included and were not needed in the application. To make each bone a separate object, the "add selected islands" was used to individually select each of the four finger bones. Following this, the bones were exported from 3D Slicer as an FBX file that consisted of 17 individual objects (Fig. 2.10) that were imported into ZBrush shown in Fig. 2.11. Each bone was smoothed using the "Smooth" brush to remove any imperfections (Fig. 2.12). Then using the ZRemesher tool with "Same" and "Adapt" applied, each bone was remeshed to ensure each bone had similar geometry. Finally, the bones were imported into a Substance Painter, and each bone was applied with "Bone Material." The bone material was made in Adobe Substance Sampler using "Starter Asset" materials modifying the color and adding a damage filter to create a natural displacement of the pattern.

The modeling of the arteries, nerves, tendons, and veins was performed using the same steps in ZBrush. This included appending cylinders which were stretched and modified using the "Move" brush to ensure the position in the hand was anatomically correct. These objects were evaluated by Dr. Scott Loewenstein for anatomical correctness, and refinements were made. These changes included ensuring the veins were on the dorsal side of the hand, adding the cruciform part of the fibrous sheath, as well as ensuring the nerves were branching from the median nerve. At this stage, the model was exported as an FBX file from ZBrush and was imported into 3ds Max for better control of the geometry of the objects (Fig. 2.13). Then in 3ds Max, using the

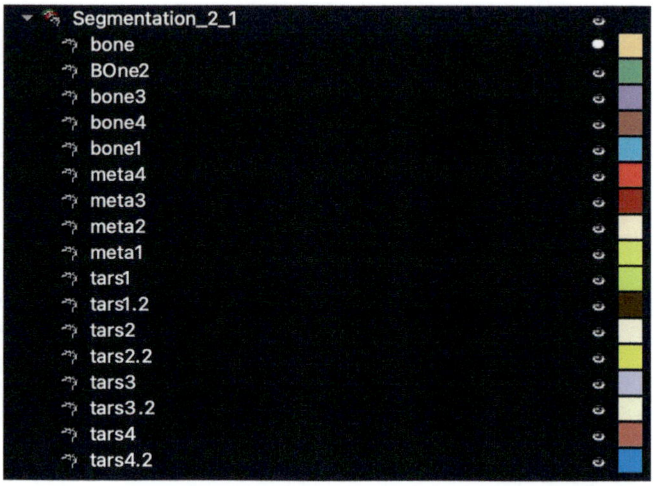

Fig. 2.10 The "Segmentation" group of all the individual bones objects

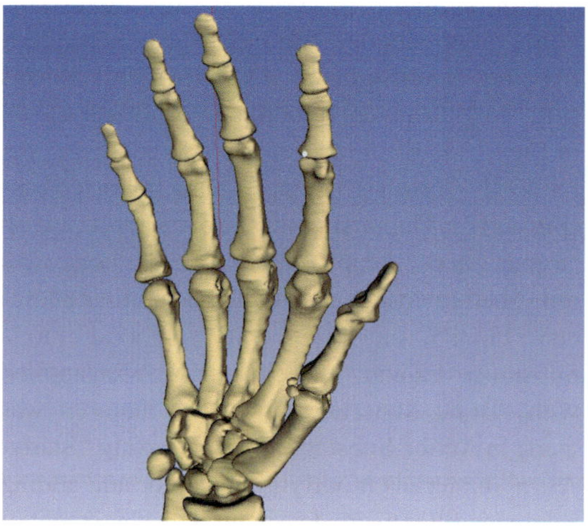

Fig. 2.11 Bones after segmentation process in Slicer 3D

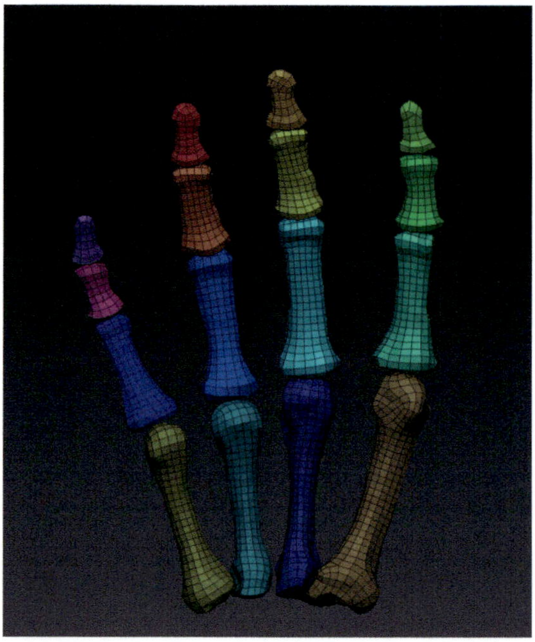

Fig. 2.12 Bone objects after retouch in ZBrush

line tool, traced the previous objects to ensure correct sizing and placement. The lines were then made into 3D cylinders and further shaped by moving the vertices with the move tool in 3D max. These steps were repeated for the arteries, nerves, tendons, and veins.

The abductor pollicis brevis muscle and the flexor pollicis brevis were the two muscles modeled at the base of the thumb. The abductor digiti minimi muscle and the palmaris brevis muscle were the two muscles modeled at the base of the fifth digit. These four muscles were included as the tendons, arteries, nerves, and veins have unique anatomy compared to the three middle fingers of the hand. As the application focuses on injuries to the index, middle, and ring finger, the choice to model the four muscles at the base of the fifth digit and thumb is to provide additional anatomical structures for the user to better orient themselves when looking at the hand anatomy. In ZBrush, a circle 3D object was appended to the

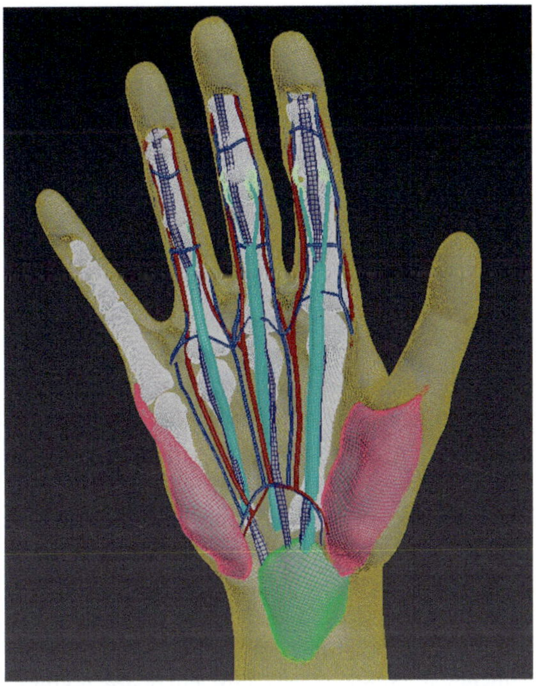

Fig. 2.13 Stage where components of the hand are added together

model. It was shaped by using the "Move" brush to form them. The two muscles on either side of the hand were modeled as separate objects but were merged using the "Merge Down" modifier. This modifier merges the currently selected object with the object that is below it in the hierarchy of objects. This was done because they needed to function as one object in the application. Once Unwrapped, they were imported into Substance Painter. The texture was baked and painted in color and smoothness layers.

In ZBrush, a circle 3D object was appended to the hand object model and was shaped by using the "Move" brush and "Smoothing" brush. This was done to create a flatter appearance to the shape and ensure it remained thick enough to envelop the flexor tendons of the digits.

Once Unwrapped it was imported into Substance Painter. The material made in Substance Painter includes a light pink base color and various pattern displacement layers as well as a texture layer to add dimension to the object.

The Articular capsules of the interphalangeal joints of the index, middle, and ring finger were created by appending a terrain 3D object, shaping, shaping it around the joint, duplicating the object, and rotating to fit the other side of the joint so it was on either side of the joint. The one-joint capsule was then duplicated twice and placed on all three fingers. Following this, the object was imported into Substance Painter and given a single color, opacity, and roughness layer. This was a white color with a slight blue tint, 80% opacity, and 50% roughness to closely resemble cartilage.

All the injured finger models were modeled using image data as the reference. The right-hand model was used by masking the ring finger in ZBrush using the "Separate Masked" Modifier. Following this, the finger and the hand were on separate layers. On the finger object, using the "Modify Geometry" tool and the "Close Holes" modifier, the hole where it was separated from the hand was closed. The rest of the modeling process was a combination of these steps; modifying the finger by using the "Move," "Smooth," "Deco," and "Standard Pen" brushes to sculpt the injury and using the "ZRemesher" tool to refine the mesh of the object (Fig. 2.14). The finger models all follow similar patterns for texturing in Substance Painter. This was done to ensure the finger injuries and the hand models all have consistent materials throughout the application.

Once the fingers were sculpted and checked for accuracy, they were exported from ZBrush and imported into 3Ds Max to be retopologized and UV unwrapped. The models were then imported into Substance Painter where the textures were baked (Fig. 2.15). First, the "skin" material was applied to the "Layers" menu. Following this, the laceration on each of the fingers was painted using the "Basic Soft" brush on a dark red and shiny fill layer that had a "Black Mask" applied. A "Blur" and "Height Adjust" filter was applied to blur the edges of the red to make the strokes more natural. An opaque fill layer was added, and the color was chosen by using the color dropper on the finger object. A "Black Mask" was then applied, and the "Basic Soft" brush was painted onto a part of the skin that was damaged and thin hanging at the edge of the laceration. Lastly, a black fill layer was added,

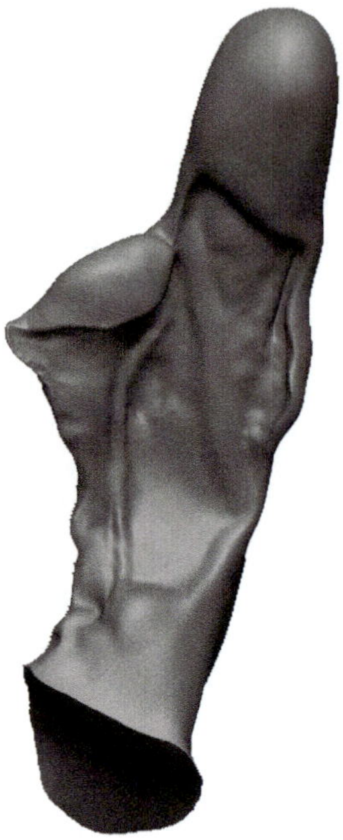

Fig. 2.14 Injury five without the vein model

and a "Black Mask" was applied. A "Curvature" generator was applied; this applies a thin layer of black in the areas of the model that have curvature. This enhances the details that were sculpted in ZBrush as well as additional dimensions and shadows (Fig. 2.15).

The injured finger model was built by using the "Mask" brush in ZBrush to separate the finger from the hand. Once the finger was separated, the details of the injury were sculpted using the "Deco," "Move," and "Smooth" brushes in ZBrush. This injury has a flexor tendon rupture; on the finger model, the laceration of the tendon is visible this was modeled by pulling shaping, and remeshing the existing geometry of the object to accurately represent the image data. It was then checked for anatomical accuracy prior to it being exported from ZBrush and into 3Ds Max.

Finally, all the other objects were imported to Substance Painter separately but were textured

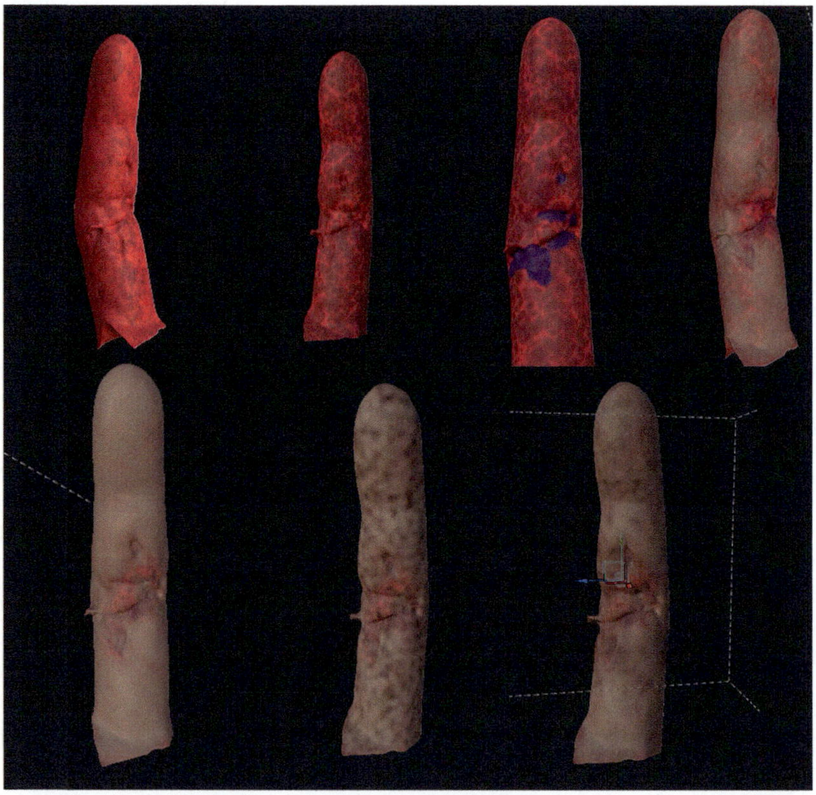

Fig. 2.15 Finger one being painted in Substance Painter. Top left is the start of the process, and the bottom right is the final stages

following the same procedure. This process entailed baking the textures and applying the "skin" material prefab to the "Layers" menu. Following this, a dark red color layer that had low roughness settings was painted using various standard Substance Painter brushes. A "Blur" and "Height Adjust" filter was applied to blur the edges of the red to make the strokes more natural. Finally, "Curvature" generator was applied; this applied a thin layer of black in the areas of the model that have curvature. This enhances the details that were sculpted in ZBrush as well as additional dimensions and shadows.

The visible tendon on the finger model and the visible proximal phalange of the index finger were painted with the "Basic Soft" brush with an off-white layer, giving the tendon a white and shiny look.

To create the animations of the ring avulsion injuries happening in the "Simulation" scene, all the models of the anatomical components of the hand, the hand, and the ring models were imported into Blender. Using the "Shape Key" modifier, a key was added to each object; this enables the ability to deform the object for animation.

With this applied to each object, animating the ring to deform simulates the pull and crush of a ring. In "Edit" and "Vertices" mode each vertex was carefully selected and moved using the "Move" tool to adjust the position and rotation of the ring to accurately simulate a crush and pull. The shape key tracks the movements of the vertices as they are being adjusted, giving a natural-looking animation. Once the ring in each scene was accurately representing a crushed and pulled ring the "Tab" button was pressed to turn off the "Shape Key." Following this, the object has tracked the mesh deformation of the object and has placed it on a value scale from 0 to 1, as this is adjusted the animation frames are adjusted accordingly. These steps were repeated for each structure in the finger which included the arteries, nerves, cruciform part of the fibrous sheath, synovial sheath, and veins.

2.3.7 Application Design

The design for the application was inspired by the original storyboard, where a flowchart of the scene uses and flow was created (Fig. 2.16). The application was developed using Unity 3D, where the Oculus integration and the XR Plugin Manager packages were downloaded from the Unity Asset Store and installed into Unity. Android was selected as the development platform, and Oculus Quest was chosen as the deployment device. The application used the OVR Camera Rig, the OVR Hand, and PointableCanvas Prefabs. The main camera used in the application was the "center eye anchor" camera component. The OVR hand prefab was required to enable hand tracking. The PointableCanvasModule handles event management for all Pointable Canvases in the scene, a Pointable Canvas must be attached to the UI canvas, as well as each canvas must also have a GraphicRaycaster component attached for it to be converted into IPointable events. The canvases must be set to World Space and have a Render Mode attached. The "Curved Unity Canvas"

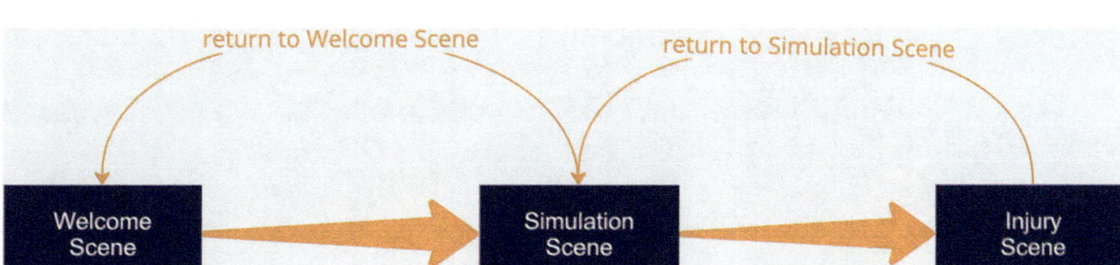

Fig. 2.16 Application development

Prefab was used for all the UI components in the application. Once these components were functioning when using the Oculus, testing of the vital interactions was next.

The "Curved Unity Canvas" is A UI panel that enables the user to select among three buttons; "How To Use" button opens a canvas with a "Video Player" component attached to visually explain how best to use the interface of the application, a "Project Information" button that opens a canvas with background information on the project and researches as well as a "Move On" button that allows the user to move on to the next scene.

The other interaction functionality that was tested aims to enable making the anatomical structures of the hand opaque/transparent. This included importing all the components of the hand and applying simple unity textures to visualize whether using the UI slider could control the opacity. There were issues in scene 3 with making the skin layers of the injured hands opaque. With the help of Dr. Matthieu Poyade, a C# class was developed to control the opacity of each of the anatomical components of the hand.

Scene 3 required the ability for the viewer to have the injured hand in front of them at a size that allows the microstructures such as the nerves and arteries, to be viewed. In this scene, there are five injuries the user can change as they please. In order to be able to press a button and show a new injured hand, a script is needed to remove the currently visible hand object and activate an inactive hand object. Ultimately there needed to be a script that had an inventory or a list of all the 3D game objects in the scene that activated them in order as a button was pressed. A GameObject array was used to store the objects from the scene. Scene 3 needed four separate functioning array scripts to control the hand objects, finger objects, injury text panel, and opacity control panel (Fig. 2.17). It was first tested with the finger objects to ensure that there was always one of the fingers active in the scene, and when the "Change Injury" button was pressed, the next model in the array would become visible, making the previous one inactive (Fig. 2.18).

Finally, a UI slider would access a "Skinned Mesh Renderer" animation in Scene 2 to switch

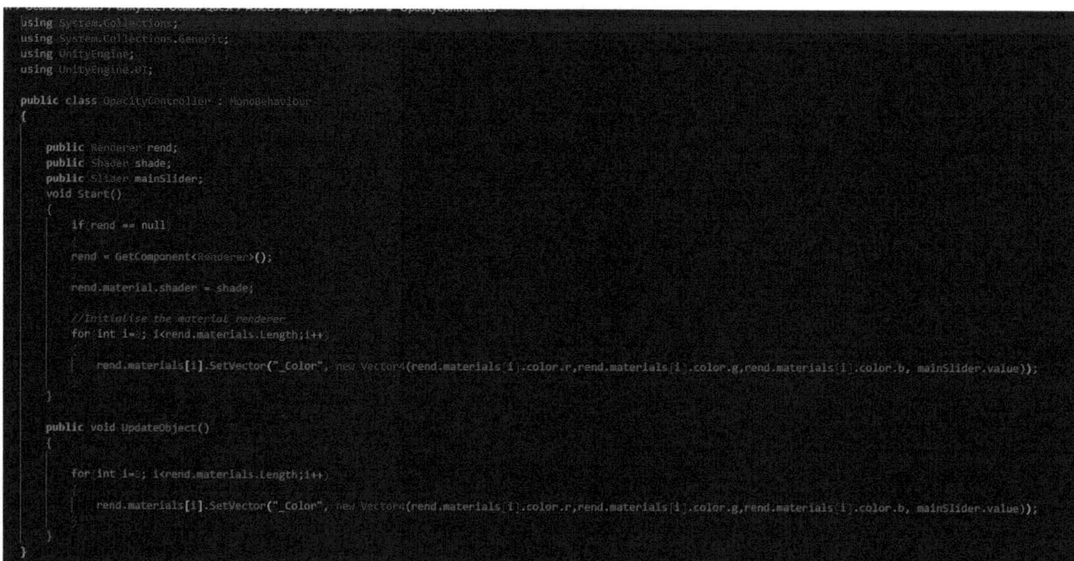

Fig. 2.17 "OpacityController" Script

```
using System.Collections;
using System.Collections.Generic;
using UnityEngine;

public class ArrayFingers : MonoBehaviour
{
    // script refrenced from 'Jimmy Vegas' on youtube video name 'HOW TO CREATE A GAME OBJECT
    //ARRAY IN C# UNITY TUTORIAL'
    //Also refrenced gamedev.stackexchange.com answer by DMGregory

    public GameObject[] handFingers;

    int _selectedObjectIndex = -1;
    //Track which object is currently selected

    public void SelectObject(int selectedIndex)
        //Disable previous selected objects if any
    {
        if(_selectedObjectIndex >= 0)
            handFingers[_selectedObjectIndex].SetActive(false);

            //update selected index and activate the corresponding objects
            _selectedObjectIndex = selectedIndex;
            handFingers[selectedIndex].SetActive(true);
    }
    void Start()
    {
        for (int i = 0; i < handFingers.Length; i++)
        {
            handFingers[i].SetActive(false);
        }

        SelectObject(0);
    }


    public void NextPrefab_ButtonClick()
    {
        //compute the next index on the list
        //the module operator wraps the index around to zero when we pass the last obj
        int nextObjectIndex = (_selectedObjectIndex + 1) % handFingers.Length;
        SelectObject(nextObjectIndex);
    }
}
```

Fig. 2.18 "ArrayFingers" Script The "public GameObject[]" declares the "Array" and creates a space for the GameObjects to be stored

between "Pull" and "Crush" injuries. This was achieved by using an "SetValueOnSlider" in a script to access the "Skinned Mesh Renderer" component attached to the object as well as setting the "BlendShapeWeight" to 0 (no mesh deformation) and the maximum value on the slider would bring the "BlendShapeWeight" to 100 (maximum mesh deformation in animation).

2.4 Results

2.4.1 Scene 1

In Scene 1, the user can find background information and navigation directions via the scene's main page (Fig. 2.19). It is intended for users to begin with simple interactions to practice using

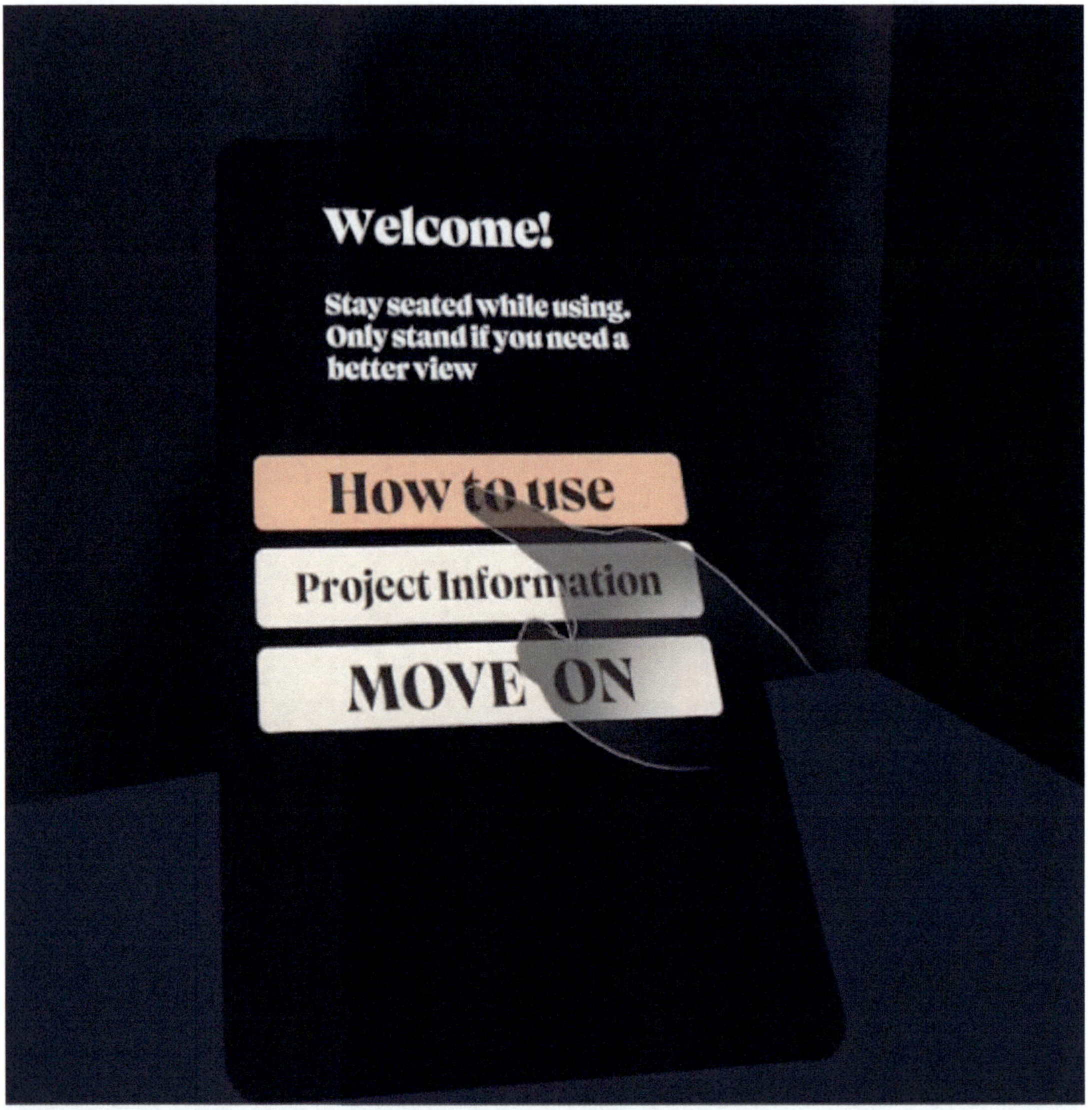
Welcome!
Stay seated while using. Only stand if you need a better view
How to use
Project Information
MOVE ON

Fig. 2.19 View of Scene One

the VR application and interface before proceeding to more complicated settings. A hand with a ring avulsion injury spins on the Y axis in the center of the scene, underneath the app branding. A UI panel to the right, and associated logos to the left (Figs. 2.20).

2.4.2 Scene Two

This scene's main function is to simulate a pull and crush injury to the ring finger; this allows the viewer to control the speed, opacity, and severity of the injury to better understand the mechanics of the injury as well as the affected anatomy (Fig. 2.21). In this scene, there is an uninjured right hand that slowly spins in the middle of the scene, to the left of the hand, there is a UI interface that explains what to expect from the scene as well as how to navigate the interface. On the right of the hand, there is another "Curved Unity Canvas" that has a "Pull" and "Crush" button. Depending on which is pressed, three sliders are activated underneath the respective button,

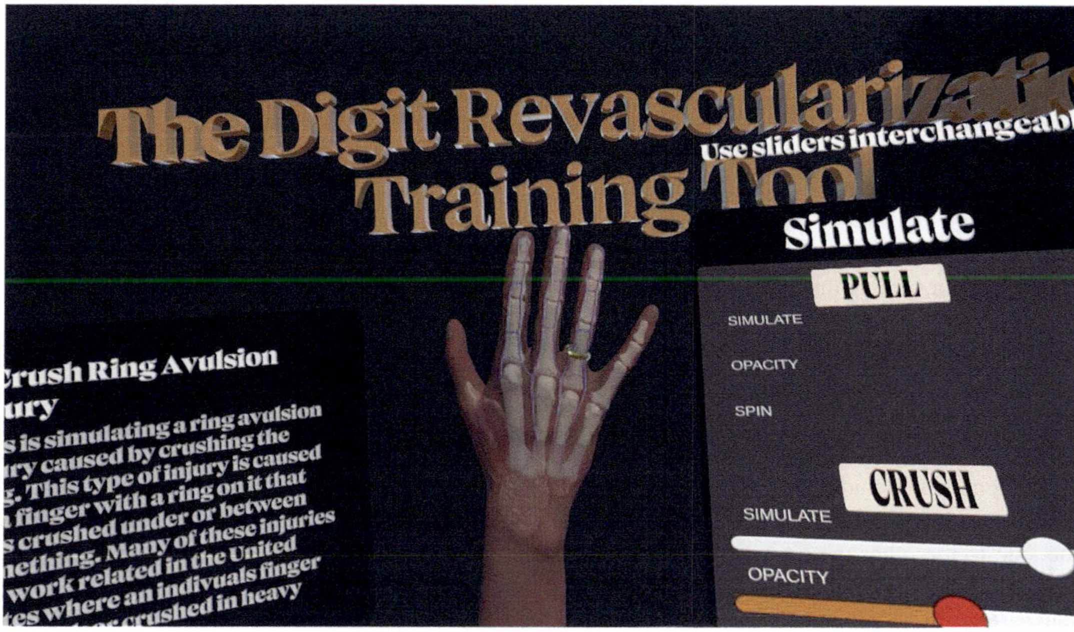

Fig. 2.20 Example of the finished UI panel in Scene One

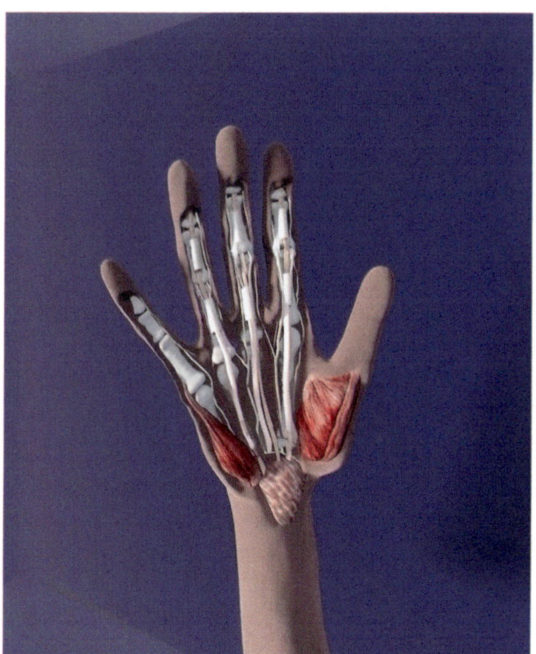

Fig. 2.21 Scene Two "Crush" injury being simulated

with the following titles "Simulate," "Opacity," and "Spin." Text that reads "Use Sliders Interchangeably" appears above the UI panel to inform the users that all three sliders can be used at the same time. These sliders are controlled interchangeably by the user enabling the ability to watch the simulation, stop and start at any stage, manage the transparency of the hand to reveal the internal anatomical structures, and simulate each component deformation as the injury occurs.

2.4.3 Injury Scene

Scene 3 is where the user can engage with the anatomy affected by ring avulsion injuries. In this scene, there is a panel on the left that explains the Urbaniak Classification system. In the middle of the scene, there is a text panel that appears on the wall behind the injured hand that explains how each injury occurred. Next to this panel, there is a 2D white frame, inside this frame is each injured finger object that is constantly spinning. The injured hand object is in the center of the scene and has two panels to the right.

The first panel has a button called "Change Injury." This button, when pressed, changes the injured hand displayed in the scene. There are five injured hands in this scene, and once the user has gone through each five injuries it starts back at the beginning with "Injury 1." This button, when pressed, also changes the description of the injury information on the text canvas behind the hand model, all five injuries have unique descriptions that are relevant to the injury showcased. The first canvas also has a UI Slider that is responsible for turning the injured hand object on its Y axis to better allow the viewer to see the anatomy from the back, front, and side depending on what structures they needed to visualize.

The second panel has the title "Scroll" at the top and lists 11 sliders for each of the 11 anatomical components included in the hand object for all five injuries. When the slider is moved from one side to the other the opacity of the selected object changes from completely opaque to transparent.

2.4.4 User Testing

2.4.4.1 Participants

Seven participants were recruited—3 surgeons/medical professionals and or experts in anatomy and 4 surgical device training and manufacturing specialists were recruited (6 Females and 1 Male), all aged between 24 and 66 years (Mean = 40.71 ± 11.92 (SD)). The participants were recruited via Dr. Jenny Clancy from the University of Glasgow and Matt Burke from Medtronic Corporation to take part in the experiment. All participants were informed of the purpose of the study and provided with a consent form as well as an Oculus Quest Health and Safety form. All participants confirmed consent, and signed consent forms were submitted for review and approved. .

All participants held a degree or a professional qualification in the medical, anatomy, or medical device and training field. Four of the participants have a background in surgical training and devices and three of the participants had an anatomy background. The participants reported their computer literacy which showed 4 out of 7 reported "intermediate," 1 reported "basic," and 1 reported "expert" computer experience. Most of the participants had not had previous experience with a VR application as 4 out of the 7 participants reported no knowledge of VR.

2.4.4.2 Apparatus

The evaluation took place in a controlled environment at the University of Glasgow, and was also undertaken in Minneapolis, USA, in a similar fashion under the supervision of Matt Burke, Medtronic, during which participants explored the interactive VR Application through an Oculus Quest 2 Head Mounted Display.

2.4.4.3 Procedure

The immersive application brought participants into two virtual rooms. The first allowed them to simulate the injury and view the effects at macro and micro levels. The second presented them with five different avulsion injuries, from which they could control each anatomical component to engage and visualize their characteristics. The participants were expected to interact and freely explore the application prior to answering the questionnaire.

Before and after each participant, the Oculus Quest 2 was wiped down and cleaned using an anti-bacterial wipe, in accordance with GSA's safety guidelines. Afterwards, participants were invited to rate a series of standardized statements using Likert scales, complete a bespoke questionnaire, and answer a series of open questions. (Figs. 2.22 and 2.23).

2.4.4.4 Data Analysis

The ITC-Sense of Presence Inventory Questionnaire (ITC-SOPI) is a standardized questionnaire (Lessiter et al. 2001) that tests the users' psychological involvement when using the application as well face and content validities. The rating scale for the ITC-SOPI questionnaire used a 5-point Likert scale using 1 (strongly disagree) to 5 (strongly agree). Presence is assessed using 44 questions organized in two sections; Section A has 6 questions to report on user sensation after the experience, and Section B has 38 questions to report on sensation during the experience. The results were collated in Microsoft Excel, and descriptive statistics were calculated

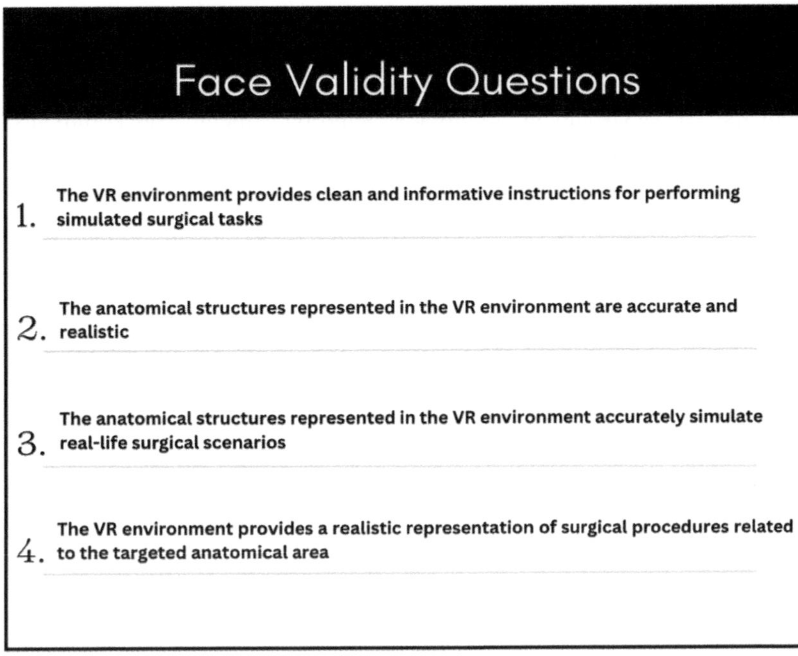

Fig. 2.22 Face Validity Questions

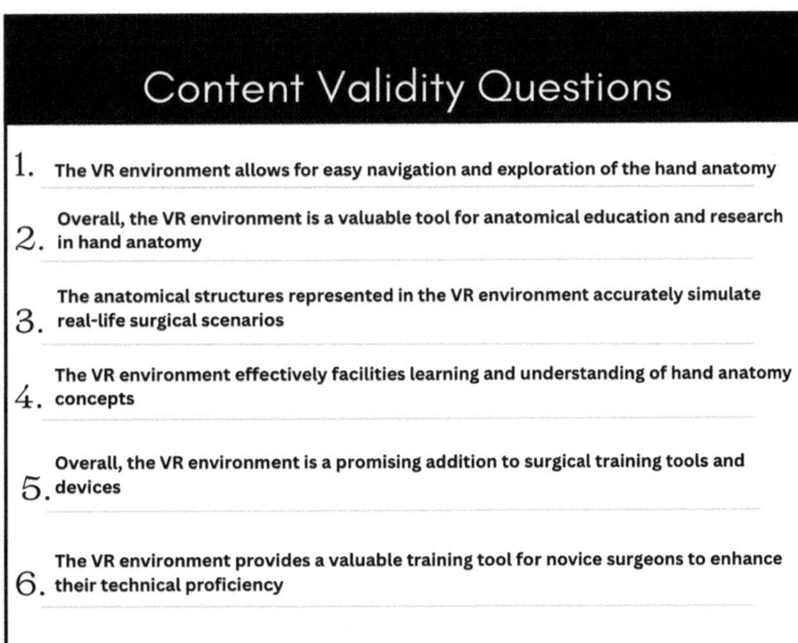

Fig. 2.23 Content Validity Questions

for the 4 constructs emanating from the ITC-SOPI questionnaire. The ITC-SOPI Questionnaire also provides a space at the end of the questionnaire for participants to leave any additional positive or negative comments about the experience. The ITC SOPI scoring was arranged into the 4 factors: "Engagement," "Negative Effects," "Ecological Validity/Naturalness," and "Spatial Presence" which measures the fidelity of the VR application. Assessing spatial presence considers two key elements of presence. The spatial presence concept is testing the sense of physical placement and control over the components within the VR environment. Engagement is testing the psychological sense of being involved with the VR environment. Ecological Validity/ Naturalness's testing how realistic the VR environment is. Finally, negative effects measure the negative psychological reactions to the VR environment.

A bespoke face validity questionnaire explored the anatomical accuracy of the models within the VR application (Figs. 2.22 and 2.23).

A bespoke content validity questionnaire explored the potential training validity of the VR application.

2.4.4.5 Ethics

Ethical Approval for this study was granted by The Glasgow School of Art's Learning and Teaching office.

2.4.5 Experimental Outcomes

2.4.5.1 Sense of Perceived Presence

The results of the ITC-SOPI Questionnaire positive for engagement (M = 4.46 ± 0.42(SD)), positive results for the ecological validity/naturalness (M = 4.24 ± 0.51(SD)), reasonably good results for the spatial presence (M = 3.98 ± 1.05(SD)), slight negative effects were reported (M = 1.48 ± 0.51(SD)) (Fig. 2.24).

Four out of the seven participants left a comment. The comments were assessed to gain a deeper understanding of what aspects of the application need further consideration and which aspects were done well. Overall, the written feedback highlighted the users felt "fully immersed" with "great detail" and "learned something about the classifications of finger crush injuries." Some issues regarding the usability of the application were expressed, such as adding "Add audio to what is happening while I moved some of the dials" sounds to the UI sliders as well as adding the ability to zoom in and out of the hand model.

The comment by one participant regarding the potential use of the application stated "As an emergency physician, I think this modality could be useful in the emergency department (A&E)," further explaining that the inclusion of "3D demonstration of ring removal techniques" would be a useful addition to the application.

2.4.5.2 Face Validity

The results shown in Fig. 2.25 show the participants felt the VR application had a high level of face validity. Question 1 tested the validity of the visual details within the VR environment and

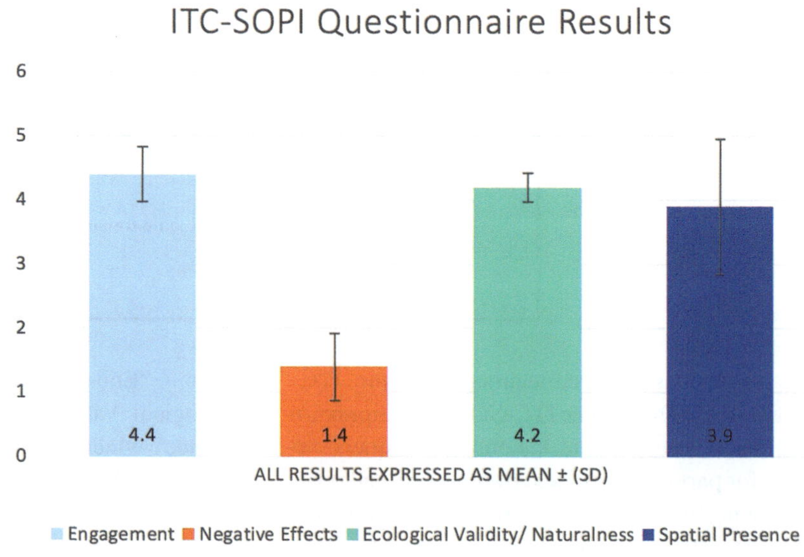

Fig. 2.24 ITC-SOPI Questionnaire Results. The chart shows the sense of presence in the VR application tested by 7 participants and the standard deviation of the answers given

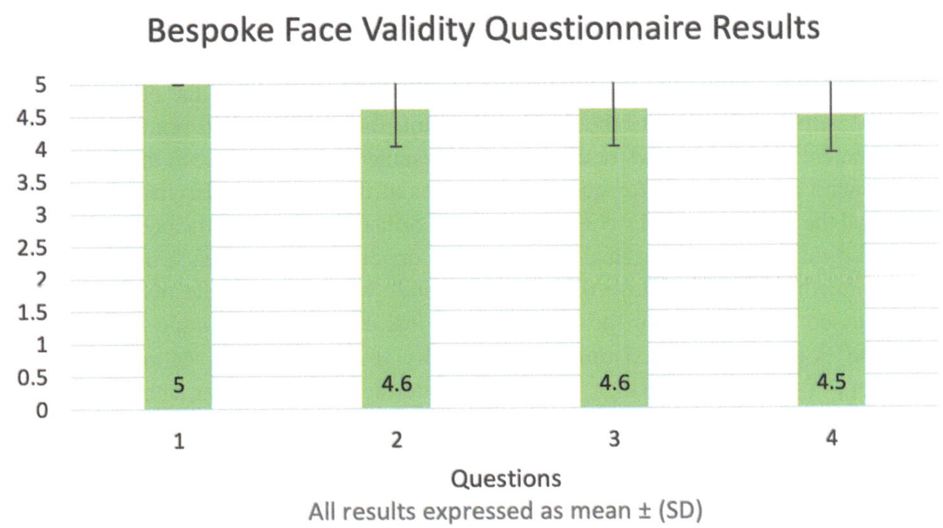

Fig. 2.25 Bespoke Face Validity Questionnaire Results. This chart shows the face validity questionnaire results and the standard deviation of the answers given by the 7 participants

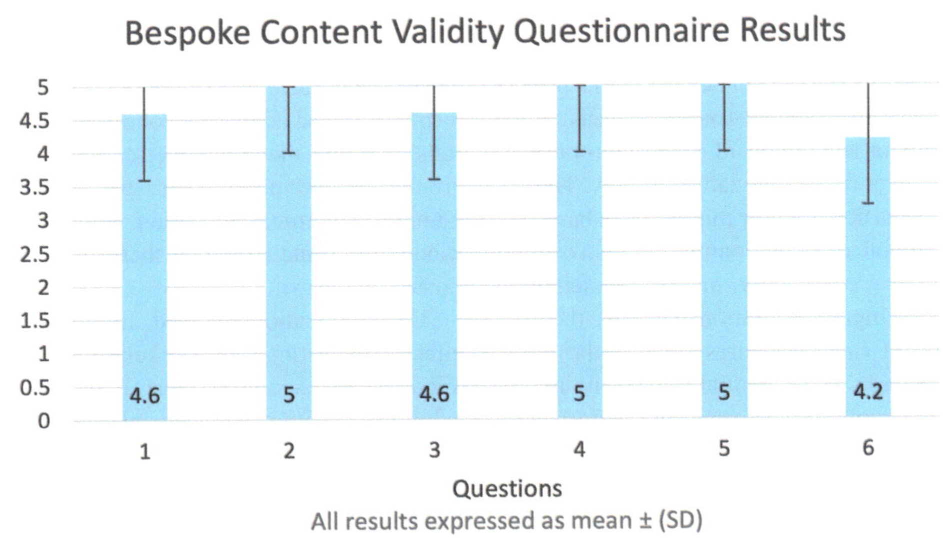

Fig. 2.26 Bespoke Content Validity Questionnaire Results. The chart shows the content validity of the VR application as well as the standard deviation of the 7 participants' answers

whether they enhance the overall experience with good results (M = 5 ± 0(SD)), Question 2 tested whether the anatomical structures within the VR environment are accurately and realistically represented with encouraging results of (M = 4.6 ± 0.57(SD)), question 3 and question 4 both were testing if the simulations depicted within the VR environment are real-life surgical scenarios with encouraging results for question 3 with (M = 4.6 ± 0.57(SD)) and question 4 (M = 4.5 ± 0.57(SD)).

2.4.5.3 Content Validity

The results in Fig. 2.26 show the participants reported the VR application having high levels of content validity. Question 1 tested the validity of the application's ability to explore the hand anatomy with an encouraging result (M = 4.6 ± 0.56(SD)), and question 2 and question 4 tested the validity of the use of the application for anatomical education and research in hand anatomy with a good result for question 2 and 4 as they had the same result (M = 5 ± 0(SD)), question 3 tested the validity of surgical simulations with a promising result (M = 4.6 ± 0.5(SD)), question 5 assessed the validity for the application within the context of pre-existing surgical simulators with promising results (M = 5 ± 0(SD)). Question 6 assessed the validity of the VR application used to train novice surgeons on their technical proficiency with a mean score of (M = 4.2 ± 0.95(SD)).

2.5 Discussion

There were a number of challenges encountered during the data and development of the VR application. One of the main challenges of this project was the lack of available source datasets in the form of CT or MRI scans of a digit pre- or post-replantation or revascularization surgery. The CT and MRI data acquired for this research has often low resolution or poor contrast which, overall, increased the complexity of the segmentation tasks. With higher resolution datasets, the segmentation of finer structures such as the blood supply, tendons and potentially even the nerves would have allowed generating anatomically accurate 3D models and potentially speeding up the modeling work. As it is, all the models presented in the application, apart from the bones, were created using photo and video references of digit revascularization and replantation procedures validated by the surgical advisor on this project.

Additional challenges were encountered throughout the development of the "Injury Scene." The user could control the opacity of each anatomical structure in the scene. Initially, the goal was to have the injured finger and hand objects opaque with the ability to make it semi-transparent to reveal the injured structures underneath. However, once the finger and hand model had a texture from Substance Painter attached, the UI slider would not allow control of the opacity from the material of the object anymore. As a result, the object would remain opaque, despite the same script working on the anatomical structures of the hand that also had materials made in the Substance Painter attached to them. Although the opacity control of each object in the "Injury Scene" was effective, the research associated to the resolution of that issue resulted was especially time-consuming. Moreover, most of the modeling and animation techniques used in this application such as photogrammetry, Blender, and Substance Painter required time and practice to gain proficiency and confidence with the technology.

The study's findings, based on the responses of seven participants to the ITC-SOPI questionnaire, indicate a positive engagement with the VR content. This aligns with the theory proposed by Lessiter et al. (2001), suggesting that content tailored to participants' interests can enhance engagement levels. Although the emotional response varied across the cohort of participants, It is possible that the diverse academic background of the participants, particularly those without anatomical education, might have contributed to some extent to these different emotional responses.

The application showed minimal negative effects, suggesting a lesser likelihood of inducing VR-induced discomfort. Overall, the participants exhibited positive engagement within the VR application, appreciating its immersive capabilities and content. The realism of the VR environment was acknowledged by participants. However, the VR application's limitation in engaging all sensory perceptions was evident. A clear link between user's perceived presence in VR and the provision of sensory information on different cues has been acknowledge in previous research (Dinh et al. 1999; Cooper et al. 2015). Despite this, the overall spatial presence was found acceptable, though including auditory cues could further enhance the experience.

The original questionnaire by Lessiter et al. (2001) emphasized that higher scores in presence support a higher degree of immersion. The presence of photorealistic models within the VR application might hypothetically have contributed to increasing the anatomical authenticity of the digital models within the app. Although this would need to be verified through further research.

This study underscores the importance of enhancing sensory immersion in VR while emphasizing the application's credibility attributed to its photorealistic components.

The content validity was preliminarily assessed through six questions (Fig. 2.23f), which indicated that participants found the content relevant for a surgical simulation tool. Despite the limited data, the anatomical and surgical training components within the VR application were deemed pertinent for hand surgery training.

Overall, the feedback received from participants was helpful in providing details on how this application could be used for Accident and Emergency Departments (A&E). It was highlighted that in the A&E department, access to specialty hand trauma microsurgeons is limited (Cho et al. (2018). Providing a resource for A&E doctors to acquire knowledge and skills independently on ring avulsion classifications and ring cutting techniques could potentially close the gap between the limited access to micro-hand surgeons and ensuring prompt and correct treatment is accessible to every patient, regardless of the location of the emergency room.

Finally, the validity of the presented experimental outcomes is limited by the small size of participants, and the remote nature of testing. Future experimental research should consider engaging with a larger, more diverse cohort, which includes more professionals with microsurgery expertise.

2.6 Conclusion

This chapter presented a VR application that showcases interactable ring avulsion injuries and evaluated the potential of VR to become a tool for preserving knowledge on digit revascularization and replantation. Digit revascularization and replantation care in the USA is a procedure most performed at high-volume hand trauma centers; however, traumatic hand injuries happen all over the USA and will present to both high- and low-volume hospitals. Although the medical professionals at the low-volume centers may not be performing the revascularization, they must have a stable understanding of the injury and indicators for replantation or amputation. Access to specialty microsurgeons let alone hand surgeons is very limited making it increasingly important that practitioners in the USA are provided with accessible tools that can enable them to be self-sufficient in their ability to correctly identify replantation candidates.

With the advent of affordable mobile VR technologies, interactive VR tools have gained traction in medical training, offering immersive and validated methods to educate professionals. The absence of scientific evidence and studies about the presence and effectiveness of similar implementations suggests a gap in research in the specific field of finger replantation. This project underscores the potential of VR in microsurgery training, especially for rare and complex injuries. VR has the potential to bridge the knowledge gap and ensure that even professionals in remote areas can identify and manage traumatic hand injuries effectively. This VR application was designed and developed to support healthcare professionals in peripheral hospitals to maintain their expertise.

Future VR applications should prioritize user interactivity, providing access to intuitive and natural interaction paradigms. Additionally, it is believed that enhancing the realism of injury simulations could be beneficial. Although interactive VR surgical simulation tools have been shown to be an effective and high-validity way to inform medical professionals, the application of VR within microsurgery has been limited. This project highlights the importance and relevance for the use of VR as an interactive way to familiarize and train practitioners on rare challenging injuries.

References

Abi-Rafeh J et al (2019) Nonbiological microsurgery simulators in plastic surgery training: a systematic review, plastic and reconstructive surgery. Available at: https://pubmed.ncbi.nlm.nih.gov/31461050/. Accessed 12 June 2023

Barbato B, Salsac A-V (2020) Finger and thumb replantation: from biomechanics to practical surgical applications. Hand Surg Rehabil 39(2):77–91. https://doi.org/10.1016/j.hansur.2019.10.198

Bowman DA, McMahan RP (2007) Virtual reality: how much immersion is enough? Computer 40(7):36–43. https://doi.org/10.1109/MC.2007.257

Breahna A, Siddiqui A, Fitzgerald O'Connor E, Iwuagwu FC (2016) Replantation of digits: a review of predictive factors for survival. J Hand Surg Eur Vol 41(7):753–757. https://doi.org/10.1177/1753193415624663

Brown M et al (2017) Annual hospital volume and success of digital replantation. Plast Reconstr Surg 139(3):672–680. https://doi.org/10.1097/prs.0000000000003087

Chiu DTW, Matthew MK, Patel A (2019) The impact of microsurgery on the treatment of ring avulsion injuries. Plast Reconstr Surg 144(6):1351–1357. https://doi.org/10.1097/prs.0000000000006276

Cho HE, Zhong L, Kotsis SV, Chung KC (2018) Finger replantation optimization study (FRONT): update on National Trends. J Hand Surg 43(10):903–912.e1. https://doi.org/10.1016/j.jhsa.2018.07.021

Cho HE, Kotsis SV, Chung KC (2019) Outcomes following replantation/revascularization in the hand, Hand clinics. Available at: https://www.ncbi.nlm.nih.gov/pmc/articles/PMC6446589/. Accessed 6 June 2023

Cipresso P, Giglioli IAC, Raya MA, Riva G (2018) The past, present, and future of virtual and augmented reality research: a network and cluster analysis of the literature. Front Psychol 9:2086. https://doi.org/10.3389/fpsyg.2018.02086

Cooper N, Milella F, Cant I, Pinto C, White M, Meyer G (2015) The effects of multisensory cues on the sense of presence and task performance in a virtual reality environment. In: EuroVR 2015, 2015-10-15 – 2015-10-16, Lecco, Italy

Cullen S, Joyce K, Theopold C (2022) Temporoparietal fascial flap for primary reconstruction of complex ring avulsion injury: a case report, JPRAS Open. Available at: https://www.sciencedirect.com/science/article/pii/S2352587822000262. Accessed 29 June 2023

Davis Sears E, Chung KC (2011) Replantation of finger avulsion injuries: a systematic review of survival and functional outcomes. J Hand Surg Am 36(4):686–694. https://doi.org/10.1016/j.jhsa.2010.12.023

Dinh HQ, Walker N, Hodges LF, Song C, Kobayashi A (1999, March) Evaluating the importance of multisensory input on memory and the sense of presence in virtual environments. In: Proceedings IEEE virtual reality (cat. No. 99CB36316) (pp. 222–228). IEEE

Egger J et al (2016) HTC Vive Mevislab integration via openvr for medical applications, PLOS ONE. Available at https://journals.plos.org/plosone/article?id=10.1371%2Fjournal.pone.0173972. Accessed 13 June 2023

Elliott RM, Baldwin KD, Foroohar A, Levin LS (2012) The impact of residency and fellowship training on the practice of microsurgery by members of the American Society for Surgery of the Hand. Ann Plast Surg 69:451. https://doi.org/10.1097/SAP.0b013e318248036d

Fufa D et al (2013) Digit replantation. J Bone Joint Surg 95(23):2127–2134. https://doi.org/10.2106/jbjs.l.01219

Giladi AM, McGlinn EP, Shauver MJ, Voice TP, Chung KC (2014) Measuring outcomes and determining long-term disability after revision amputation for treatment of traumatic finger and thumb amputation injuries. Plast Reconstr Surg 134:746e. https://doi.org/10.1097/PRS.0000000000000591

Guillery M (2023a) Hand injury examples. [Digital illustration]

Guillery M (2023b) Urbaniak classification system illustration

Hudaib A et al (2018) Requirements prioritization techniques comparison. Available at https://www.researchgate.net/publication/322487895_Requirements_Prioritization_Techniques_Comparison. Accessed 19 June 2023

Hustedt JW, Bohl DD, Champagne L (2016) The detrimental effect of decentralization in digital replantation in the United States: 15 years of evidence from the National Inpatient Sample. J Hand Surg Am 41(5):593–601. https://doi.org/10.1016/j.jhsa.2016.02.011

Jewett CA, Uppuganti S, Desai MJ (2021) Avoiding ring avulsion injuries with silicone rings: a biomechanical study. J Hand Surg 46(11):1030.e1–1030.e5. https://doi.org/10.1016/j.jhsa.2021.02.025

Jones M, Gujral S (2016) Ring avulsion injuries. Eplasty, [online] 16, p.ic5. Available at https://www.ncbi.nlm.nih.gov/pmc/articles/PMC4753839/. Accessed 10 Dec 2022

Kakar S, Bakri K, Shin AY (2012) Survey of hand surgeons regarding their perceived needs for an expanded upper extremity fellowship. J Hand Surg 37:2374–2380.e1-3. https://doi.org/10.1016/j.jhsa.2012.08.013

Kohan J, Mangan J, Patel A (2022) Access to reconstructive hand surgery in the United States ..., Access to reconstructive hand surgery in the United States—investigating the obstacles: a scoping review. Available at https://journals.sagepub.com. https://doi.org/10.1177/15589447221131853. Accessed 1 Aug 2023

Konczalik W, Michno D, Kang N (2019) 8.4 Reconstruction of the digit. In: Hand trauma in clinical practice. Springer, Cham, pp 100–104

Lessiter J, Freeman J, Keogh E, Davidoff J (2001) A cross-media presence questionnaire: the ITC-sense of presence inventory. Presence 10:282–297. https://doi.org/10.1162/105474601300343612

Long C, Suarez PA, Hernandez-Boussard T, Curtin C (2019) Disparities in access to care following traumatic digit amputation. Hand:155894471882470. https://doi.org/10.1177/1558944718824700

Mahmoudi E, Chung KC (2017) Effect of hospital volume on success of thumb replantation. J Hand Surg Am 42(2). https://doi.org/10.1016/j.jhsa.2016.11.020

Meehan M, Razzaque S, Whitton MC, Brooks FP (2003) Effect of latency on presence in stressful virtual environments, IEEE virtual reality. Proceedings, Los Angeles, CA, USA, pp 141–148. https://doi.org/10.1109/VR.2003.1191132

Odobescu A, Goodwin I, Berbiche D, BouMerhi J, Harris PG, Danino MA (2018) High Fidelity microsurgical simulation: the Thiel model and evaluation instrument. Plastic Surgery 27(2):118–124. https://doi.org/10.1177/2292550318800324

Overview of Hand Surgery [WWW Document] (2021). https://www.hopkinsmedicine.org/health/treatment-tests-and-therapies/overview-of-hand-surgery. Accessed 27 Oct 23

Sebastin S, Chung K (2013) Challenges in measuring outcomes following digital replantation. Semin Plast Surg 27(04):174–181. https://doi.org/10.1055/s-0033-1360584

Struckmann VF, Gaus S, Schilling T, Bickert B, Kneser U, Harhaus L (2020) Digital avulsion injuries: epidemiology and factors influencing finger preservation. Arch Orthop Trauma Surg 140(10):1575–1583. https://doi.org/10.1007/s00402-020-03576-3

Urbaniak JR, Evans JP, Bright DS (1981) Microvascular management of ring avulsion injuries. J Hand Surg Am 6(1):25–30. https://doi.org/10.1016/S0363-5023(81)80006-8

Winter JM, Petropolis C (2021) A novel silicone simulation model for microvascular anastomosis. Plast Surg 30(2):113–116. https://doi.org/10.1177/22925503211003835

Yeung AWK et al (2021) Virtual and augmented reality applications in medicine: analysis of the scientific literature. J Med Internet Res. Available at: https://www.ncbi.nlm.nih.gov/pmc/articles/PMC7904394/. Accessed 13 June 2023

Yoon AP, Kane RL, Wang L, Wang L, Chung KC (2021) Variation in surgeon proficiency scores and association with digit replantation outcomes. JAMA Netw Open 4(10):e2128765. https://doi.org/10.1001/jamanetworkopen.2021.28765

MyoSITE: A Site-Specific Mixed Reality Educational Tool for Life Sciences

3

Mirja Koponen, Matthieu Poyade, and Craig Daly

Abstract

The MyoSITE project explored how to design a digital site-specific life-sciences educational tool that encompasses both the physical and digital sphere and how to present in this space a digital whole-cell model that accurately reflects the dense and differentiated environment of cellular mesoscales. A large animated digital cell model was created to fit the University of Glasgow Advanced Research Centre ARC-XR exhibition space. The mixed reality approach was used to explore the digital content of the model (heartbeat and its regulation within the cell), employing a hand tracking-enabled head-mounted display (HMD). Various types of immersion and interactions were explored for co-opting the digital material whilst retaining access to the outside of the digital environment. The application featured several magnification layers, allowing the user to examine and interact with differently sized molecular structures. The user experience in terms of usability and the educational potential of the application were probed as a part of the project. The multi-user aspect, site-specificity, and scalar handling of the material were well received by the specialist panel. The MyoSITE application showed great potential as a proof-of-concept, and the project effectively illustrated the benefits of using extended reality (XR) technologies in life sciences education, emphasizing the importance of further research into mixed reality for this field.

Keywords

Mixed reality · Virtual reality · Life sciences education · E-learning · Whole-cell modelling

3.1 Introduction

Digital technologies are transforming the speed and range of theoretical research and providing entirely new methods for engaging with this research. For scientific visualization, extended reality (XR) serves as a comprehensive term encompassing all immersive technologies, rep-

M. Koponen (✉)
School of Medicine, Dentistry and Nursing, College of Medical, Dentistry and Nursing, University of Glasgow, Glasgow, UK

School of Innovation and Technology, Glasgow School of Art, Glasgow, UK
e-mail: mk@ergodic.org.uk

M. Poyade
School of Innovation and Technology, Glasgow School of Art, Glasgow, UK
e-mail: M.Poyade@gsa.ac.uk

C. Daly
School of Cardiovascular and Metabolic Health, University of Glasgow, Glasgow, UK
e-mail: Craig.Daly@glasgow.ac.uk

J. Clancy, M. Poyade (eds.), *Medical Visualization and Applications of Technology – Volume 2*, Biomedical Visualization 5, https://doi.org/10.1007/978-3-031-63463-5_3

resenting a range of experiences that merge elements of the physical and virtual worlds. The most familiar modes of XR are augmented reality (AR) and virtual reality (VR). AR superimposes digital information like images, sounds, or 3D models onto the real world through smartphones or AR glasses whereas VR encloses the user into an entirely fabricated, computer-generated, interactive environment using head-mounted displays (HMD) (McDonnell 2019; Lee and Takenaka 2022). However, most recent hardware developments are increasingly amalgamating aspects of both the physical and virtual realms in mixed reality (MR) settings, enabling interaction with digital content whilst staying anchored in the real environment. MR allows users to engage with virtual objects as if they seamlessly coexisted in the same physical space. These technologies find diverse applications across various fields, including gaming, education, and healthcare (Sutherland et al. 2019; Barteit et al. 2021; Curran et al. 2023).

Visualizing biological processes can be challenging due to the wide variation in the size of participating agents. MyoSITE was an experimental project that investigated the potential of developing a site-specific mixed reality (MR) application for life sciences. It presented accurately scaled structures of an individual cell to foster a more authentic perception of cellular mesoscales—a space of processes, interactions, and reagents spanning from the molecular to the cellular level. The project was established to construct a cell model as an educational resource, using the MR approach to create a digital learning environment, fitted within a physical space where the model could be experienced in a scaled manner and where its various attributes could be further explored. The use of both MR and VR scenes was designed to allow interaction with users of several headsets simultaneously, thus enabling multi-user engagement with the content in the form of a 'digital classroom', run on unconnected headsets without the need for a single overarching system.

3.1.1 MyoSITE as a Whole Cell Model

The project was motivated by the ambition to create a comprehensive simulation of a whole cell (WC modelling), a goal that has long eluded the scientific community (Goodsell et al. 2020). Challenges have included the diverse and scattered nature of the source data and the computationally intensive modelling process (Daly 2019; Maritan et al. 2022). However, the increasing availability of data-driven models has made it feasible to build more complete simulations that emulate real-life instances. In certain cases, this has provided fresh insights into specific processes or structures (Shen et al. 2019; Burbaum et al. 2021). To gain a comprehensive understanding of larger-scale systems, it is essential to have a multi-level depiction of their structures, especially for projects that encompass the mesoscale range (Goodsell et al. 2020; Maritan et al. 2022). However, access to accurate models can be a particular problem in molecular and cell biology, where the materials can be heterogeneous. The authors of a recent pioneering project, which aimed to construct a complete model of a Mycoplasma genitalium cell, highlighted the difficulties they faced in handling various databanks, file formats, and gaps in available data (Maritan et al. 2022). The process involved meticulously curating the material and generating numerous homologous models and part-models from various sources, which were then painstakingly assembled, often manually, to create a comprehensive structure representing an entire cell. Indeed, many researchers point out that achieving a fully functional, interactive, 3D whole-cell presentation based solely on data is still a challenge (Johnston et al. 2017; Daly 2019; Maritan et al. 2022). Whilst many have expressed a preference for medical scanner or microscopy-derived models as opposed to manually generated, 'artist-modelled' ones (Johnston et al. 2017; Maritan et al. 2022), these approaches can currently be seen as overlapping, leveraging the advantages of both: utilizing data-derived material for scientific precision and verisimilitude, and resorting to manual modelling in cases where data sources are lacking or when simplification is warranted (Johnston et al. 2017; Goodsell et al. 2020; Maritan et al. 2022).

Visualizing scalar conditions in 3D at both the molecular and cellular levels has fundamentally altered our general comprehension of biological processes (Safadel and White 2019; Goodsell et al. 2020). Encountering these models in three dimensions holds significant importance for both the specialist researchers and the broader public in enhancing understanding of the material world, and a key challenge for this project was to develop a digital classroom with practical utility in both contexts.

3.1.2 MyoSITE as an Educational Model

Utilizing XR technologies within the science classroom settings provides a range of advantages. It enables hands-on interaction and the ability to observe and manipulate the materials in 3D (Logeswaran et al. 2021; Venkatesan et al. 2021; Liu et al. 2022). In the learning process, engaging with various sensory aspects of the material, such as size, texture, and movement, enhances theoretical understanding and facilitates the comprehension of complex processes (Venkatesan et al. 2021).

Conveying complex 3D dynamics is a challenge in science education, and the traditional manner in which science material has been delivered, using pictures and physical models, has significant limitations (Levy 2013; Bernholt et al. 2019; Liu et al. 2022). Whilst animations are seen as somewhat helpful, they are still essentially 2D presentations where the depth information is crucially lacking (Johnston et al. 2017). As XR allows full 3D animation, time-based processes can be observed in a more realistic way. Another aspect of ready scalability is the ability to handle material that could be not practically possible or even dangerous to handle. Classic examples of this are VR scenes and applications, presenting interactive anatomy models of a beating heart including valve function, electrophysiology, and blood flow while placing the user inside the small-scale anatomical structures. In 2018, Fujitsu together with Tokyo University developed a high-accuracy VR heart simulator for use in medical training, where the user was able to place interactive electrodes on the surface of a virtual body and by altering the voltage to observe both the ECG and the excitation effect on the high-detail 3D heart model (Fujitsu 2018). Many simpler simulations are available in a real or lecture form in the public domain, where the use of the VR scenes can be observed, such as 360 degree VR animation of a beating heart by Hybrid Medical Animation (2015), pulse-to-blood flow visualiser by LudicWorlds (2022), and lecture videos by Acadicus (2021) and MedicalholodeckAcademy (2023).

In the field of chemistry, challenges for students and researchers alike can arise due to the utilization of three representation levels—macroscopic, sub-microscopic, and symbolic—and the relationships between them (Levy 2013; Wu et al. 2021; Liu et al. 2022). While the shift between symbolic and non-symbolic or material representation is a linguistic mechanism, the practices of presenting material in a cross-scalar manner, where interactions are seamlessly explored across a range of scales (from macroscopic to sub-microscopic), have been constrained by traditional disciplinary boundaries and available research tools. XR provides a distinct advantage in reducing the abstraction level by making previously unseen materials visible (Stefani et al. 2018; Barrow et al. 2019) and offering multiple ways to refocus the complex multiscale material.

Due to its adaptability to scaling, XR is especially well-suited for the educational exploration of cellular mesoscales. (Daly 2019; Goodsell et al. 2020). Hence, there is an ongoing need for research into educational methods for presenting data-based cell structures with these technologies (Daly 2019). Using XR, spatial relationships and concepts can be explored in a novel way that not only reduces abstraction but, in a way, echoes the original conditions of natural sciences, where an important part of the process was empirical—physical or even sensory—observation. The engendered sense of empirics can provide meaningful, contextual, situated learning experiences. As a proof-of-concept, the MyoSITE project investigated the development of interactive scenes that capitalize on the multimodal and multimedia capabilities of MR for presentation, observation, interaction, and learning.

3.1.3 MyoSITE as a Site-Specific Model

The premise for project MyoSITE was to present the confocal microscope-derived cardiomyocyte model as a site-specific application. This served two primary purposes. Firstly, aligning the scales with the actual dimensions of the exhibition space provided a rationale for the range of scales that could be investigated. In this instance, the Glasgow University Advanced Research Centre (ARC) XR room set the limit for the cell size. This, in turn, enabled exploration of the sizes of other cellular and molecular structures within these defined boundaries, all in accurate relation to the cell size.

Secondly, basing the project on a tangible location allowed probing the potential for integration and interaction between the physical and digital space. Whilst the application could be used by a single user, MR approach supported the creation of a 'digital classroom' as a collaborative space with fluid boundaries. In the MyoSITE application, this involved exploring digital scenes and interactions built upon existing data-derived models where feasible and experimenting with various MR scene types using hand tracking-enabled HMD (Oculus Quest 2). Both approaches served to investigate ARC-XR as a space for development and to establish a precedent for future site-specific work.

The selected cell model was a cardiac myocyte for several reasons. The dimensions of a cardiomyocyte, being long and thin, could be adjusted to match the proportions of the ARC-XR research space, which is a longitudinal room. The muscle cell contents are highly organized (sarcomeres), enabling the replication of structures to convey a tightly packed cellular interior. Lastly, myocytes are contractile, a trait that can be effectively illustrated within an MR setting.

3.1.4 Aims and Objectives

The primary aim of this project was to assess the feasibility of constructing a site-specific digital MR model of a cell with accurate scalar representation. This aim was accomplished by completing the following objectives:

- Sourcing and modelling a set of digital protein models characteristic of a myocyte.
- Designing a Unity-based interactive application for Oculus Quest 2, exploring molecular aspects of heartbeat regulation.
- Deploying the application within a real-world setting as a MR production, utilizing physical space, light, and sound.
- Designing and conducting user testing of the site-specific application.

The research questions explored were:

- How can a data-derived digital representation of the structure of a single cell be created as an interactive application while maintaining realistic scalar proportions of the material?
- How can a site-specific MR approach enhance the learning experience and the application content?
- How can the model be utilized for group learning?

The subsequent section describes the materials and workflow of the application development.

3.2 Materials and Methods

3.2.1 Project Materials

The software and hardware used in the application development for the project are listed in Table 3.1, including the game engine (Unity),

Table 3.1 Software and hardware used in the development of the application

Software	Purpose	Produced by
MeshLab	Software used for cleaning, repairing, and editing the high polycount molecular models	ISTI–CNR https://www.meshlab.net
3DStudio Max	Software used for modelling, retopologizing, and texturing the 3D models	Autodesk, Inc. https://www.autodesk.co.uk/products/3ds-max/overview
Unity	Software used for developing the application structure, interactions, texturing, and animations	Unity Technologies https://unity3d.com/unity
Visual Studio	Software used in conjunction with Unity for developing C# code for interactions within the application	Microsoft Corporation https://visualstudio.microsoft.com/
Photoshop 2022	Software used for creating and editing images and textures	Adobe Systems, Inc. https://www.adobe.com/uk/

(continued)

Table 3.1 (continued)

Software	Purpose	Produced by
Audacity	Used for audio editing and file format conversion for sound assets	Audacity Team https://www.audacityteam.org
Zbrush	Software used for repair and closing holes in high-poly meshes.	Pixologic Inc., Maxon https://www.maxon.net/en/zbrush
RCSB Protein Data Bank	The online tools used in aid of the scaling of the models	https://www.rcsb.org
Midjourney, Inc.	Image generative AI tool, used to assist in generating moodboard images	Midjourney.com
Hardware	**Purpose**	**Produced by**
PC system Intel 11th Gen Intel Core i5 @ 2.6 GHz 16GB Ram GPU: NVIDIA GeForce RTX 3060	PC used for application development	Intel, Nvidia, Gigabyte
MacBook Pro (Retina, 13-in., 2018)	PC used for design (texture and image processing)	Apple
Oculus	The application was developed with and for display on Oculus Quest 2 hardware (Oculus Quest 2 Oculus Insight tracking, 1832 × 1920 resolution, 6DOF)	Meta Quest (https://www.oculus.com)

modelling software packages (Meshlab, Autodesk 3ds Max, and ZBrush), and the development and display hardware. (Intel IntelCore i5 PC with Nvidia GeForce GPU and Oculus Quest2 VR Headset.) All the data file sources for models, audio, textures, and VR plugin packages are itemized in Table 3.2.

3.2.2 Project Workflow

The application's overall development followed the workflow described in the chart in Fig. 3.1. After the initial development of the mood- and storyboards, a functional model application was developed concurrently with asset modelling and

Table 3.2 Data files sourced for the development of the application

Data	Purpose/content	Accessed at:
RCSB Protein Data Bank	Source for molecular models: 7UTI Actin 7UTL Actin 7BTS Beta 1 Receptor, adrenaline 4MQS Muscarinic receptor	https://www.rcsb.org; all models are available under the CC0 1.0 Universal (CC0 1.0) Public Domain Dedication Rynkiewicz MJ, Pavadai E, Lehman W. Alternative modeling of tropomyosin in human cardiac thin filament in the calcium bound state (2022) https://doi.org/10.2210/pdb7uti/pdb Rynkiewicz MJ, Pavadai E, Lehman W. Alternative modeling of tropomyosin in human cardiac thin filament in the calcium bound state (2022) https://doi.org/10.2210/pdb7utl/pdb Xu X, Kaindl J, Clark M, Hubner H, Hirata K, Sunahara R, Gmeiner P, Kobilka B K, Liu X. Structure of human beta1 adrenergic receptor bound to epinephrine and nanobody 6B9. (2020) https://doi.org/10.2210/pdb7bts/pdb Kruse A C, Ring A M, Manglik A, Hu J, Hu K, Eitel K, Huebner H, Pardon E, Valant C, Sexton P M, Christopoulos A, Felder C C, Gmeiner P, Steyaert J, Weis W I, Garcia K C, Wess J, Kobilka B K. Structure of active human M2 muscarinic acetylcholine receptor bound to the agonist iperoxo (2013) DOI: https://doi.org/10.2210/pdb4mqs/pdb
National Center for Biotechnology Information PubChem	4946 Propranolol, stick view 247704 Adrenaline, stick view	Structure of active human M2 muscarinic acetylcholine receptor bound to the agonist iperoxo National Center for Biotechnology Information. PubChem Compound Summary for CID 4946, Propranolol. https://pubchem.ncbi.nlm.nih.gov/compound/Propranolol. Accessed Jan. 9, 2024 National Center for Biotechnology Information. PubChem Compound Summary for CID 247704, (S)-adrenaline. https://pubchem.ncbi.nlm.nih.gov/compound/S_-adrenaline. Accessed Jan. 9, 2024
Source for the myocyte—XR Life Sciences	The myocyte cell membrane mesh	https://skfb.ly/oG69D

(continued)

Table 3.2 (continued)

Data	Purpose/content	Accessed at:
Texture file: palm_tree_bark ground_wet_003	Files used to texture the assets	Polyhaven.com https://polyhaven.com/a/palm_tree_bark Cilliers R, Savva C Licence CC0 3D textures https://3dtextures.me/2020/06/01/ground-wet-003/ Licence CC0
369017__patobottos__heartbeats-61.wav	Sound of heartbeat—mixed to 60 bpm and sped to 90 bpm	Patobottos; Accessed at freesound.org: Heartbeats 61.wav by patobottos I License: Creative Commons 0 I Timestamp: 2023-06-14 14:31:54.226261
686823__erokia__ambient-wave-75.wav	Background sound—shortened and remixed	Erokia; Accessed at freesound.org: Ambient Wave 75.flac by Erokia I License: Attribution NonCommercial 4.0 I Timestamp: 2023-06-26 21:21:29.326447
104006__rutgermuller__wood_scrape_soft_close.aiff 369730__joedl__gurgling-non-human.wav 588305_wolfowi__horror-gurgling-crunching-owi.wav 366819__michaelvelo__bubbles-in-water-popping.wav	Local sounds inside the model—remixed	Rutgermuller: Wood_Scrape_Soft_Close.Aif by RutgerMuller I License: Creative Commons 0 I Timestamp: 2023-07-20 11:59:25.724930 Joedl: Gurgling (non human).wav by joedl I License: Creative Commons 0 I Timestamp: 2023-07-20 12:01:18.918721 Wolfovi: Horror Gurgling Crunching OWI by WolfOWI I License: Attribution NonCommercial 3.0 I Timestamp: 2023-07-20 12:01:55.840746 MichaelVelo: Bubbles in water popping.wav by Michaelvelo I License: Attribution NonCommercial 3.0 I Timestamp: 2023-07-20 11:55:34.718603 All accessed at freesound.org
Oculus XR Plugin	OVR camera rig, OVR synthetic hands	Unity Technologies https://unity.com/

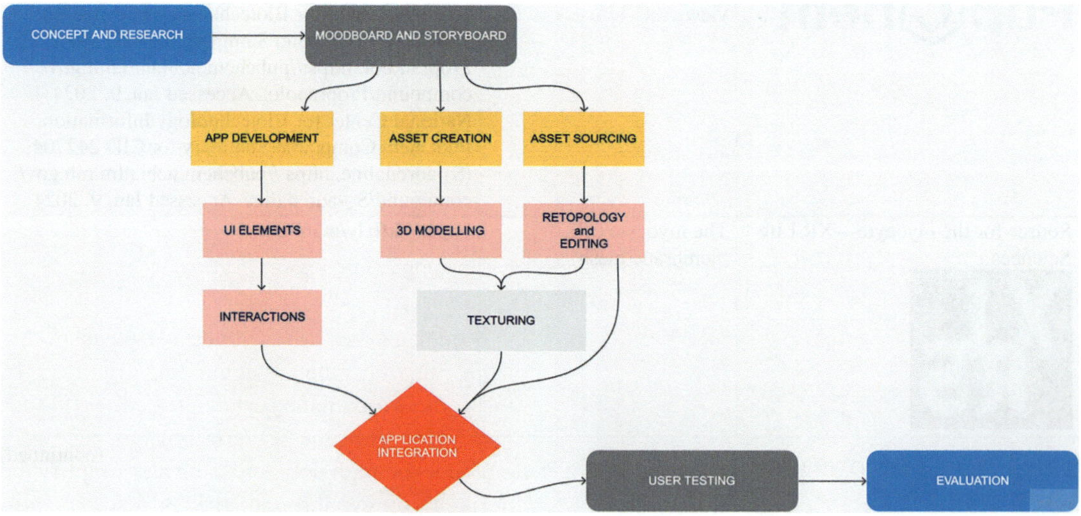

Fig. 3.1 MyoSITE Design and development workflow

sourcing. After this, the assets were incorporated into the application structure, the functionalities adjusted, and the application tested. After the first testing, improvements were implemented to the application user interface based on the initial testing results, and testing was repeated with round 2.

3.2.3 Design Concept

The MyoSITE project aimed to present a whole cell alongside models of its internal structures, allowing users to explore them at their correct relative scale. The application was designed for both group and individual use. Based on this concept, several design features were implemented. A MR approach was used to create a 'social space' that would foster natural group interaction and movement, allowing users to view a sizable digital object from different perspectives by walking around. This was realized by using the Pass-through feature of the Oculus Quest 2 HMD. The integrated hand tracking functionality was used as the preferred interaction method, enabling intuitive and natural manipulation of digital objects through hand gestures. The presence of menus and other digital elements, such as texts and labels, was minimized to maintain focus on the digital objects appearing in the real space. The soundtrack was simple, emphasizing a sense of space while complementing the digital content.

The storyboard was designed around the idea of one main scene, which would serve as the central area for user navigation, accompanied by several 'close-up' scenes for more detailed interactions, functioning as 'desktop study stations' (Fig. 3.2).

The narrative of MyoSITE explored the regulation of the heartbeat, featuring elements such as adrenaline and the drug propranolol. Also included were animated models of actin filaments, integral components of sarcomeres, as these cellular microstructures play a crucial role in contraction and consequently a vital part in heart function.

A moodboard was created to guide the overall aesthetics of the project (Fig. 3.3). The project drew inspiration from current research on

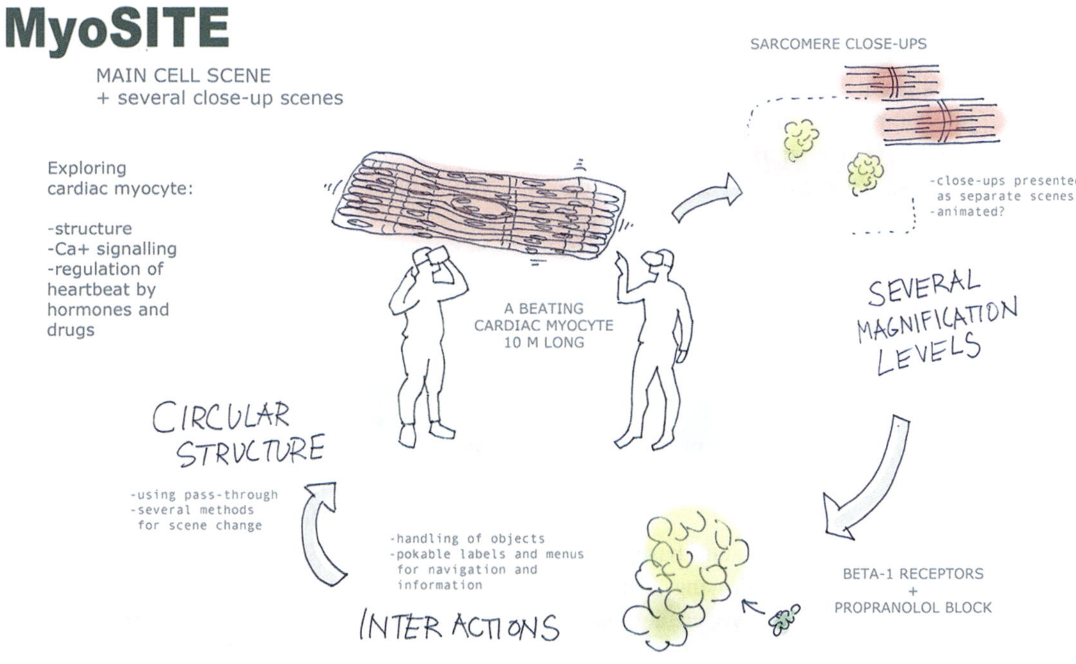

Fig. 3.2 MyoSITE storyboard showing the circular structure of the application design, with one central scene and several close-up scenes

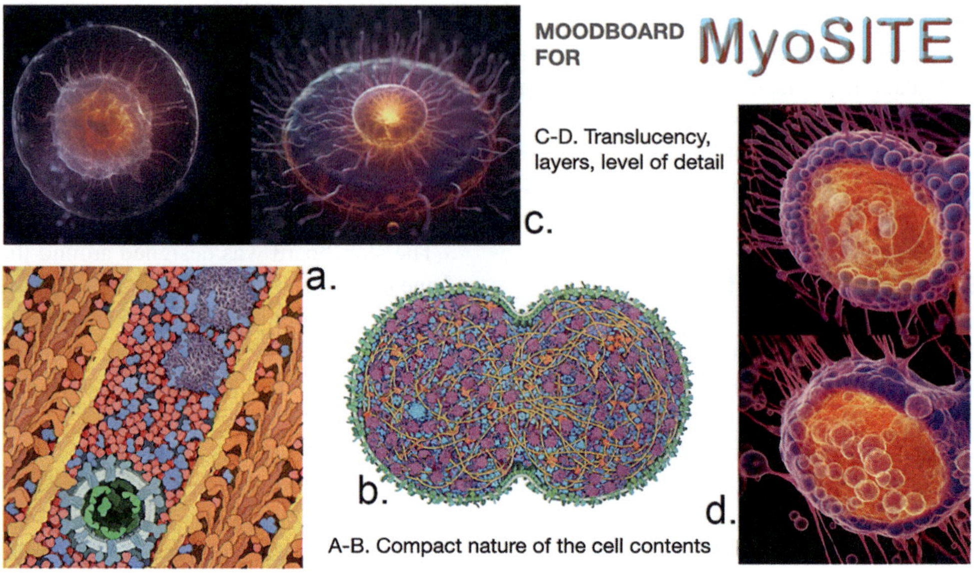

Fig. 3.3 MyoSITE moodboard (Reproduced from **a** Goodsell 2021; **b** Goodsell 2022; **c–d** Midjourney 2023)

whole-cell modelling (Goodsell et al. 2020; Maritan et al. 2022), utilizing visual and artistic materials sourced from the open-source Protein Data Bank (PDB; Table 3.2) as a significant reference for moodboard imagery.

In addition to Internet sourcing for relevant material, generative AI (Midjourney 2023) was employed to create visuals using specific prompts (such as: 'translucent cell anatomy structure with nucleus, golgi apparatus, mitochondria, sarcoplasmic reticulum visible' and). Some of the generated outcomes successfully conveyed the desired textures and lighting for mood board communication (Fig. 3.3c, d). However, it is essential to note that these images were not realistic, indicating the need for further refinement of AI-assisted mood board generation.

3.2.4 Development of the 3D Models

The MyoSITE application used data-based models whenever possible. The following structures were selected for inclusion: a myocyte cell membrane, a nucleus, myofibrils, mitochondria, muscarinic receptor and beta1-adrenoceptor, drugs propranolol and adrenaline, and the Actin-troponin complex in two versions, one with Ca + and one without. Of these, the cell membrane, mitochondria, receptors, and drug molecules were available as data-based models.

One of the project's objectives was to maintain the accurate relative scale of all structures, commencing from the dimensions of the exhibition room and the largest model, the cardiomyocyte, which was set to a length of 10 m. The sizes for the rest of the 3D models were referenced from Levick (2008) and the Protein Data Bank (Table 3.2; Fig. 3.4),

The project adhered to the following sizing (Table 3.3):

Only the main scene was scaled corresponding to the ARC-XR space (first five entries in Table 3.3), where the components were scaled to be accurate for the 10 m model. The pop-up scene models had components that were already in relative scale as parts of the downloaded models, and this ratio was preserved, while the scene was not set to specific magnification level; therefore, sizing and magnification level data for these entries in the Table 3.3 is given as n/a.

3.2.4.1 Extraction and Preparation of Data-Based Models

A set of models was downloaded using available source material from online data banks, and these had to be processed for inclusion into the interac-

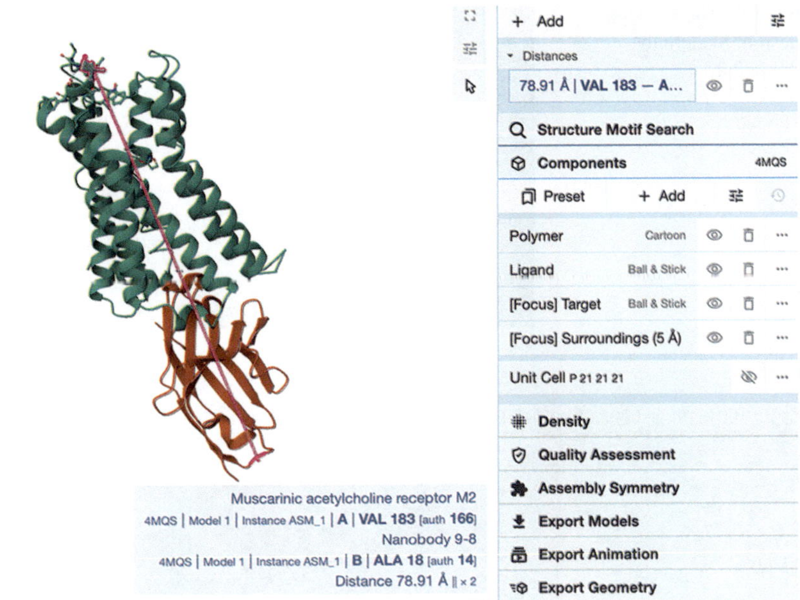

Fig. 3.4 Measuring the Muscarinic Receptor (with its nanobody) in PDB. Image from the RCSB PDB (RCSB.org; Table 3.2) of PDB ID 4MQS (Kruse et al. 2013)

Table 3.3 MyoSITE model sizing chart

Model	PDB/PubChem ID no	Real size length	(Real size diameter)	Length in app	Magnification level
Myocyte	-	100 μm	25 μm	10 m	X 100,s000
Myofibrils	-	100 μm	1 μm	10 m	
Mitochondrion	-	1 μm	n/a	10 cm (variable)	
Nucleus	-	10 μm	n/a	1 m	
B-1 receptor scene 2	7BTS	67.4 Å	n/a	0.67 mm	
B-1 receptor scene 3–4	7BTS	67.4 Å	n/a	n/a	n/a
Muscarinic receptor	4MQS	78.9 Å	n/a	n/a	n/a
Propranolol	4946	n/a	n/a	n/a	n/a
Adrenaline	247704	n/a	n/a	n/a	n/a
Actin–myosin filament animated	7UTI 7UTL	506.2 Å	n/a	n/a	n/a

tive application. The goal was to maintain the highest level of detail while creating a mesh that is clean and has minimal polygons.

3.2.4.1.1 The Myocyte Cell Membrane

The myocyte cell membrane was obtained from the XR Life Sciences Sketchfab site (Table 3.2, Fig. 3.5). The model had a relatively low polygon count of 4.7 k and 2.4 k vertices, requiring no further retopology.

In 3ds Max, the Open Subdiv modifier was applied to refine the geometry. A scaling box of 10 m × 2.5 m × 1.5 m was generated, and the model was adjusted to match this size. A UVW map (box) was applied, and the model was exported into Unity. Here, the cell membrane was duplicated for a layered effect. Both layers were configured for transparent rendering, with the inner layer receiving a texture map to simulate a generic biomaterial.

3.2.4.1.2 The Muscarinic Receptor

The muscarinic receptor, retrieved from the Protein Data Bank (Table 3.2; file 4MQS), was converted into an STL file, and imported into 3ds Max for further processing. The model included embedded molecules, which were initially separated into layers. This was done within 3ds Max

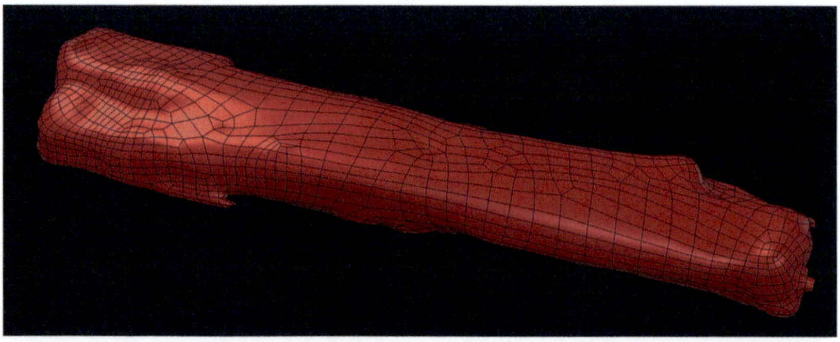

Fig. 3.5 The myocyte mesh in Sketchfab (Table 3.2)

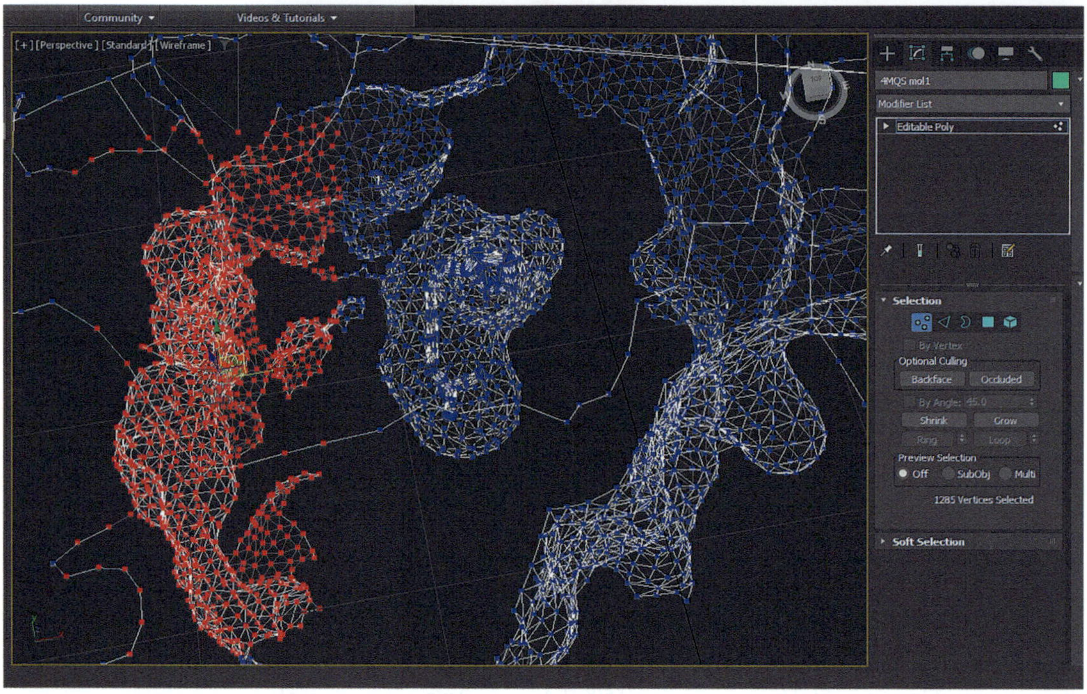

Fig. 3.6 Removing embedded molecules from the muscarinic receptor

manually by cutting and removing the main mesh (Fig. 3.6) in order to retain the ligand position within the mesh. Triangular remnants were identified, detached, and removed. The molecule component was then reinstated to its original scale and position within the receptor mesh.

With a polygon count of 49,974, retopologizing the receptor mesh was necessary to allow digital models to be smoothly rendered through the HMD. Initial attempts in 3ds Max using the automatic retopology modifier yielded unsatisfactory results due to multiple holes in the mesh. The model was then transferred to ZBrush, where the topology was adjusted by closing the gaps. Although ZRemesher was attempted for retopology, it proved unsuccessful, causing the application to stall. Returning to 3ds Max, the ProOptimizer modifier was applied at 80%, reducing the mesh to a level suitable for retopology. The final polygon count was reduced to 20 k, resulting in a satisfactory mesh structure composed of quads (Fig. 3.7).

3.2.4.1.3 The Beta1-Adrenoceptor

The beta1-adrenoceptor, obtained from the Protein Data Bank (Table 3.2; file 7BTS), underwent a similar process of download and conversion into an STL file. Four embedded molecules were extracted in 3DS Max by cutting and eliminating the surrounding mesh (See Fig. 3.8a).

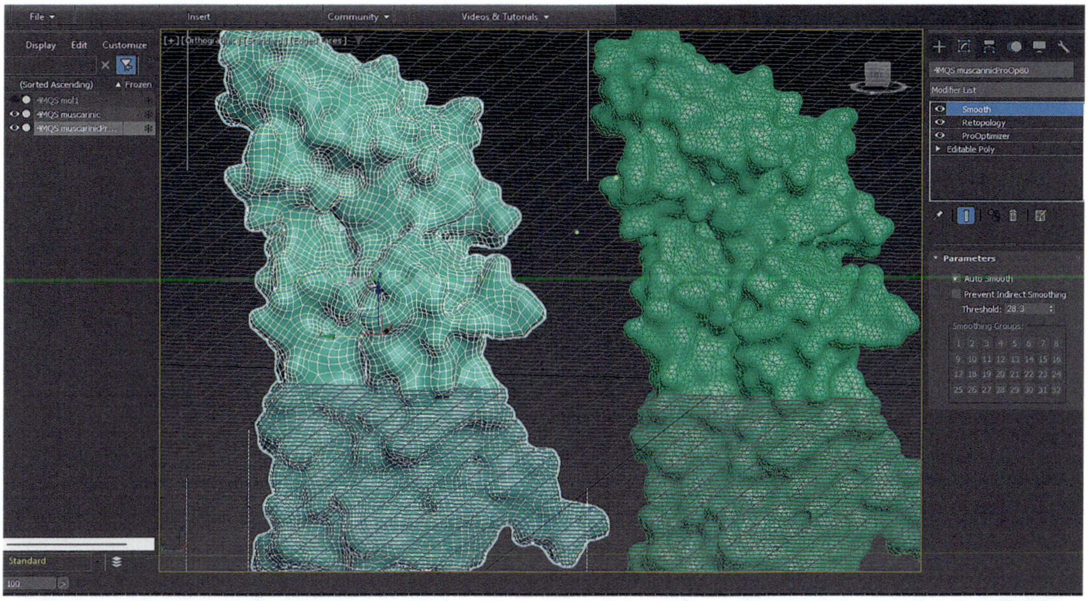

Fig. 3.7 Muscarinic receptor mesh before retopology (right) and after (left)

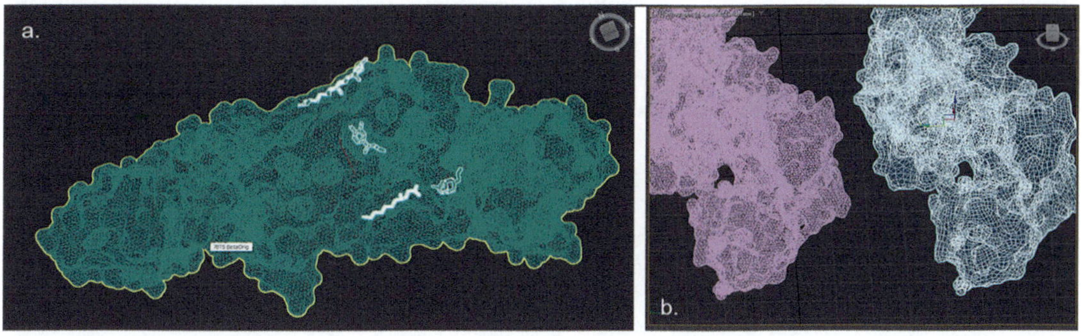

Fig. 3.8 (**a**) Beta1-adrenoceptor with four embedded molecules. (**b**) Beta1-adrenoceptor before retopology (left) and after it (right)

Subsequently, a duplicate of the receptor was reconstructed by removing the molecules vertex by vertex.

The triangular gaps within the receptor mesh were sealed using ZBrush, and the model was subsequently processed within 3ds Max with the ProOptimizer modifier set at 80% and with a retopology modifier. This process resulted in the reduction of the final model's polygon count from 79,780 to a satisfactory 17 k (Fig. 3.8b).

3.2.4.1.4 Adrenaline

An adrenaline molecule was initially identified within the PDB (Table 3.2) beta1-adrenoceptor model. The extracted molecule's mesh was of low quality (Fig. 3.9a), thus prompting the acquisition of a replacement through the PubChem website (Table 3.2; model number 247704).

The size and placement of the adrenaline within the beta1-adrenoceptor was then matched with the original one (Fig. 3.9b).

3.2.4.1.5 Propranolol

Propranolol structure was downloaded through the National Institute of Health PubChem databank (Table 3.2; model number 4946, see Fig. 3.10).

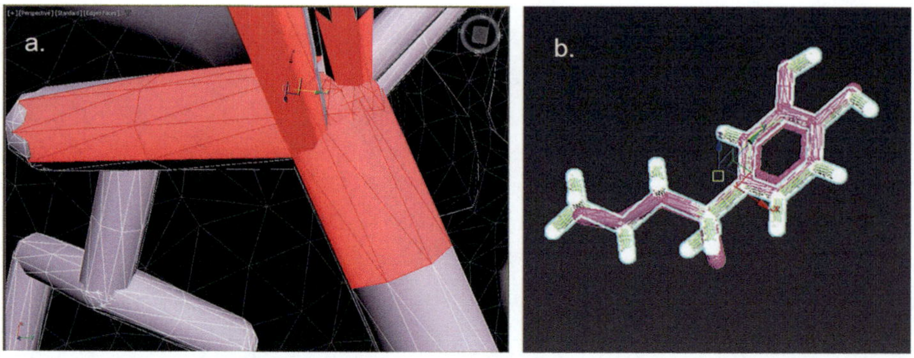

Fig. 3.9 (**a**) Close-up of the adrenaline molecule showing poor quality of the mesh. (**b**) The new adrenaline molecule (white) is lined up with the original (pink), in position in 3ds Max

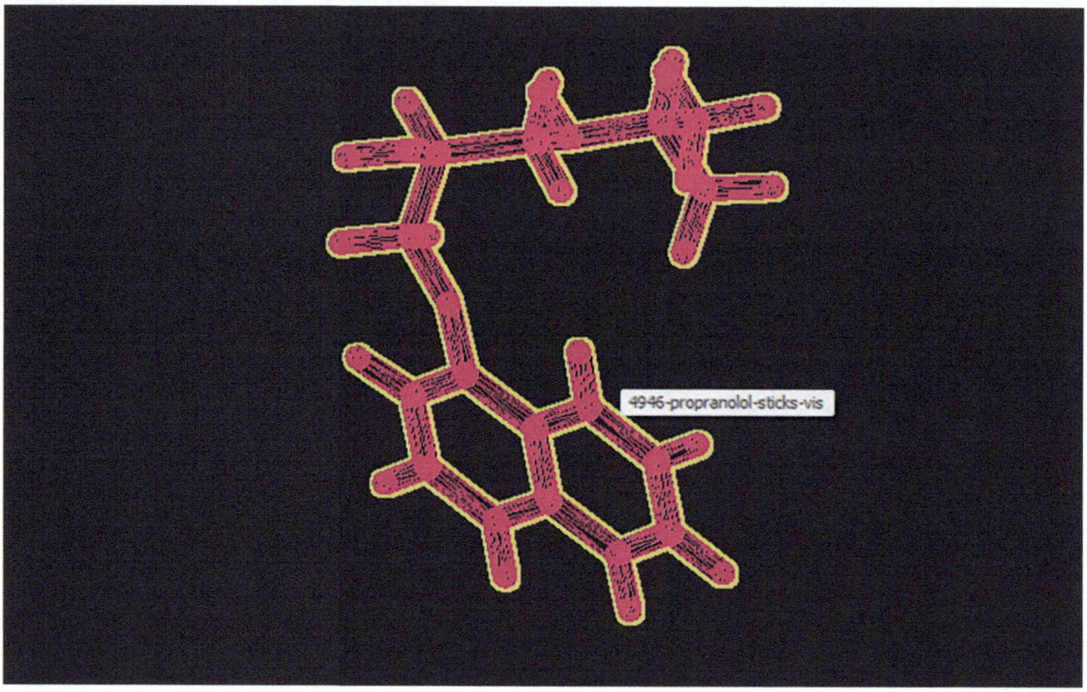

Fig. 3.10 Propranolol molecule, model 4946

3.2.4.1.6 The Actin–Troponin Filament

The Actin–Troponin filament models were procured from the PDB (Table 3.2; 7UTL and 7UTI). Both models were characterized by high polygon counts and were in a state of disrepair, exhibiting numerous gaps and non-manifold features (see Fig. 3.11a).

The Actin–troponin model incorporating Calcium (7UTI) had an unclean mesh with a polygon count of 1,222,080. The model presented a challenge for 3ds Max and ZRemesher, requiring initial processing within MeshLab. The polygon count was halved via the Quadric Edge Mesh Decimation, followed by a mesh repair, cleansing, and restoration (Fig. 3.11b). Fixing non-manifold edges re-introduced aberrant polygons, but after several iterations of fixing and healing commands, the algorithm returned a cleaned mesh.

The model was subsequently exported into 3ds Max at 300 k vertices and subjected to the ProOptimizer modifier at varying percentages. The version was then re-imported, cleansed, further reduced in MeshLab, and processed again in 3ds Max. Final iterations of cleaning and restora-

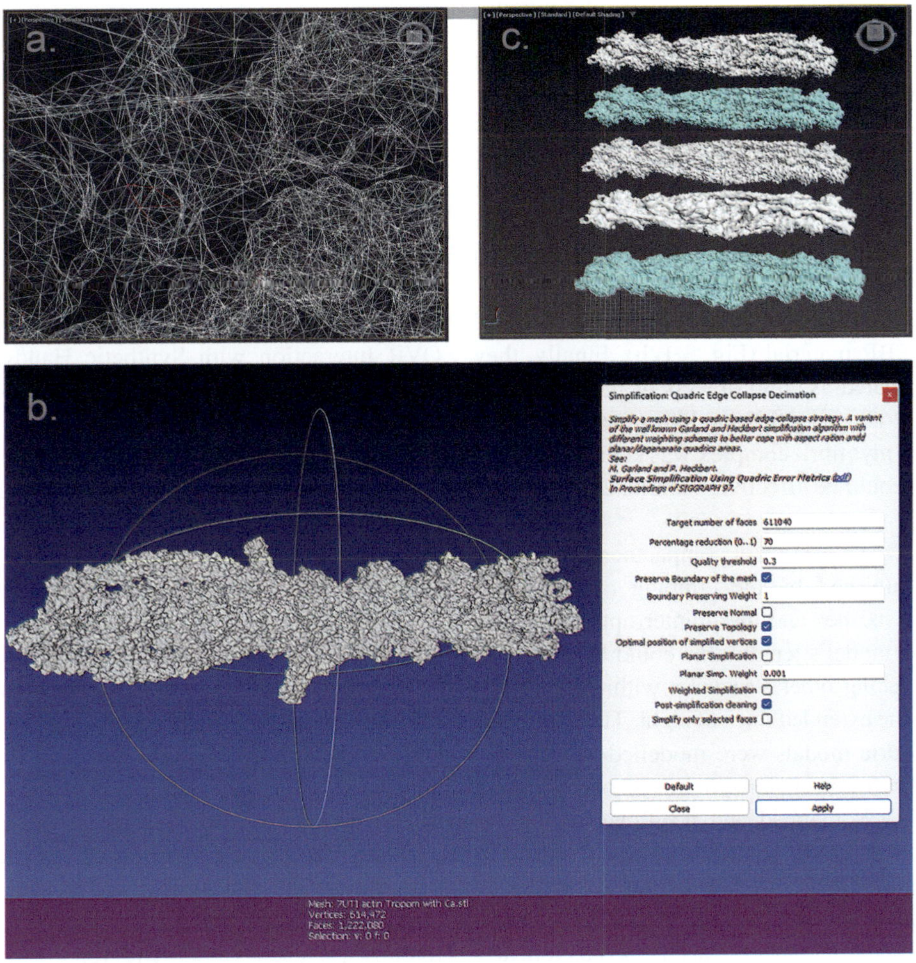

Fig. 3.11 (**a**) Close Up of 7UTI mesh with holes and aberrations (**b**) The model 7UTI in MeshLab, polygons halved (**c**) Versions of reduced meshes of actin–troponin filament model, with the original in the centre, the final one on the bottom

tion were conducted back within MeshLab. In the most successful run, the cleaned mesh was processed with the 3ds Max ProOptimizer modifier set at 5% and with retopology modifiers, resulting in 50 k faces (Fig. 3.11c). In this version, most of the high poly model's original detail was successfully retained, yielding a sufficiently clean and repaired mesh ready for import into Unity.

Model 7UTL exhibited similar characteristics, with numerous aberrations and a high polygon count of 1,373,564. A comparable process was applied, involving a succession of stages including reduction, mending, and cleansing of the mesh, alternating between MeshLab and 3ds Max. This iterative process ultimately yielded a visually satisfactory model with a significantly reduced polygon count of 49,191 faces.

3.2.4.2 Modelling of Assets

In order to create a context for the data-derived models, certain structures were created using 3ds Max and scaled to the correct proportions. These served as a framework that would allow visualizing the relative placement and movement of the intracellular structures. To convey a sense of compactness within the cell, it was densely populated with cell-long, 10-m myofibrils that closely followed the irregular contours of the membrane. These structures had a diameter of 10 cm and were intended to exhibit a striated appearance that would resemble sarcomeres, each approximately 20 cm long within the MyoSITE scale. The myofibril tubules were created by elongated prime hexagonal cylinders with uniform smoothing groups. These cylinders were then shaped to conform to the cell membrane outline using the FFD modifier with a 15 × 6 × 5 control point grid (Fig. 3.12a).

Subsequently, they were collapsed into an editable mesh, subjected to UVW mapping, exported as FBX files into Unity, and textured using a PBR material (Fig. 3.12b). Finally, they were animated as child objects of the cell membrane. By adopting this modelling approach, the extensive myofibril complex was kept less expensive and could be effectively animated within the headset.

Whilst the sensation of compactness was somewhat diminished by the clipping of individual myofibril meshes and the uninterrupted visibility along the model's length, this could be mitigated by introducing other structures within the cell to obstruct the extended lines of sight. The simplified mitochondria models were modelled in 3ds Max as clusters of irregularized boxes of 10 cm in length, UVW mapped and positioned along the myofibrils in Unity. The nucleus was constructed from a prime sphere, set to 1 m long, and imported into Unity as an FBX file. In the close-up scenes, the cell membrane model was shaped as a nearly flat box, with mesh vertices manipulated for a more organic appearance and curvature achieved through smooth selection. Lastly, the two actin–tropomyosin filament models were aligned in 3ds Max (See Fig. 3.13).

3.2.5 Development of the Immersive Experience

The MR application was developed on Oculus Integration Software Development Kit, making use of the Pass-through capabilities of Oculus Quest 2 headsets. The game was set up to use the integrated Oculus hand tracking for interactions. The primary interactive setup involved using an OVR Camera Rig with a Centre Eye Anchor, an OVR Interaction with Synthetic Hands configured for both hand grab and poke functionalities, and a Pointable Canvas Module.

Each scene contained stationary information user interface (UI) panels positioned in world space and a hand menu following the user's movements within the physical space. Initially, the idea was to implement a pop-up menu on the raised left palm, but this proved challenging within the installed SDK version due to issues related to the visibility of different layers of panels and buttons, conflicts in material properties, and render queue values, and an alternative approach was devised. A bespoke script, ManageMenuVisibility(), caused a cube to appear at the centre marker of the left palm upon palm movement. When triggered, it brought up a UI menu that was duplicated and configured differently for each scene. The versions provided access to model layers and pop-up UI panels with additional information about the model. All these functionalities were managed through the button options in the inspector, with an additional 'toggle' script added to the functionalities that needed

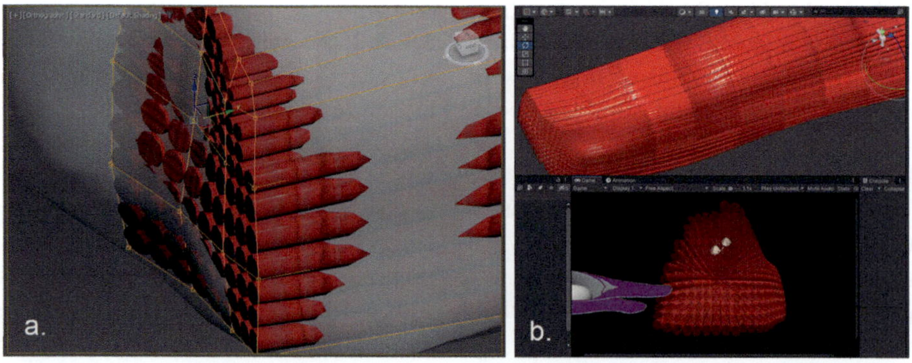

Fig. 3.12 (**a**) Using the FFD grid in shaping the myofibrils (**b**) Myofibril set imported into Unity

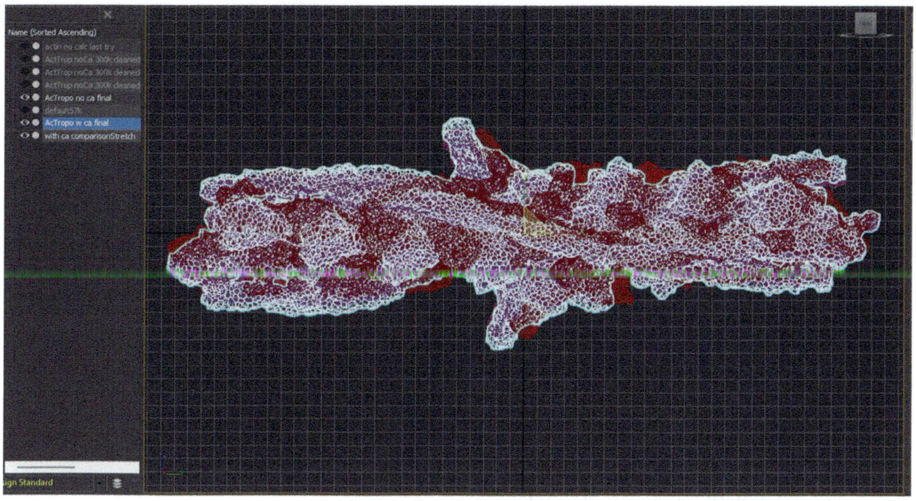

Fig. 3.13 Actin filaments lined up, the model with calcium in white and scaling widget in yellow

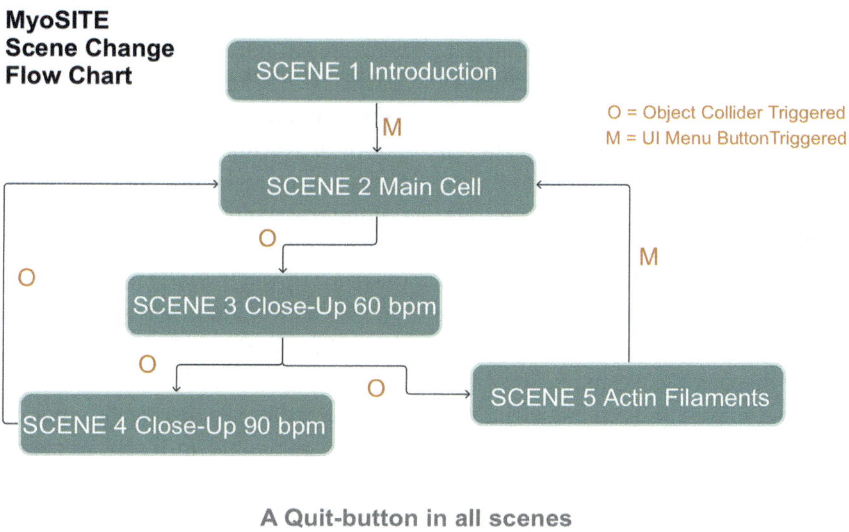

Fig. 3.14 MyoSITE Scene Flow Chart

to be activated and deactivated repeatedly from the same button in a Boolean manner.

The transitions between scenes were facilitated either by menu buttons or a script for scene transitions that was activated by a collider on an object or within the space. The flow of scene changes is illustrated in Fig. 3.14.

The three stationary 'pop-up' scenes (scenes 3, 4, and 5) needed to open in front of the user regardless of their position within the physical room. To preserve the user's positioning data for the ambulatory main scene, all the game objects of these 'desktop' scenes were enclosed within a parent game object and positioned at a specific distance in front of the camera. To implement this, a script named MoveObjectOnStart() was developed (Fig. 3.15).

Specific models were designed to be interacted with for both observation and handling, including propranolol and adrenaline molecules in scenes 1, 3, and 4, as well as actin filaments in scene 5. The OVR synthetic hands were paired with game objects that had attached scripts to enable handling (HandGrabFreeTransformer(),

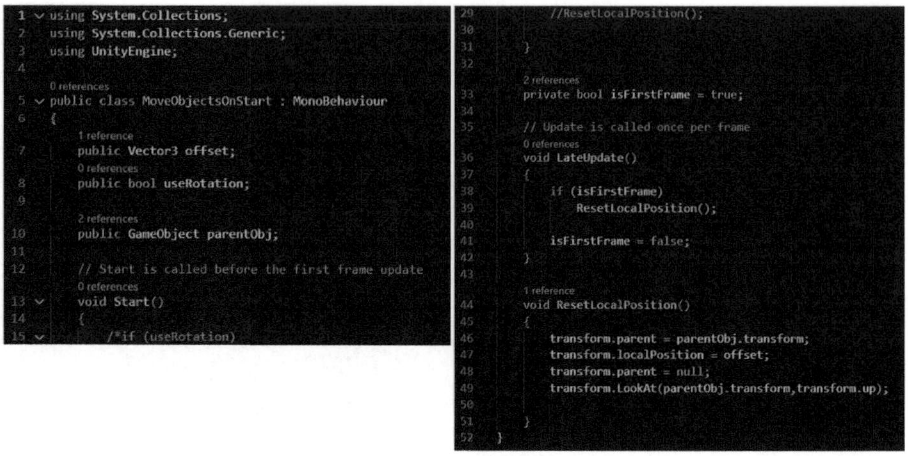

```
using System.Collections;
using System.Collections.Generic;
using UnityEngine;

0 references
public class MoveObjectsOnStart : MonoBehaviour
{
    1 reference
    public Vector3 offset;
    0 references
    public bool useRotation;

    2 references
    public GameObject parentObj;

    // Start is called before the first frame update
    0 references
    void Start()
    {
        /*if (useRotation)
```

```
        //ResetLocalPosition();

    }

    2 references
    private bool isFirstFrame = true;

    // Update is called once per frame
    0 references
    void LateUpdate()
    {
        if (isFirstFrame)
            ResetLocalPosition();

        isFirstFrame = false;
    }

    1 reference
    void ResetLocalPosition()
    {
        transform.parent = parentObj.transform;
        transform.localPosition = offset;
        transform.parent = null;
        transform.LookAt(parentObj.transform,transform.up);

    }
}
```

Fig. 3.15 MoveObjectOnStart() script for MyoSITE

Grabbable(), and TouchHandGrabInteractable() from Oculus Sample Scenes). In scenes 3 and 4, game objects were also employed for collision-triggered scene changes.

A generic ambient soundtrack was chosen from freesound.org for the background to establish a serene and expansive atmosphere. For scenes 2–5, a human heartbeat sound was modified into a one-beat-per-second clip within Audacity. This clip served as a timing guide for setting the animations. In scene 4, the clip was accelerated in the inspector to 1.5 times for a heart rate of 90 beats per minute. For an enhanced visceral experience, four audio clips were distributed along the cell model for localized sounds audible in scene 2 when entering the myocyte (for details on all audio clips and sources, see Table 3.2).

Since the scenes featured molecular material, many assets incorporated some level of animation. The myocyte cell model was animated using the Unity animation system, employing a one-second-long scaling animation to simulate a 60 beats-per-minute heartbeat audio. The cell's contents were configured as children of the cell mesh to be animated in sync with it.

All texturing work was performed within Unity. Molecular models were assigned simple colour materials, as texture maps were unnecessary to emphasize the inherent complexity of these meshes. Custom materials were generated for the cell membranes, nucleus, myofibrils, and mitochondria. The membranes were given an organic textured appearance by combining medical colour maps with separately sourced normal maps and utilizing transparent rendering. The myofibril texture necessitated a striated effect, achieved by modifying diffuse and normal maps of a palm trunk in Photoshop to resemble a textured, striped, glossy red muscle surface. These maps were then tiled in Unity to repeat closely along the length of the cylinder mesh (Fig. 3.16).

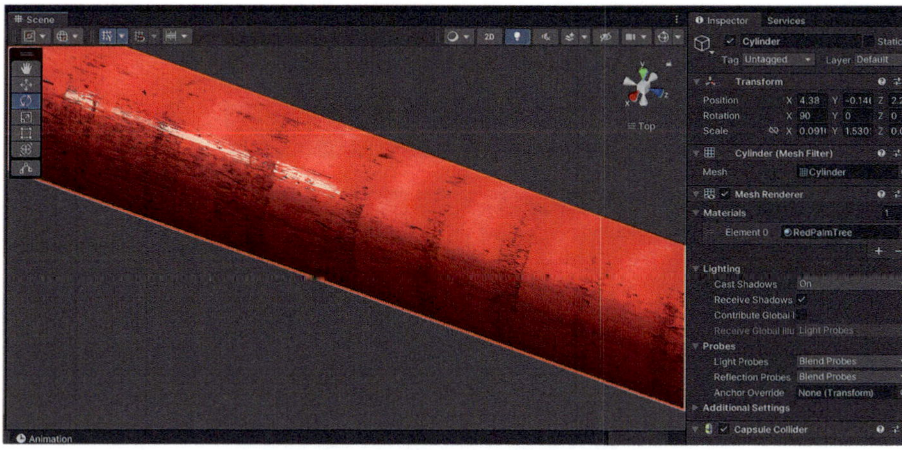

Fig. 3.16 Close-up of the red palm-trunk texture for myofibrils before tiling

3.3 Results of the Development

The chart below illustrates the application's final flow, content, and interactions (Fig. 3.17).

The application was intended for presentation in the ARC-XR space at the University of Glasgow Advanced Research Centre. It was exhibited on a maximum of four headsets simultaneously. Given that the largest model, the myocyte mesh, was tailored to fit the room in a specific manner, the application was set to initiate in the headsets at designated positions. These positions were marked in the room at both ends with a cross on the floor, ensuring that subsequent users experienced the myocyte model in their headset with the correct spatial configuration.

The MyoSITE opening scene 1 provides a brief welcome and an introduction to the project. The user is encouraged to familiarize themselves with the VR hands and locate the palm menu, which can be accessed by poking a cube on their left palm. A pink grabbable adrenaline model is suspended in front of the user, along with accompanying text inviting them to practise grabbing it with their fingers. They can then proceed to load the main scene via the 'Load MyoSITE' button on the palm menu (see Fig. 3.18). This welcome scene allows the user to acclimate to movement in VR and, optionally, receive additional guidance from a staff member in group settings.

Scene 2 is the main scene of the application, and it opens in full pass-through mode, displaying the exhibition room and other occupants. The pass-through mode is rendered in Oculus 2 with grey tones, against which the digital objects stand out in colour. In the centre of the room, a 10-m-long, red, beating cardiac myocyte model is suspended 1.4 m above the ground. It pulsates in sync with a 60 beats-per-minute human heart audio track. Two text panels in the space offer information about the scene and the application. It is important to note that the pass-through feature cannot currently (at the time of the writing) be natively recorded on Oculus Quest 2 and is represented in generic documentation in black; below is both in-headset documentation and an artistic rendering of the cell in the ARC-XR room, providing a sense of the real-life scale and appearance of the pass-through scene (Fig. 3.19b).

The user is encouraged to freely explore and move around the model, observing the movement and scale of various elements. Inside the model, localized sounds can be heard. The palm menu (Fig. 3.20a) enables the user to activate circles that help locate the 0.47-mm beta1-adrenoceptor on the cell membrane. By finding and tapping these receptors, the user can transition to the subsequent close-up scene (Fig. 3.20b).

Scene 3 emerges as a 'pop-up' scene 1 m in front of the user, featuring a portion of a cell membrane with two embedded beta1-adrenocep-

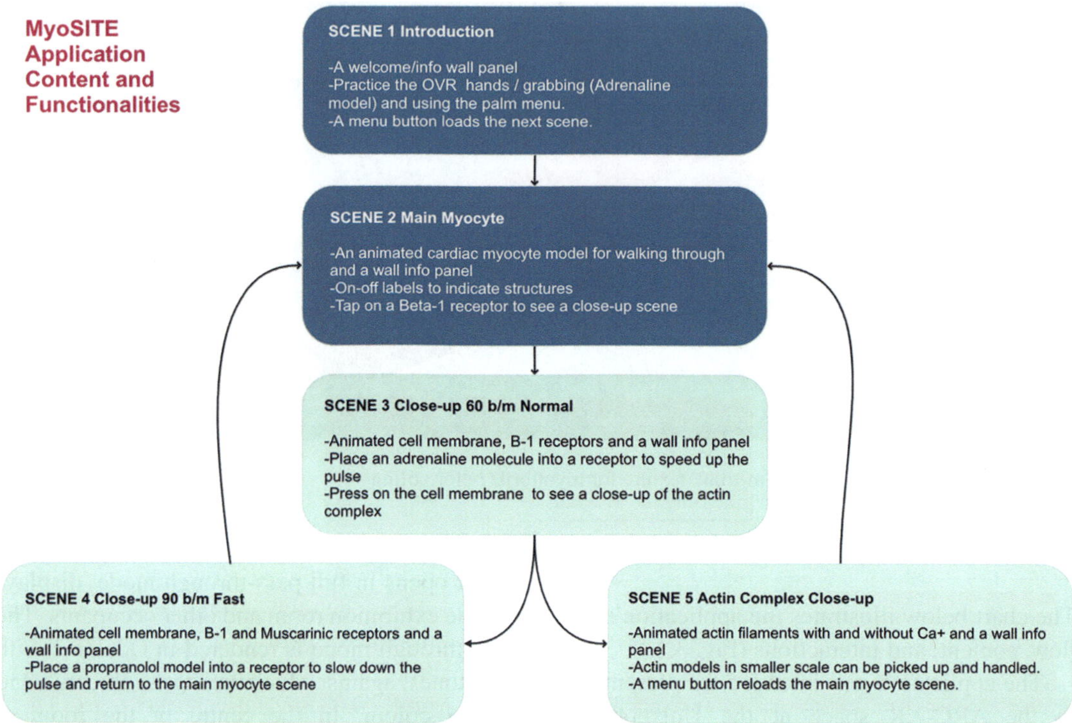

Fig. 3.17 Application Content and Functionalities

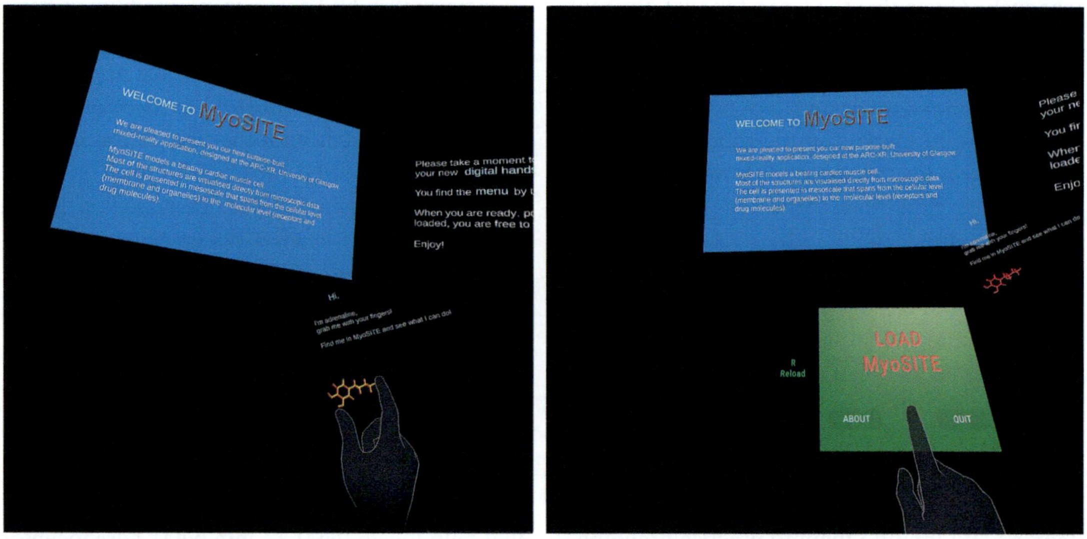

Fig. 3.18 Scene 1 with the pop-up menu

tor models, animated in synchronization with the heartbeat audio (Fig. 3.21).

The user can speed up the heartbeat by grabbing a small, suspended adrenaline molecule and placing it in the beta1-adrenoceptor (Scene 4; Fig. 3.22).

Scene 4 is likewise a 'pop-up' scene (Fig. 3.23). The adrenaline molecule is visible within the B-1 receptor, and the animation and heartbeat audio are now faster (90 bpm) due to the effects of the hormone.

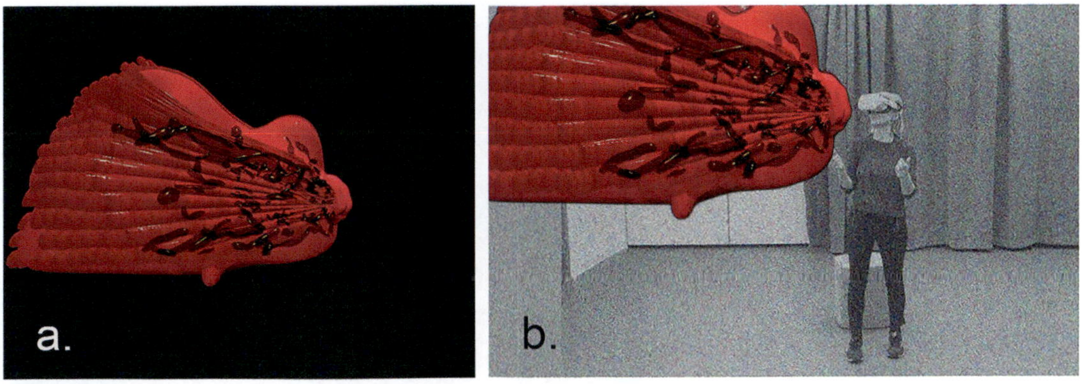

Fig. 3.19 (**a**) MyoSITE scene 2. The main pass-through scene, headset documentation (**b**) The pass-through scene, artist rendering

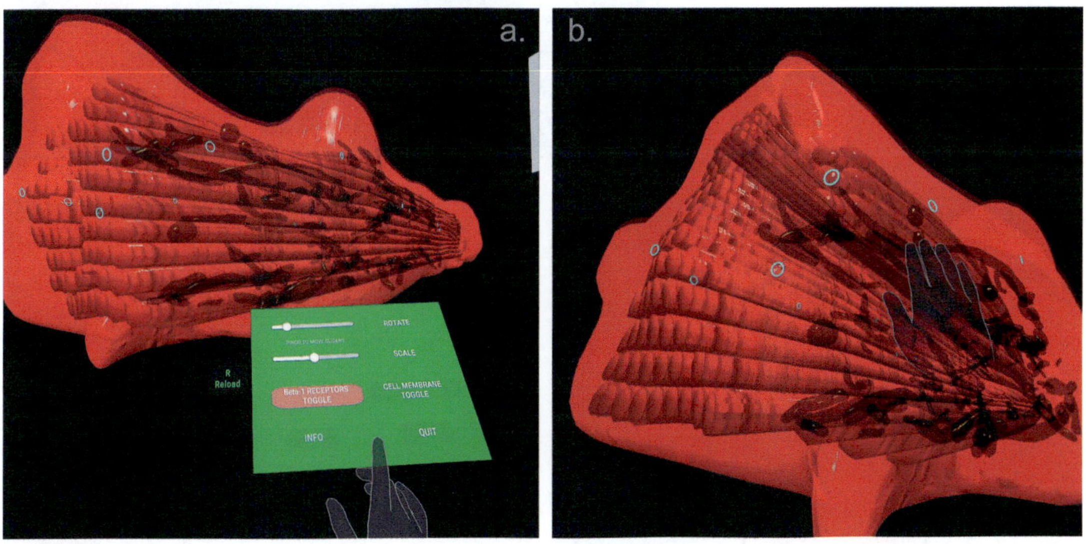

Fig. 3.20 (**a**) MyoSITE scene 2. Palm menu (**b**) Circles indicating location of the beta1-adrenoreceptors

By replacing the adrenaline in the beta1-adrenoceptor with the beta blocker propranolol, the user can slow down the heartbeat and return to the main scene with a slower 60 bpm pulse (Fig. 3.24).

From scene 3, the user also has access to a close-up of the actin filaments in scene 5, another non-passthrough pop-up. In front of the user, a large-scale suspended animation displays a detailed model of an actin–tropomyosin filament segment, transitioning between calcium-rich and calcium-free states (Fig. 3.25).

The animation is synchronized with the 60-bpm heartbeat audio. Handleable models of both rods are suspended to the user's right, accompanied by text indicating the calcium status. The user can learn more about the actin models and view a filament diagram in the pop-up informational panel. A palm menu button allows the user to return to scene 2.

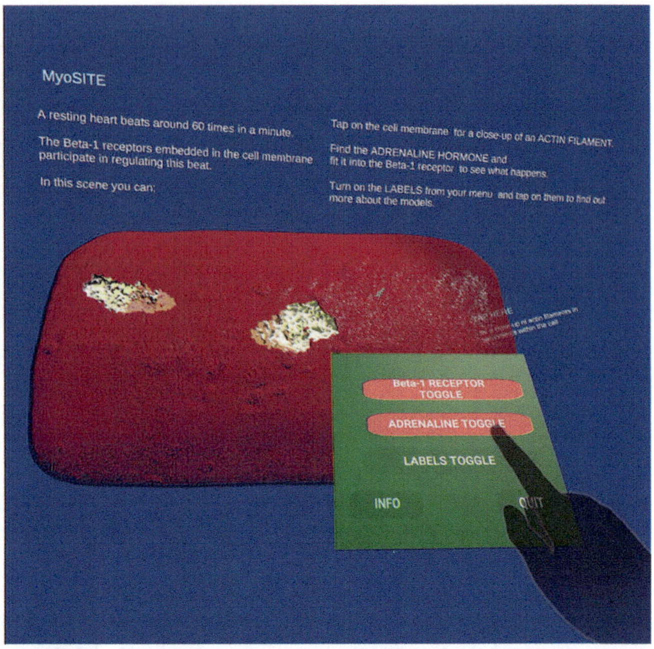

Fig. 3.21 MyoSITE scene 3

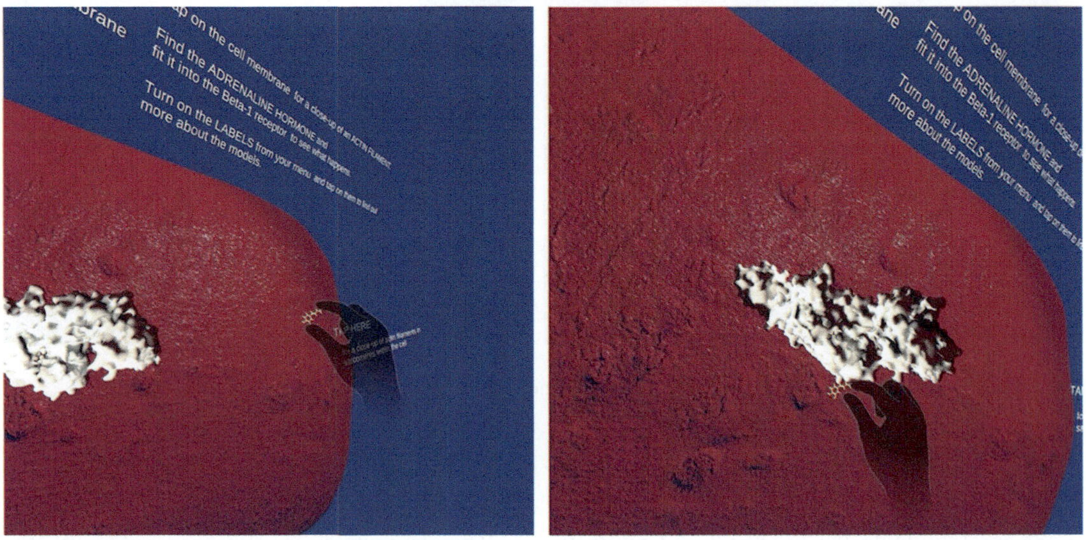

Fig. 3.22 Scene 3, interaction with adrenaline

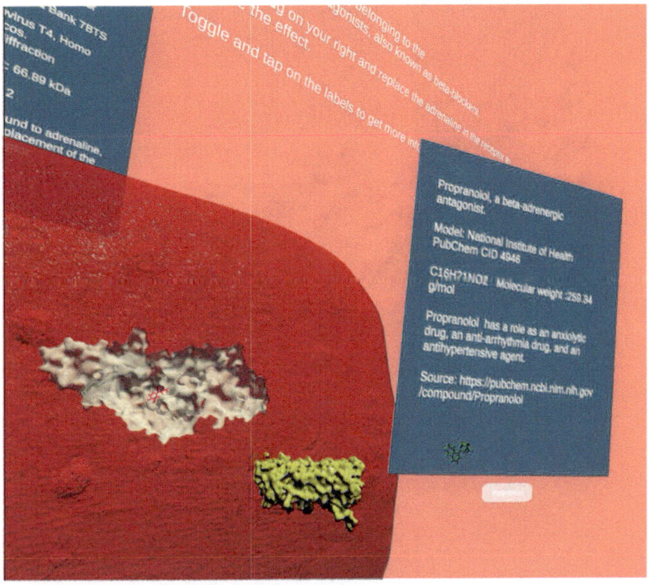
Toggle and tap on the labels to get more
Propranolol, a beta-adrenergic antagonist.
Model: National Institute of Health PubChem CID 4946
Propranolol has a role as an anxiolytic drug, an anti-arrhythmia drug, and an antihypertensive agent.
Source: https://pubchem.ncbi.nlm.nih.gov /compound/Propranolol

Fig. 3.23 MyoSITE scene 4, showing adrenaline (pink) in beta1-adrenoceptor (white) and an example of a pop-up panel for model info (data source: Kim et al. 2023)

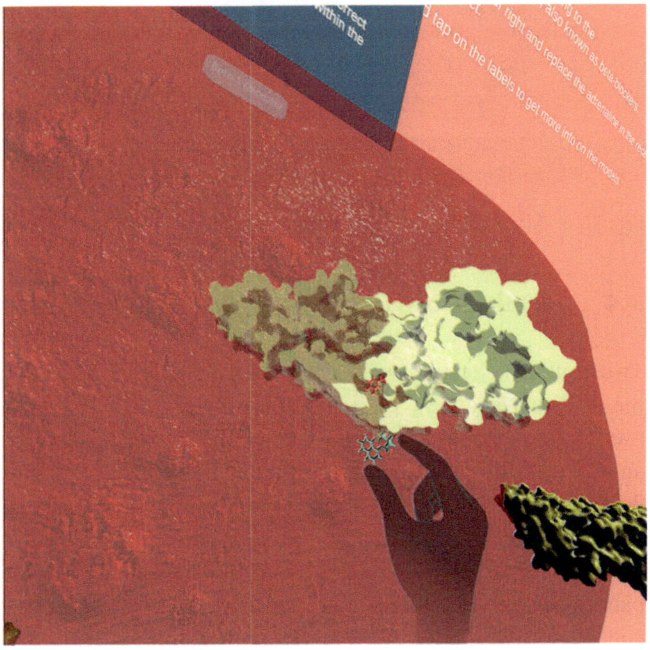

Fig. 3.24 Scene 4 interaction

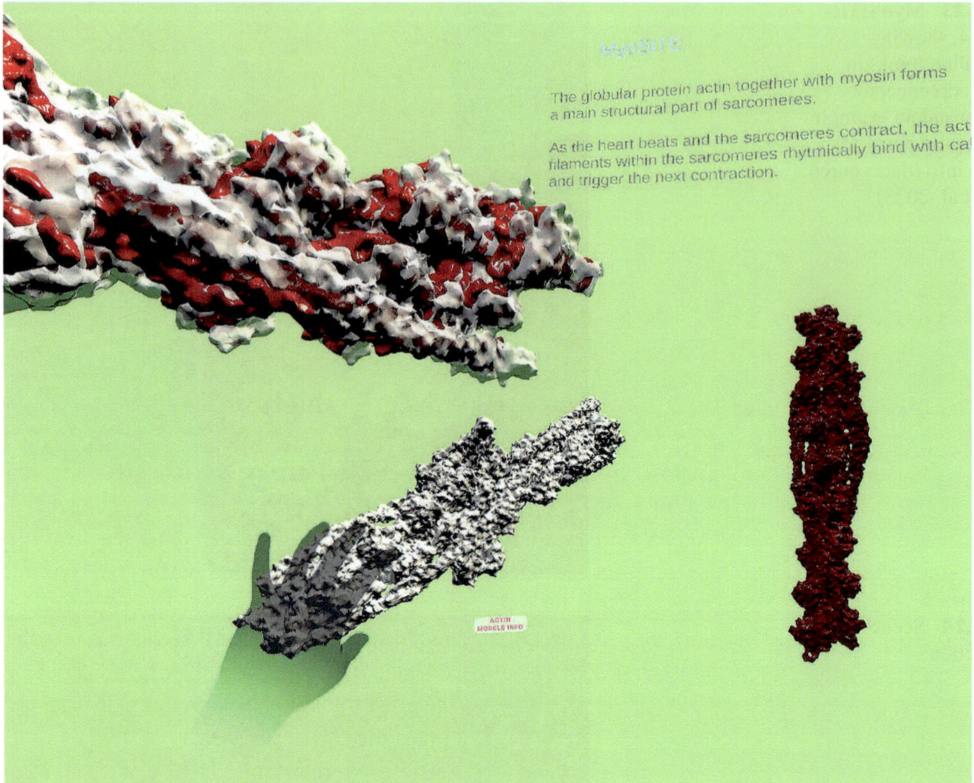

Fig. 3.25 MyoSITE scene 5, showing interaction with actin rod

3.4 Evaluation

Two rounds of testing were conducted to assess the MR experience's overall usability and its proof-of-concept merits. The testing consisted of an initial exploratory round 1, followed by round 2 which assessed usability of a refined application, where alterations had been made based on the feedback from the first cohort of test participants. The second round employed a new test cohort, not familiar with the application, in order to get an accurate usability assessment from first-time users.

The evaluation focused on two main factors: (1) The usability and content of the current application and (2) the potential of the application for educational scenarios, including its suitability for use by multiple participants. These evaluations aimed to examine how specialists in Life Sciences would perceive the app's site-specific nature (allowing for real-world scaling) and the inclusion of both pass-through and 'desktop' close-up scenes. Ethical approval (tier 1) was granted by the Glasgow School of Art.

3.4.1 Participants

The specialist participants were recruited from the School of Cardiovascular and Metabolic Health, the School of Humanities and the Advanced Research Centre at the University of Glasgow. Nine individuals participated in the round 1 study. The participants' ages ranged from 35 to 62 ($M = 47 \pm 11.8$). Among them, 5 identified as female and 4 as male. Seven participants listed their field of expertise in life sciences, two specializing in cardiovascular sciences. The group included three individuals with expertise in computer use, of which one was a researcher in XR, with previous experience in VR development. Four participants had no prior experience with VR equipment or computer games. Three further individuals participated in the round 2 testing. Two were 31 years old, and one was 24. Two identified as female, and one as male. Two participants specialized in cardiovascular sciences, while one had a background in philosophy and XR research.

3.4.2 Procedure

During the exploratory round 1, the testing environment was controlled but informal. The application's origin was set in the Oculus Quest 2 headsets and the workspace was aligned with the room's dimensions. The participants were received in space a maximum of three at a time. Each participant was provided with a headset, escorted to the designated starting position, provided with a verbal overview of the testing process, and encouraged to freely explore the VR environment and its features at their own pace. The multi-user format facilitated participants in discussing and asking questions. Assistance with equipment usage was also provided. This approach aligned with the expected social nature of a pass-through multi-user experience. The round 2 of testing was conducted with minimum interaction for the standardized usability assessment.

3.4.2.1 Data Analysis

The exploratory testing round 1 covered a standardized set of usability questions (System Usability Score, SUS; Brooke 1995) and questions on the user's perception of visual impact and accuracy, aspects of the user interface, movement and scene features, and the application's potential for educational use. Input text boxes for additional comments were also provided.

The 10 SUS questions were rated on a 5-point Likert scale and analysed according to the SUS Scoring Method (Brooke 1995), with the SUS median benchmark value of 68. For the remaining 5-point Likert scale questions about user's perception of visual impact and accuracy, descriptive statistics (Mean values and standard deviations) were computed. Percentages were calculated for the multiple-choice questions. The open-ended commentary served to qualify perceived strengths and areas for improvement and to capture any potential outlier issues.

The second round of testing involved the SUS questionnaire exclusively, without qualifying questions. The round was conducted after implementing improvements to the application instructions and navigation. A SUS questionnaire is used in testing a system's usability in terms of not only user satisfaction but also the effectiveness and efficiency of using it for the desired outcome (Brooke 1995). Therefore, a fresh cohort of testing subjects was recruited for this round to avoid any effect of familiarity that comes with a previous use of the application.

3.4.3 Experimental Outcomes

The exploratory round 1 canvassed the participants for user and content experience of the MyoSITE app. Overall, the specialist participants ($N = 9$) found the visual content to be engaging ($Mean = 4.56 \pm 0.73$), with a high degree of realism ($Mean = 4.22 \pm 0.67$) and logically proportioned scaling ($Mean = 4.33 \pm 0.71$). Other positive aspects mentioned were the soundscape of the application ($N = 5/9$), interactions ($N = 5/9$), observing models at scale ($N = 4/9$), informative content ($N = 2/9$), and a sense of immersion ($N = 2/9$).

The participants generally found navigating the virtual environment intuitive ($M = 4.00 \pm 0.71$). The MR pass-through aspect of the main scene was not found to be distracting from viewing the digital content and, indeed, when preference was expressed, it was deemed more preferential to the full VR-scenes ($N = 3/9$ to $N = 1/9$, respectively, with $N = 5/9$ expressing no preference). One participant noted that seeing others removed anxiety about bumping into them and provided a sense of presence without physical interference. However, there was less confidence in some other UI features, such as the hand menu, the app's navigation, or the use of digital hands ($M = 3.89 \pm 1.05$).

The testing also probed the participants' expert evaluation of the educational potential of the application. They were asked to assign scores for the perceived importance of various features of MyoSITE for educational contexts, ranging from not important at all (1) to very important (5). In order of preference, the scores were:

- Text/information panels (M = 4.56 ± 0.73)
- Handling interaction (M = 4.56 ± 0.73)
- Ability to see and communicate with others during use (M = 4.22 ± 0.44)
- Controllable visual layers in models (M = 4.11 ± 0.78) and
- Ability to block off others and focus on in-app instructions (M = 3.56 ± 0.88)

There was unanimous agreement on the significance of the pass-through features ('seeing and communicating with others') for educational use, with 100% of respondents agreeing or strongly agreeing. Regarding their preference for the kind of information to focus on, none of the participants prioritized information on the models used (such as the type and origin of the data). Five participants (N = 5/9) favoured explanations of the scene content, while four expressed no preference (N = 4/9). Most participants considered the application suitable for public engagement (M = 4.44 ± 0.73), and all deemed it appropriate for higher education classrooms (M = 4.56 ± 0.53).

All experts also completed the SUS questionnaire, in round 1 (N = 9). Round 1 resulted in an overall SUS score of 67.5 (Fig. 3.26).

The result falls slightly below the SUS standard score of 68, which is considered marginally acceptable (Bangor et al. 2008). While a relatively large portion of participants had no prior experience with XR (N = 4/9), potentially contributing to user apprehension, there were evident areas needing improvement, as was also clearly highlighted in responses to user experience questions.

Consequently, a series of improvements were implemented before the second round of testing. The information panels were adjusted to aid in navigation. The capsule colliders on the B-1 receptors, which triggered the scene change, were enlarged for ease of use, and some receptors were lowered for improved access. The receptors were highlighted by blue rings, toggled from the

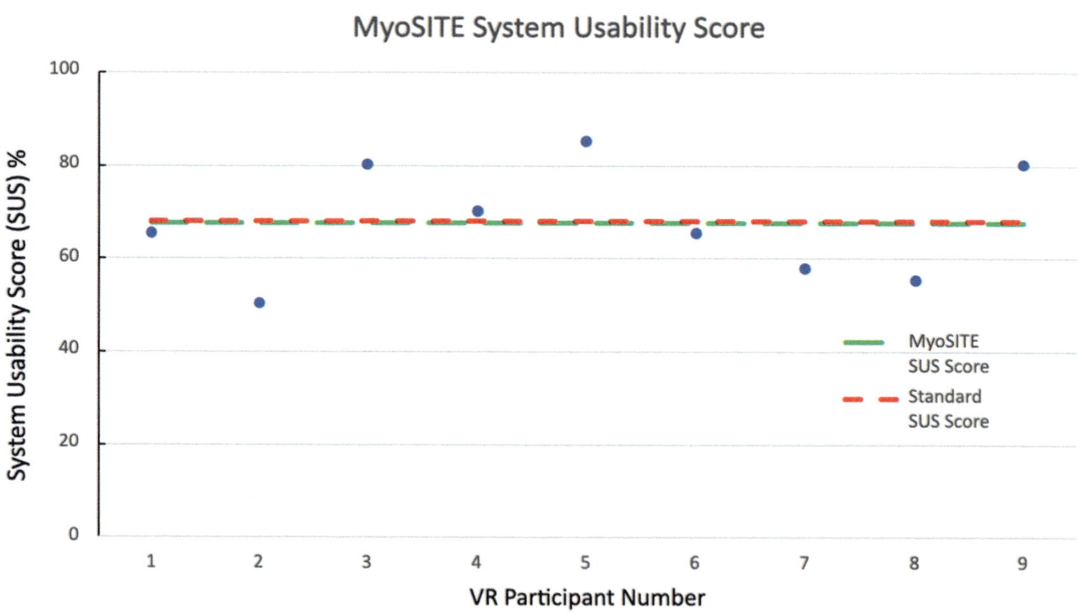

Fig. 3.26 Round 1 testing System Usability Score

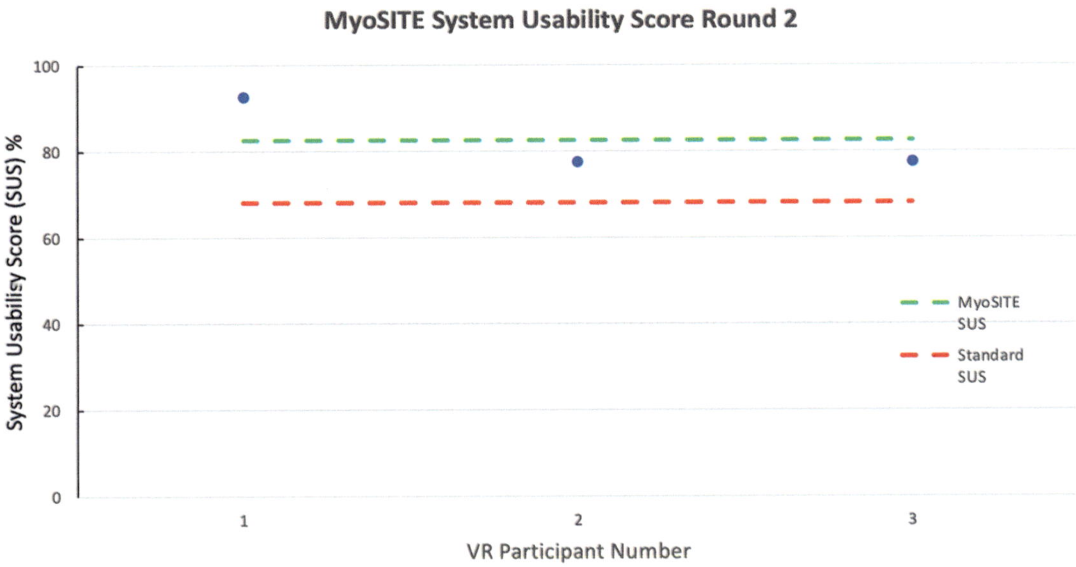

Fig. 3.27 Round 2 testing System Usability Score

palm menu. Adjustments were also made to the hand menu 'Quit' function text to prevent accidental exits.

The round 2 testing (N = 3) involved only SUS questions and yielded a score of 82.5, which is considered an excellent outcome (Bangor et al. 2008; Fig. 3.27).

3.4.4 Discussion

Overall, the test participants awarded the highest scores for engagement with visual content and comfort during pass-through scenes. Conversely, the lowest scores were given for ease of navigation, digital hand usage, and hand menu navigation. In the second round, although 2 out of the 3 participants were using immersive technologies for the first time, the user scores were notably higher at 82.5. The improved score places the application's usability at an excellent level, indicating a successful implementation of the improvements made after the first round. The improved score in round 2 elevates the application usability from a marginal to an acceptable category and moves its associated Net Promoter Score from Detractor to Promoter (Sauro 2018), suggesting that users are more inclined to recommend it. However, further SUS testing with a larger participant pool would be beneficial, given the limited size of the test group.

A distinctive feature of MyoSITE was prioritizing 'real' models derived from X-ray diffraction, electron and confocal microscopy over illustrative ones in an interactive environment. Indeed, two participants commended the visual content and the 'wow-factor' of the experience (N = 2/9), supporting the idea that these structures, familiar from their research, could now be visually explored. The fact that none of the participants favoured information about the source data over more traditional narrative explanations of the scene and interactions suggests that using the application primarily as a 3D viewer with access to data provenance might be less valuable than utilizing it as a credible tool for understanding structure and processes. Immersive VR-based viewers for microscopic data in 3D, such as inViewR (arivis AG 2023) or ConfocalVR (Stefani et al. 2018), are typically configured to visualize a single stack or data set at a time and permit the manipulation of various viewing parameters. However, as research tools, they focus on exploring a single volumetric data stack and are not designed to integrate data from multiple sources or employ additional interactive elements, animations, gamified tasks, or annotations that could be customized to address specific educational needs.

The modular structure, as tested with MyoSITE, incorporating a central pass-through scene and several in-depth pop-up VR scenes, provides considerable flexibility in focusing on different aspects of the cellular mesoscale, including relative scales and processes. It also supports user communication. Emphasizing the importance of scientific collaboration, the ConfocalVR project introduced virtual avatars for user representation. However, the entire interaction occurs exclusively within the VR environment, and while it allows multi-user interaction, it is detached from the physical environment. The introduction of a mixed reality approach, as with MyoSITE, can be used to retain a sense of the conventional classroom setting while interacting with digital content.

Overall, the results of MyoSITE testing were highly encouraging. Participants found the application engaging and invested significant time in exploring its contents, something that could be measured in testing future versions of the app alongside a more detailed user assessment of the time spent and the level of engagement with different scenes and features of the app. The assessment of the content was positive, and the usability scores for the current version were elevated to an excellent level following the improvements. The project's concept, featuring a shared central scene with breakout focused scenes, was well received, and effectively utilized in practice, with multiple users exploring the model through their headsets concurrently. All expert participants deemed the application suitable for both public engagement and higher education classrooms.

A logical progression in testing would involve conducting SUS usability testing with a broader participant pool and implementing further standardized assessments—such as the cross-media presence questionnaire ITC-Sense of Presence Inventory (ITC-SOPI) or Presence Questionnaire (PQ) (Moinnereau et al. 2022)—to delve deeper into the sense of spatial presence and engagement, particularly in relation to the two distinct scene types, employing a varied level of immersion. The related concepts of sense of presence (a psychological and emotional sense of the user being within the virtual environment) and immersion (a sense of being absorbed by the experience) that are characteristic of XR learning situations (Interaction Design Foundation—IxDF 2023) have shown to enhance the learning process through increased engagement, better spatial understanding, and contextualized learning. (Logeswaran et al. 2021; Goodsell et al. 2020; Venkatesan et al. 2021; McGowin et al. 2021; Curran et al. 2023) MyoSITE presents within one application two different levels of immersion, each with their own affordances; pass-through scenes that facilitate interaction and ground the user in the natural physical environment, and full immersion VR scenes that can engender total immersion (Venkatesan et al. 2021) and emphasize individual work and future testing could be done on assessing this aspect of the application.

3.5 Summary, Limitations, Future Directions

The MyoSITE project embarked on the development of a site-specific life science application prototype and assessed its feasibility on three key aspects: modelling an entire cell, investigating affordances and challenges when tied to a specific site, and exploring the educational potential of a mixed reality model using the pass-through feature as a design principle.

In general, the feedback indicated that several design objectives were successfully met. The sense of scale at the cellular mesoscales, a key project goal, was well-received by users, and the preference for pass-through scenes and the recognition of shared space as valuable for educational purposes support the design concept. The MyoSITE application was tailored for the ARC-XR space and included five scenes, one of which featured full pass-through. The site-specific approach allowed for large scale, which minimized the need for zooming, enabling users to successfully explore the whole cell with models of internal structures at a proportional scale. The mixed reality scene introduced the possibility for multi-user interaction within the shared space whilst effectively mitigating some of the HMD-based digital experience drawbacks—a sense of isolation and motion sickness. Indeed, the criticism often raised about VR experiences is that they are isolating experiences (Venkatesan et al. 2021). However, the sociability of the use situation was readily observable as the users addressed each other in the pass-through scene, highlighting the potential for collaborative use of the application. The user interaction permits knowledge dissemination whilst using the app, and so can support collaboration essential in scientific research due to increasingly intricate problems and rapidly expanding, highly specialized knowledge base (Hara et al. 2003). The benefits of collaboration in learning are well established (Panitz and Panitz 1998; Laal and Ghodsi 2012; Glaister et al. 2023). However, collaborative learning in XR is currently not well-researched (van der Meer et al. 2023). Furthermore, an overwhelming portion (90%) of the research has been conducted on non-HMD-based systems, not on headset-based use (van der Meer et al. 2023). Therefore, an exploration into HMD-based collaborative learning using the app could present a fruitful avenue for future study.

The development process of MyoSITE involved acquiring, processing, and modelling cellular structure meshes and integrating them into an interactive application using the Unity game engine. A challenge encountered was the uneven quality of the source meshes, which were not originally designed for this purpose. However, a working process was developed to overcome these challenges and allow for various source materials from both confocal and electron microscopy to be effectively transferred into a digital, mixed-reality, interactive 3D viewing environment.

The application underwent iterative development and testing involving limited cohorts of cardiovascular sciences and XR specialists from the University of Glasgow. The two rounds of evaluation provided encouraging feedback that resulted in immediate improvements to the application. While the expert cohorts due to the time constraints of the project were inevitably small, the following evaluation phase should involve a larger participant pool. Additionally, other forms of standardized testing, including investigations into the sense of presence experienced while using the app, would be beneficial. Nonetheless, it can be said that the MyoSITE app serves as a promising initial step for visualizing such a complex dataset.

During the project, several key limitations came to light. Firstly, while the research questions pertain to XR development broadly, the application itself was developed for a specific technology (Oculus 2), which may introduce constraints in future use when the technology is updated. It also presents other tech-specific challenges, such as the difficulty of capturing pass-through, which is not natively supported and has required third-party software, unavailable for this project. Another technology-related limitation was experienced with the guardrail, the use of which has since been simplified in the consecutive versions of the head-mounted device (HMD) software. This is especially important in the future development of mixed reality applications for use in large spaces, such as MyoSITE. As the tailoring of an application to fit a particular space can be done in two ways (designed into the app as a development concern and also offered to the application user through various UI scaling and rotation options), the ability to access and use guardrail more flexibly could be a useful feature for large installations, particularly in mixed-use spaces. Secondly, as the technology matures, the synchronization of the development platform (in this case, the Unity game engine) with the HMD will similarly present an evolving array of conditions for the development process. In the case of MyoSITE, the spatial configuration of the application and its behaviour within the headset presented an ongoing challenge. However, these concerns are likely mitigated by future improvements to the spatial mapping and camera systems of the HMD. Further application development could include explorations of site-specificity, including the use of real-world objects, and aspects regarding usability, including optimization and menu functionality, to boost the learning experience. Designing interactive MR scenes with varying orientations towards the physical space presents another area that warrants further exploration.

3.6 Conclusion

We have presented a methodological and technological framework tailored for the development of a mixed reality application, MyoSITE, specifically designed for life sciences. There is educational potential of the application as a multiscale cellular model, envisioning it as an interactive, collaborative digital classroom based on the use of individual, unconnected HMDs. Additionally, the processing and presentation of complex molecular data needed to construct a multiscale interactive digital environment were investigated.

Since its inception, the MyoSITE app has been requested and distributed to higher education institutions in Scotland, England, and Ireland. The application was well received by the users and, as a proof-of-concept, holds significant promise. The multi-use aspect and site-specificity proved effective, and further design considerations in this direction could be productive. This might involve exploring varied levels of immersion, tailoring the application for other specific locations with the aim of providing user controls for spatial calibration, and employing the app in different single and multi-use educational situations.

The ability to view a variety of biological structures at the mesoscale was well-received among specialist evaluators. The positive feedback demonstrated that XR engagement can be a valuable tool for life sciences education, and continued research into mixed reality holds exciting potential for the field of life sciences.

References

Acadicus (2021) Heart Anatomy and Flow by Dr. Nick Slamon. In: YouTube. https://www.youtube.com/watch?v=SE9MFFjJW8A&list=PL2ZhoWMzZvMfghXGQcUlcij6ldDo1Rea3&index=30&t=77s. Accessed 2 Jan 2024

arivis AG (2023, April 07) Observing 3D microscopic images using virtual reality. News-Med. Retrieved on 11 Jan 2024 from https://www.news-medical.net/news/20191219/Observing-3D-Microscopic-Images-using-Virtual-Reality.aspx

Bangor A, Kortum P, Miller J (2008) An empirical evaluation of the system usability scale. Int J Hum Comput Interact 24(6):574–594

Barrow J, Sands A, Hurst W (2019) Augmented Reality for Enhancing Life Science Education. Paper presented at VISUAL 2019, the 4th international conference on application and systems of visual paradigms, Rome, Italy, 30 June–4 July 2019

Barteit S, Lanfermann L, Bärnighausen T et al (2021) Augmented, mixed, and virtual reality-based head-mounted devices for medical education: systematic review. JMIR Ser Games 9(3):e29080. https://doi.org/10.2196/29080

Bernholt S, Broman K, Siebert S et al (2019) Digitising teaching and learning–additional perspectives for chemistry education. Israel J Chem 59(6–7):554–564

Brooke J (1995) SUS: a quick and dirty usability scale. Usability Eval Ind 189

Burbaum L, Schneider J, Scholze S et al (2021) Molecular-scale visualization of sarcomere contraction within native cardiomyocytes. Nat Commun 12(1):4086. https://doi.org/10.1038/s41467-021-24049-0

Curran VR, Xu X, Aydin MY et al (2023) Use of extended reality in medical education: an integrative review. Med Sci Edu 33:275–286. https://doi.org/10.1007/s40670-022-01698-4

Daly CJ (2019) From confocal microscope to virtual reality and computer games; technical and educational considerations. Infocus Mag 54:51–59

Fujitsu (2018) Fujitsu launches "Heart Explorer" to study heart behavior. https://www.fujitsu.com/global/about/resources/news/press-releases/2018/0411-01.html. Accessed 27 Dec 2023

Glaister C et al (2023) Informal collaborative learning (ICL)—student perspectives on the role of informal collaborative learning ICL in higher education. Teach High Educ. https://doi.org/10.1080/13562517.2023.2177843

Goodsell DS (2021) Myoglobin in a whale muscle cell. In: RCSB Protein Data Bank. https://doi.org/10.2210/rcsb_pdb/goodsell-gallery-032

Goodsell DS (2022) JCVI-syn3A minimal cell. In: RCSB Protein Data Bank. https://doi.org/10.2210/rcsb_pdb/goodsell-gallery-042

Goodsell DS, Olson AJ, Forli S (2020) Art and science of the cellular mesoscale. Trends Biochem Sci 45(6):472–483. https://doi.org/10.1016/j.tibs.2020.02.010

Hara N et al (2003) An emerging view of scientific collaboration: Scientists' perspectives on collaboration and factors that impact collaboration. J Am Soc Inf Sci Technol 54(10):952–965. https://doi.org/10.1002/asi.10291

HybridMedical (2015) 360° VR animation I inside a beating heart. In: YouTube. https://www.hybridmedicalanimation.com/work/interactive/360-degree-inside-a-beating-heart/. Accessed 16 Apr 2023

Interaction Design Foundation—IxDF (2023, November 16) What is Immersion in Extended Reality (XR)? Interaction Design Foundation—IxDF. https://www.interaction-design.org/literature/topics/immersion

Johnston APR, Rae J, Ariotti N et al (2017) Journey to the centre of the cell: virtual reality immersion into scientific data. Traffic 19:105–110. https://doi.org/10.1111/tra.12538

Kim S, Chen J, Cheng T et al (2023) PubChem 2023 update. Nucleic Acids Res 51(D1):D1373–D1380. https://doi.org/10.1093/nar/gkac956

Kruse A, Ring A, Manglik A et al (2013) Activation and allosteric modulation of a muscarinic acetylcholine receptor. Nature 504:101–106. https://doi.org/10.1038/nature12735

Laal M, Ghodsi S (2012) Benefits of collaborative learning. Procedia Soc Behav Sci 31:486–490. https://doi.org/10.1016/j.sbspro.2011.12.091

Lee Y, Takenaka BP (2022) Extended reality as a means to enhance public health education. Front Publ Health 10:1040018. https://doi.org/10.3389/fpubh.2022.1040018

Levick JR (2008) Introduction to cardiovascular physiology. Butterworth Heinemann, Oxford

Levy D (2013) How dynamic visualization technology can support molecular reasoning. J Sci Educ Technol 22(5):702–717

Liu Q, Ma J, Yu S, Wang Q, Xu S (2022) Effects of an augmented reality-based chemistry experiential application on student knowledge gains, learning motivation, and technology perception. J Sci Educ Technol 33:153–167. https://doi.org/10.1007/s10956-022-10014-z

Logeswaran A, Munsch C, Chong YJ et al (2021) The role of extended reality technology in healthcare education: towards a learner-centred approach. Future Healthc J 8(1):e79–e84. https://doi.org/10.7861/fhj.2020-0112

LudicWorlds (2022) Virtual blood flow, real heart beat. In: YouTube. https://www.youtube.com/watch?v=Ome2lz_sNN4. Accessed 9 Apr 2023

Maritan M, Autin L, Karr J et al (2022) Building structural models of a whole mycoplasma cell. J Mol Biol 434(2):167351. https://doi.org/10.1016/j.jmb.2021.167351

McDonnell N (2019) Immersive technology and medical visualisation: a user's guide. In: Rea P (ed) Biomedical visualisation. Series: advances in experimental medicine and biology, vol 1156. Springer, Heidelberg, pp 123–134. https://doi.org/10.1007/978-3-030-19385-0_

McGowin G et al (2021) A meta-review of learning research in immersive virtual reality. Proc Hum Factors Ergon Soc Annu Meet 65(1):894–898. https://doi.org/10.1177/1071181321651326

MedicalholodeckAcademy (2023) The human body in virtual reality: path of blood through the heart. In: YouTube. https://www.youtube.com/watch?v=2TU5E-tzg0U&list=PLLleQABuPzNyDrapiJnOWxtSMsCCpQpo-&index=13. Accessed 2 Jan 2024

Midjourney (2023) Midjourney response to Mirja Koponen, 23 May

Moinnereau MA et al (2022) Immersive media experience: a survey of existing methods and tools for human influential factors assessment. Qual User Exp 7:5. https://doi.org/10.1007/s41233-022-00052-1

Panitz T, Panitz P (1998) Encouraging the use of collaborative learning in higher education. Univ Teaching Int Perspect:161–201. https://doi.org/10.4324/9780429459092-7

Safadel P, White D (2019) Facilitating molecular biology teaching by using augmented reality (AR) and Protein Data Bank (PDB). TechTrends 63(2):188–193. https://doi.org/10.1007/s11528-018-0343-0

Sauro J (2018) 5 ways to interpret a SUS score. Available via MeasuringU. https://measuringu.com/interpret-sus-score/. Accessed 20 June 2023

Shen X, Hou Y, Colli D et al (2019) 3D dSTORM imaging reveals novel detail of ryanodine receptor localization in rat cardiac myocytes. J Physiol 597(2):399–418. https://doi.org/10.1113/JP277360

Stefani C, Lacy-Hulbert A, Skillman T (2018) ConfocalVR: immersive visualization for confocal microscopy. J Mol Biol 430(21):4028–4035. https://doi.org/10.1016/j.jmb.2018.06.035

Sutherland J, Belec J, Sheikh A et al (2019) Applying modern virtual and augmented reality technologies to medical images and models. J Digit Imaging 32(1):38–53. https://doi.org/10.1007/s10278-018-0122-7

Van der Meer N et al (2023) Front virtual real sec virtual reality and human behaviour, p 4. https://doi.org/10.3389/frvir.2023.1159905

Venkatesan M et al (2021) Virtual and augmented reality for biomedical applications. Cell Rep Med 2(7):100348. https://doi.org/10.1016/j.xcrm.2021.100348

Wu SH, Lai CL, Hwang GJ et al (2021) Research trends in technology-enhanced chemistry learning: a review of comparative research from 2010 to 2019. J Sci Educ Technol 30:496–510. https://doi.org/10.1007/s10956-020-09894-w

Creating an Intuitive Model for Translation of Preoperative Imaging to Intraoperative Visualisation in Paediatric Surgery: Leveraging Augmented Reality for Accurate Depth Perception and Inner Anatomy on Tablet AR Platform

4

Nicole Gourlay, Giuliana Torpiano,
Michael Jacovides, and Matthieu Poyade

Abstract

In the realm of surgical procedures, the integration of augmented reality (AR) stands as a promising avenue for elevating precision and refining outcomes. By superimposing digital data onto real-time surgical views, AR has the potential to offer comprehensive, three-dimensional visualisation that enhances the identification of crucial anatomical structures and optimises the surgical planning process.

This research acknowledges the challenges linked with AR implementation, particularly concerning head-mounted displays (HMDs) and the intricate matter of depth perception. While previous studies have signalled potential distractions and ergonomic issues with HMDs, the complex nature of depth perception remains a crucial factor for accurate surgical procedures that demand careful consideration and mitigation.

To illustrate the practical potential of AR in surgery, the study focuses on the development and testing of an innovative AR model utilising a tablet device, specifically tailored for paediatric surgical settings. Through System Usability Scores (SUS) and user satisfaction assessments, the model was demonstrated to be user-friendly and efficient, meeting the desired standards of usability.

Participant feedback uncovered valuable insights, revealing the application's strength in

N. Gourlay (✉)
School of Medicine, Dentistry and Nursing, College of Medical, Dentistry and Nursing, University of Glasgow, Glasgow, UK

School of Innovation and Technology, The Glasgow School of Art, The Hub, Pacific Quay, Glasgow, UK

G. Torpiano
Surgical Registrar at the Royal Hospital for Children, Glasgow, UK

Honorary Clinical Lecturer, University of Glasgow, Glasgow, UK
e-mail: Giuliana.Torpiano@ggc.scot.nhs.uk

M. Jacovides
Honorary Clinical Lecturer, University of Glasgow, Glasgow, UK

Consultant Paediatric and Neonatal Surgeon, Royal Hospital for Children, Glasgow, UK
e-mail: Michael.Jacovides@ggc.scot.nhs.uk

M. Poyade
School of Innovation and Technology, The Glasgow School of Art, The Hub, Pacific Quay, Glasgow, UK
e-mail: M.Poyade@gsa.ac.uk

J. Clancy, M. Poyade (eds.), *Medical Visualization and Applications of Technology – Volume 2*, Biomedical Visualization 5, https://doi.org/10.1007/978-3-031-63463-5_4

simplifying complex medical concepts for patients and their families, exceeding its perceived utility for the surgical team. This illuminates possibilities for improved doctor-patient communication, addressing gaps in medical interactions.

Acknowledging the need for refinements, particularly in enhancing the application's usability intraoperatively, the study emphasises the significance of smaller, less intrusive markers and additional anatomical information for seamless integration. Addressing these technical challenges is imperative to unlock the full potential of AR in surgical contexts.

This research serves as a testament to the potential of AR in enhancing surgical procedures, paving the way for the utilisation of tablet-based AR to bridge the gap between pre-operative imaging and intra-operative findings. With further developments, this innovative approach holds promise to redefine surgical practices, heighten patient care, and advance medical outcomes across diverse healthcare applications.

Keywords

Augmented reality (AR) · Three-dimensional visualisation · Depth perception · Doctor-patient communication · Paediatric surgery Tablet-based AR

4.1 Introduction

Recent advancements in medical imaging and device technologies have led to the widespread adoption of image-guided therapy in the medical field (Zhao et al. 2021). These innovations, combined with minimally invasive surgical techniques, promise enhanced precision and improved postoperative outcomes (Marescaux and Diana 2015; Prevost et al. 2019).

In conventional image-guided procedures, surgeons must mentally bridge the gap between preoperative imaging data (e.g. CT, ultrasound, and MRI) and the physical surgical site. While valuable for planning and guiding surgeons, these procedures can be challenging, particularly in paediatric surgery due to the intricate nature of paediatric anatomy (Ieiri et al. 2011; Souzaki et al. 2013). This prompts a call for exploration into navigation-assisted techniques to reduce damage to delicate structures and enhance patient outcomes.

Augmented reality (AR) technology is gaining momentum in healthcare. AR offers real-time guidance and navigation tools for surgeons (Deng et al. 2013; Pérez-Pachón et al. 2020; Zhao et al. 2021; Barcali et al. 2022). This chapter delves into the potential of a user-friendly AR application on a tablet for paediatric surgery to aid in the navigation of complex anatomical structures and improve surgical outcomes.

4.1.1 Image-Guided Surgery

Navigated surgery is a cutting-edge medical technique that combines real-time imaging technology with precise surgical procedures and has revolutionised various medical disciplines, including neurosurgery, orthopaedics, and minimally invasive surgeries (MIS) (Miner 2017; Léger et al. 2020; Lex et al. 2022). Integrating advanced imaging modalities such as MRI, CT, or ultrasound with sophisticated computing systems enables surgeons to accurately locate and target specific areas with precision, assisting in complex procedures.

Image-guided navigation system (IGNS) utilises preoperative images by tracking surgical tools and presenting their positional relationship with the patient through virtual tools displayed on the images, often on a monitor or screen (Deng et al. 2013). However, this requires a frequent shift in focus between the surgical field and the computer screen to observe the real-time alignment between surgical instruments and the patient's anatomy. This may divert the surgical focus from the physical aspects of the operation and "may also cause a certain degree of guidance error" (Deng et al. 2013).

Whilst these systems offer numerous benefits, they can occasionally become distracting or cumbersome during surgical procedures due to the abundant equipment that these computing systems require (Deng et al. 2013; Brecevich et al. 2019). This technology often requires the integration of various monitors, tracking devices, power cables, and navigation tools, which can occupy valuable space and potentially disrupt the surgical workflow.

Whilst these systems provide invaluable assistance, they also require careful management and maintenance to minimise potential distractions or challenges they may introduce.

4.1.2 Augmented Reality for IGNS

AR refers to a digital innovation that overlays virtual data, objects, or visuals onto the actual physical environment, enriching the user's experience and interaction with the world around them (Carmigniani and Furht 2011). Typically using a display device, AR allows the user to see both the physical world and virtual objects simultaneously, creating an interactive and immersive blended experience. Specialised AR head-mounted display (HMD), specifically designed to deliver interactive AR experiences, such as Microsoft HoloLens™ or Magic Leap™, often feature advanced sensors, cameras, and see-through displays which allow overlaying digital content seamlessly onto the user's point of view. Other HMDs, like Oculus Quest 1&2™ which were primarily designed for virtual reality (VR), also offer options to incorporate AR functionalities in a more limited fashion. These devices typically encompass the user's entire field of view, providing a completely immersive AR experience.

Alternatively, portable devices such as smartphones and tablets with built-in cameras are also being used as accessible platforms for AR applications (Borovanska et al. 2020; Carswell et al. 2022). The choice of device depends on the specific application, user requirements, and desired level of immersion and interaction with the augmented environment.

4.1.3 HMD AR Devices for Healthcare

Since the 1990s, HMD AR devices have emerged as a prominent tool being explored for surgical guidance (Mondal et al. 2020). Through seamlessly blending virtual elements with the real world, HMD AR devices offer real-time guidance and access to patient data in a hands-free manner by registering patient-specific data with the patient's body (Pérez-Pachón et al. 2021). HMDs can commonly be categorised as either optical see-through (OST) (e.g. Microsoft HoloLens™) or video see-through (Apple Vision Pro™). OST HMDs utilise partially transparent and reflective optical combiners to merge virtual images with the actual environment. In contrast, video see-through HMDs employ a camera attached to the HMD to capture real-time footage of the real world, which is then combined with virtual images using a scene generator (Wen et al. 2017).

Despite the growing interest in HMD devices, ongoing limitations such as limited field of view (FOV), latency, depth perception and spatial awareness, fatigue, and infection control. HMDs for IGNS are still being widely researched and adapted before approval of use in a clinical setting (Princle et al. 2018). The financial expense also poses another constraint in its adoption. Technological advancements are aimed at addressing these challenges and improving the utility and effectiveness of HMDs for AR in IGNS (Meulstee et al. 2018).

In efforts to address these challenges, Behrus Puladi et al. (2022) developed an open-source system for optical HMD devices for AR-based surgery on human cadavers. Developed through the popular game engine Unity™, the implementation of this system requires a HoloLens or other compatible HMD device. The development of IGNS systems through game engines is becoming increasingly popular due to graphical performance and rapid prototyping; however, there is still a lack of studies using these tools (Pérez-Pachón et al. 2020).

Though Behrus Puladi et al. (2022) demonstrated a promising application, the presented system was found to have some drawbacks when presented to investigators. An ill-fitting HoloLens resulted in a misalignment of virtual and real objects, causing errors in their superimposition. Furthermore, it was noted that the tracking mount used may cause obstruction concerns and could lead to tracking errors where space is limited.

Widespread adoption is still a distant goal due to existing technological limitations and human-factor challenges, such as fatigue from lack of natural eye accommodation and retinal blur effects, that hinder their practical usage and application (Mamone et al. 2020; Cutolo 2019).

4.1.4 Projected AR for Surgery

Projected AR for surgery offers a novel approach by directly projecting virtual information onto the surgical field, avoiding the need for traditional displays or HMDs. While it has advantages over HMDs in terms of comfort and spatial awareness, it is important to note that it can be affected by lighting conditions and requires advanced calibration (Mamone et al. 2020; Wen Rong et al. 2017).

4.1.5 AR Tablet Device for Surgery

AR tablet devices provide a portable and user-friendly platform for AR integration in the operating room. Rapid advancements in tablet device technology allow for the combination of AR with a handheld device, providing surgeons the tool to superimpose patient-specific virtual models generated from medical imaging onto the surface of the patient's body in a predetermined location. Wen Rong et al. (2017) present an IGNS system using tablet-based AR which consists of a tablet computer, a Microsoft Kinect v2 sensor, and a desktop workstation.

Wen Rong et al. (2017) state that prior to surgery, surgeons utilise pre-operative medical imaging to acquire anatomical information for analysis and surgical planning. During the planning phase, surgeons delineate target areas of operation, determine access points for surgical instruments, and establish trajectories. Critical structures and organs are then marked on 2D images and then segmented and exported into 3D models. The 3D models are transferred to the tablet through either a cable or a Wi-Fi. To match these models with the surgical field, the tablet's built-in camera and the Kinect device are used, employing vision-based tracking and point-model registration. The depth data captured by the Kinect Cameras is registered within the virtual world's coordinate system and then displayed on the tablet screen. During the guidance procedure, the surgeon retains the flexibility to choose the desired overlay for intraoperative surgical guidance, seamlessly switching between 2D medical images, 3D models, or a combined display of both (Wen et al. 2017). Through extensive experimentation, both in and out of the surgical environment, it was determined that the system effectively aided surgeons in visually identifying concealed anatomical landmarks and provided guidance for accurate needle insertion (Wen et al. 2017). The overall set-up time to use the technology was approximately 18 min and it was found that the system ran smoothly through testing; however, there was concern that a slowdown in computational speed when incorporating more complex vessels may affect the overall AR experience.

Whilst this technology potentially reduces the need for constant reference to external monitors or separate imaging systems, this technology could potentially increase operative time by hindering surgeons with extended set-up times and intraoperative latency delays.

Weiwei Deng et al. (2013) propose an easy-to-use Tablet-AR system which only requires a tablet PC and a wireless router to avoid previously stated complications with HMDs, cable management, and poor image quality. The purpose of this "Tablet-AR system" is to integrate pre-operative imaging information into the live surgical environment by displaying overlaid images on the tablet screen. Prior to surgery, the Tablet-AR system generates a 3D model of, in their case, an entire head or a segmented brain tumour, establishing an image coordinate system (ICS) based on the patient's pre-operative imaging data.

During surgery, the system continuously tracks the tablet's position relative to the patient's head in real time. It then projects the 3D model onto the tablet's screen coordinate system (SCS), transmitting the positional data to the tablet. The projected object position data is overlaid on the tablet's screen, which concurrently displays the real-time surgical scene captured by its back-facing camera (Deng et al. 2013).

It was found during feasibility testing that no additional navigation approach, including traditional surgical navigation, was needed before and during the surgical procedure. The device presented accurate and direct navigational information with an average alignment error of less than 6 pixels and was determined as a feasible output for AR in IGNS (Deng et al. 2013). Whilst this study provides sufficient evidence in favour of tablet-based AR for IGNS, it was concluded that further optimisation for proper clinical use must be explored—a main point of focus being depth perception.

4.1.6 Depth Perception in AR for IGNS

Depth perception is a crucial and often overlooked aspect of developing AR for surgery (Choi et al. 2015). Monocular and binocular cues enable depth perception, with HMDs offering binocular cues, and phones/tablets relying on monocular depth cues (El Jamiy and Marsh 2019). Accurate depth perception allows surgeons to accurately gauge distances and spatial relationships between the virtual objects and the real surgical field. Sielhorst et al. (2006) suggest that though data is often presented in the correct place, the actual spatial position of the visualisation is often perceived as being closer or further due to the discrepancy in the real/virtual overlay. Accurate depth perception is essential for manipulation tasks such as needle insertion and tissue handling and for navigating through anatomical structures. In contrast, inaccurate depth perception can affect spatial awareness which may overall lead to confusion and potential complications during the procedure (Kruijff et al. 2010).

In an evaluation study by 20 surgeons, it was found that frame rate proves an important factor in the overall performance (Sielhorst et al. 2006). Participants were asked to locate 20 spots per visualisation inside a body phantom using a pointer: whilst wearing an AR HMD. It was found that the volume-rendering visualisation, as opposed to the Surface Rendering, Glass Effect, and Virtual Window techniques, was preferred by surgeons in terms of depth perception; however, this resulted in frame rate and latency performance issues.

Whilst there is ongoing research dedicated to addressing depth perception in AR for surgery, the limited evidence and significant gap suggest that there are grounds for further exploration that must be understood before AR can be implemented and trusted in the operating room. Significant challenges persist in developing robust depth perception algorithms, calibrating AR systems to real-world surgical environments, and ensuring seamless integration with surgical workflows. Factors such as lighting conditions and anatomical complexity also pose additional obstacles to developing a successful AR application for surgery (Mamone et al. 2020; Wen Rong et al. 2017).

4.1.7 An Interactive Android-Based AR Application for Paediatric Surgery

Augmented reality presents a solution by seamlessly merging virtual elements with the real environment, offering live guidance and instant access to patient data. While head-mounted displays (HMDs) have limitations like spatial awareness issues and restricted field of view (Cutolo 2019; Mamone et al. 2020), tablet devices provide a practical, portable, and user-friendly platform for integrating AR in the operating room (Deng et al. 2013). Studies have demonstrated the effectiveness of tablet-based AR systems in aiding surgeons in identifying hidden structures and guiding precise needle insertion (Deng et al. 2013; Wen et al. 2017).

Our research seeks to develop and test a tailored AR tablet application for paediatric surgery. This research aims to explore how AR on a tablet device can identify concealed or obstructed structures during surgery, potentially minimising inadvertent damage to surrounding tissues. Additionally, we aim to evaluate the effectiveness of this application as an educational tool for both experienced surgeons and trainees.

This research aimed to assess the feasibility of a new Android-based AR application, "VitaSight AR Surgical," tailored for paediatric surgery. The goal was to enhance surgical outcomes by translating preoperative images into intraoperative findings. This was developed as a collaboration between the Royal Hospital for Children Glasgow, The Glasgow School of Art, and The University of Glasgow.

4.2 Materials and Methods

4.2.1 Materials

A variety of software (Table 4.1), data (Table 4.2), and hardware (Table 4.3) were used when designing and developing VitaSight AR Surgical.

Table 4.1 Software

Software	Use	Developer
Unity	Application development engine	Unity Technologies (Unity Real-Time Development Platform I 3D, 2D, VR and AR Engine)
Slicer 5.2.2	Visualisation, processing, segmentation and analysis of medical images Output of anatomical 3D models	3D Slicer (3D Slicer image computing platform I 3D Slicer)
3ds Max 2023	3D computer graphics program for 3D modelling Used for retopologising 3D models	Autodesk, Inc. (Autodesk I 3D Design, Engineering and Entertainment Software)
Adobe Substance 3D Painter	3D painting software Used to add texture and materials directly to 3D meshes in real-time	Adobe (Adobe Creative Cloud I Details and products I Adobe)
Adobe After Effects 2023	Compositing application for post-production video editing	Adobe (Adobe Creative Cloud I Details and products I Adobe)
Adobe Acrobat	View, create, and manipulate digital forms for participant testing	Adobe (Adobe Creative Cloud I Details and products I Adobe)
Procreate 5.3.4	Raster graphics editor application	Procreate (Procreate®—Sketch, Paint, Create.)
Visual Studio 2019	Source-code editor	Microsoft (Microsoft—Cloud, Computers, Apps and Gaming)
Microsoft Excel	Spreadsheet editor with data visualisation and analysis tools	Microsoft (Microsoft—Cloud, Computers, Apps and Gaming)
Color Oracle	Colour blindness simulator	Bernie Jenny, Nathaniel Vaughn Kelso (Color Oracle I Color Oracle)
Miro	Mind map notation	Miro (Miro I Online Whiteboard for Visual Collaboration)

Table 4.2 Data

Data	Use	Source
CTA Cardio	Segmentation of anatomical models	Slicer (3D Slicer image computing platform I 3D Slicer)
CTA abdomen (Panoramix)	Segmentation of anatomical models	Slicer (3D Slicer image computing platform I 3D Slicer)
TotalSegmetator plug-in	Segmentation of skin, lungs, oesophagus, heart, left and right erector spinae muscles, and iliopsoas muscles	Wasserthal et al. (2023)

Table 4.3 Hardware

Hardware	Company	Use
Samsung Galaxy Tab S5e	Samsung Electronics (https://www.samsung.com/)	Device used for application build and run throughout entirety of project
Acer Predator Triton 500 SE 16″ 16:10 display	Acer (Acer Store UK I Laptops, Desktops, Chromebooks, Monitors and more! I Acer UK Official Online Shop)	Device used to design and develop the application and supporting models

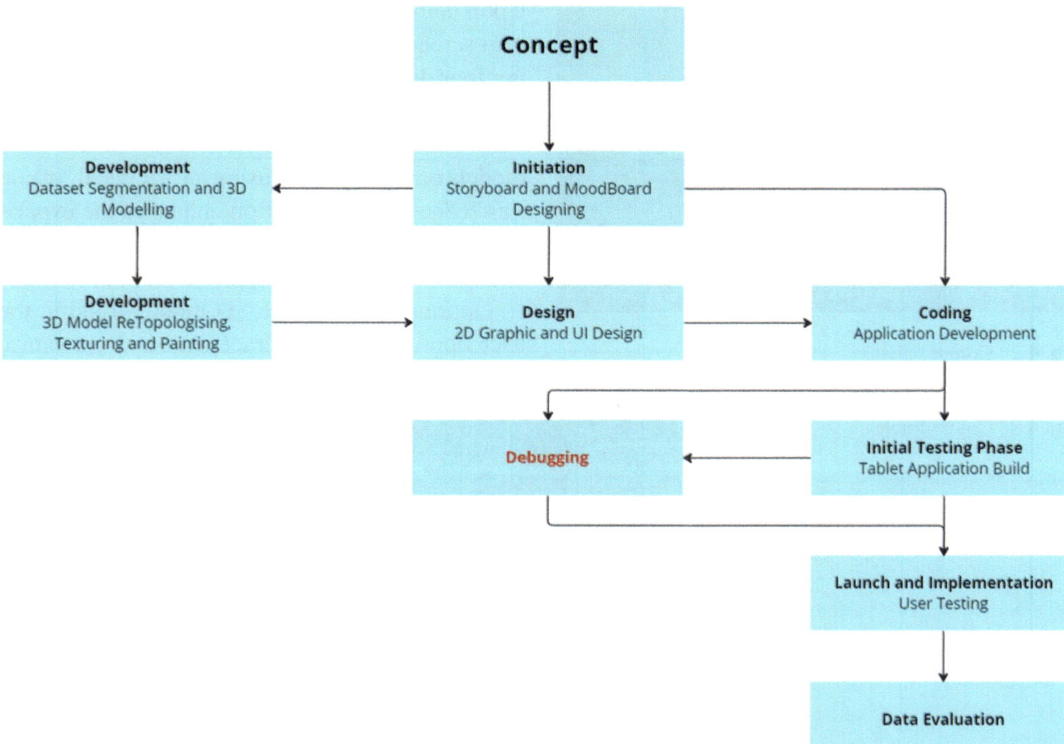

Fig. 4.1 Workflow chart

4.2.2 Concept and Workflow

The purpose of this project is to evaluate the usability and feasibility of a user-friendly model for amalgamating pre-operative images into intra-operative findings using augmented reality on a commercially available Android tablet in paediatric surgery, with the goal of improving surgical outcomes and reducing damage to surrounding structures.

Figure 4.1 shows a basic overview of the developmental workflow. The application name "VitaSight AR Surgical" was chosen to reflect the core purpose of the application.

A colour palette (Fig. 4.2) was carefully selected after testing with the Deuteranopia (Common) colour blindness setting on Color Oracle (Fig. 4.3). Navy blue and white create a stark contrast, making text and graphics easily discernible for users with various types of colour vision deficiencies. By incorporating salmon pink as an accent colour, it was ensured that important details are distinguishable without solely relying on colour differentiation.

In the early stages of the project, storyboards illustrated the entire application functionality within a single screen (Fig. 4.4), incorporating features like a medical dataset overlay option as

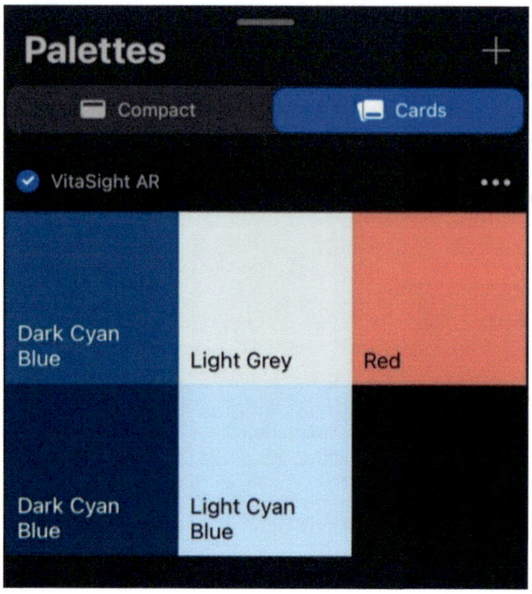

Fig. 4.2 Colour palette

well as the AR 3D Medical Visualisation. As the project evolved, these storyboarded compositions underwent refinements through an iterative process to ensure that the final application design had a better user experience.

A proposed storyboard was proposed (Fig. 4.5) keeping in mind the need to provide users with a seamless immersive experience. Upon launching the app, users are greeted with a start screen which leads to a swipe menu presenting four distinct scene options.

Option 1 offers the AR functionality which allows the user to superimpose 3D anatomical models onto the patient using an AR decal. Inside this scene, a "more" button enhances the experience further, triggering a pop-up panel that offers a range of customisation options for the AR view.

Option 2 leads to the 3D mode, granting the user opportunity to interact with and customise

Fig. 4.3 Color Oracle

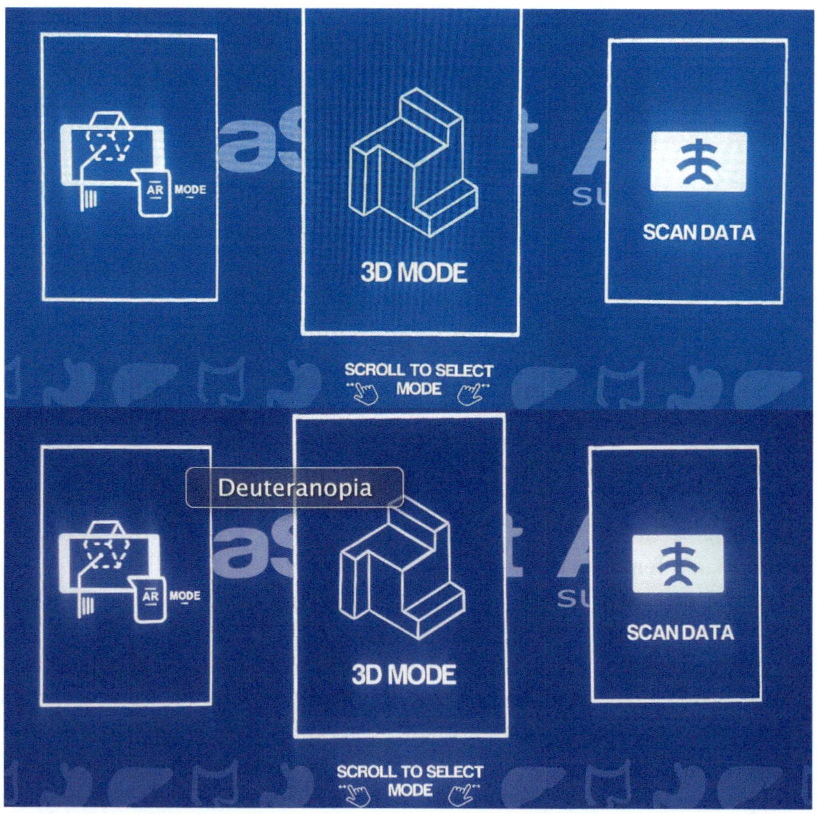

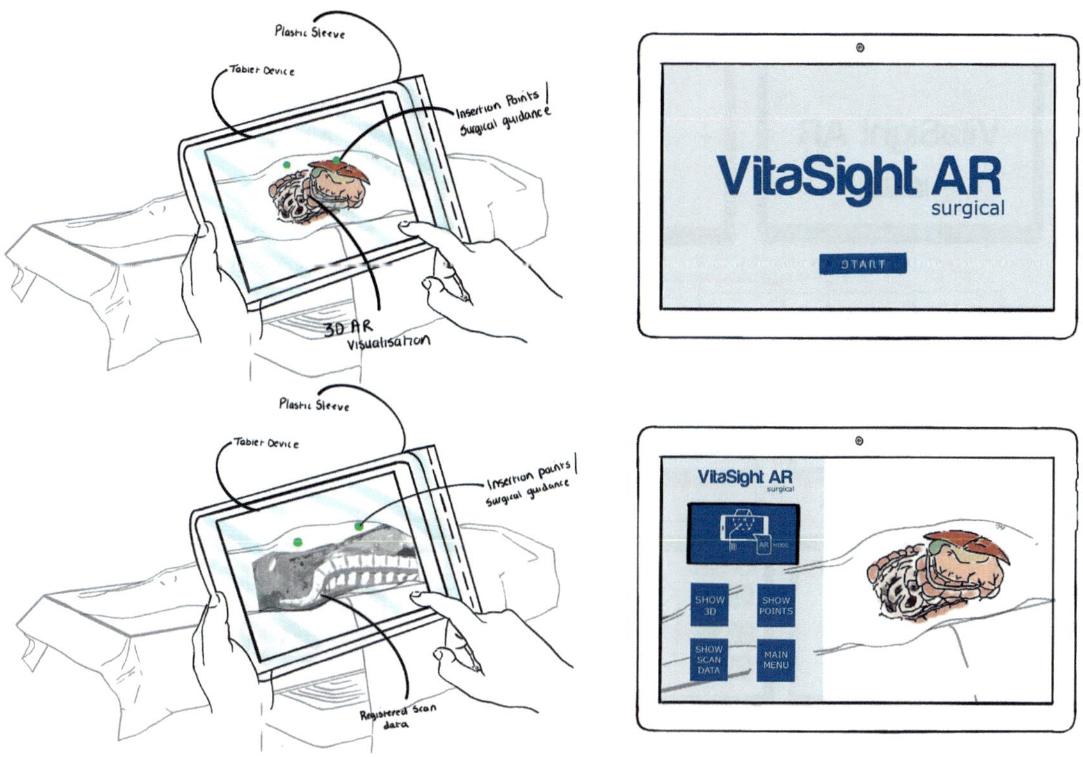

Fig. 4.4 Initial storyboard sketches with the proposal of having all functionality limited to one scene

anatomical models segmented directly from open-source CT scan data.

Option 3 unveils a scan mode, where the user can scroll through the patient-specific medical dataset and take notes for analysis and education. Option 4 directs users to an informative screen, providing them with details about the application's purpose and development.

To ensure effortless navigation, each scene includes an exit button, allowing users to quit the app conveniently. Additionally, a home button is provided, allowing the user to return to the swipe menu for seamless exploration.

4.2.3 3D Modelling

4.2.3.1 3D Content Generation

The 3D models used throughout the application were generated and textured using a combination of Slicer 5.2.2 (Open-Source Medical Dataset), Autodesk 3ds Max, and Adobe Substance Painter (Fig. 4.6).

The process of generating 3D anatomical models for the application involved a meticulous approach. Datasets were carefully selected from the Slicer 5.2.2 repository, followed by a detailed segmentation process. Challenges arose during the segmentation phase, notably when accurately delineating the liver due to its complex shape and surrounding structures. After initial attempts using the AI-driven auto segmentation tool, Segment CT Liver Plug-In, which also failed to accurately extract the liver; a shift to a different dataset, specifically the CTA Cardio (Open-Source) Medical dataset, was made. This transition resulted in significantly improved accuracy and better representation of anatomical structures relevant to the paediatric surgical context.

The segmentation process went beyond simple extraction, involving the careful alignment of organs, refinement, and the integration of

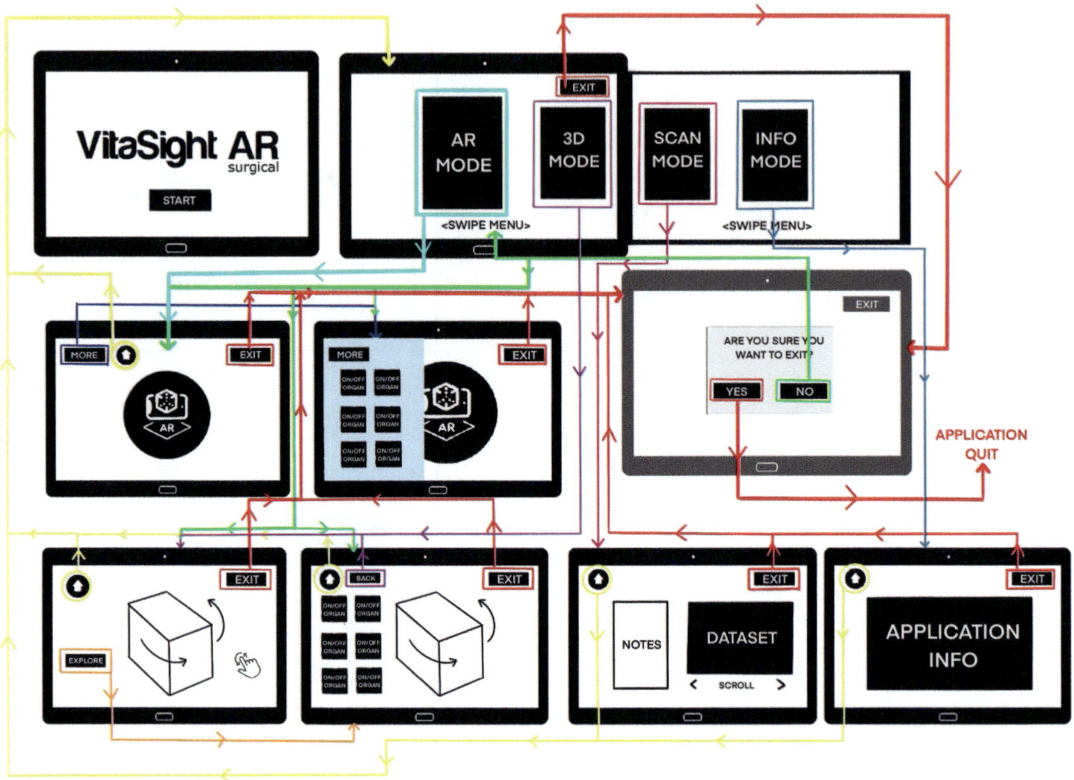

Fig. 4.5 Initial interactive application storyboard with the proposed application flow

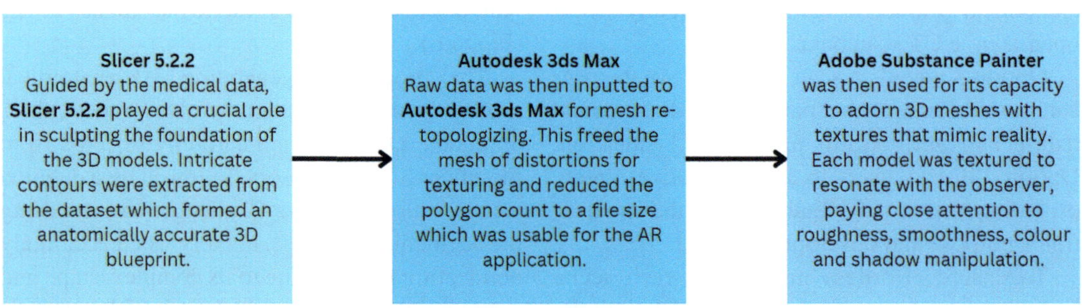

Fig. 4.6 3D content generation workflow

skin boundaries to create a truly immersive augmented reality (AR) experience. Each stage of segmentation was meticulously designed not only to achieve anatomical accuracy but also to enhance visual realism within the AR environment (Fig. 4.7).

A subsequent step involved the application of a median smoothing technique inside the segment editor. This process introduced a familiar boundary smoothing effect ranging between 2 mm and 6 mm (Table 4.4). This mitigated any residual roughness or imperfections whilst maintaining the integrity of the anatomical features (Fig. 4.8).

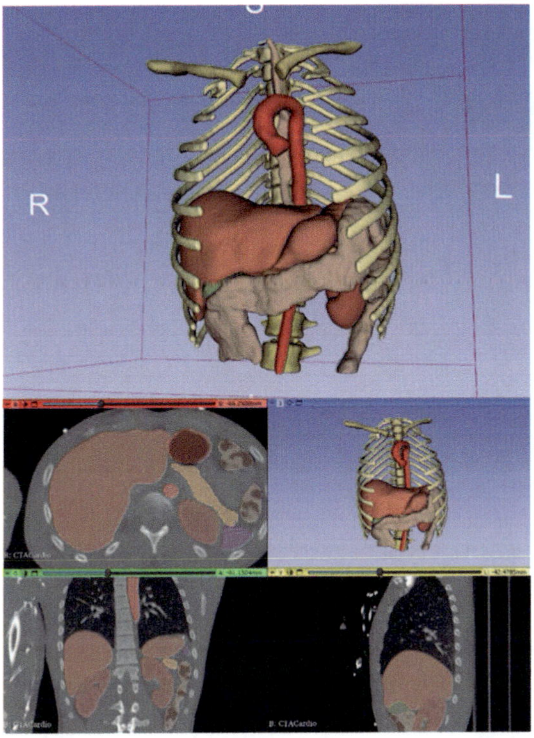

Fig. 4.7 Models from CTA Cardio dataset segmentation

Model meshes were imported and inspected inside 3ds Max, and any remaining disconnected polygons were manually deleted. To optimise models for real-time rendering, it was necessary to reduce the high polygon count and simplify the mesh topology through the 3ds Max auto-retopology tool (Table 4.5).

Further smoothing of the models tended to take place during the retopologising process in 3ds Max as a result of simplifying the mesh. Importantly, it was ensured that this step did not compromise the underlying anatomical accuracy that had been refined inside Slicer. By importing each model into 3ds Max individually, tailored retopology techniques were applied to preserve their unique shapes and sizes, preventing any loss of detail (Fig. 4.9). Vertebrae, for instance, conform naturally to the contours of the spine and therefore are shaped accordingly (Mahadevan 2018). This approach was chosen in the anticipation of the integration within the Unity game engine, as it would align with the user preferences to toggle individual models on or off within a scene.

Table 4.4 Anatomical model segmentation settings

Anatomical structure	Intensity range (threshold)	Smoothing
Liver	45–100	Settings: Median Region of calculation: 6.00 mm
Gallbladder	12–38	Settings: Median Region of calculation: 2.00 mm
Pancreas	80–120	Settings: Median Region of calculation: 3.00 mm
Stomach	(−990)–(−900)	Settings: Median Region of calculation: 4.00 mm
Colon	(−970)–45	Settings: Median Region of calculation: 6.00 mm
Spleen	65–145	Settings: Median Region of calculation: 3.00 mm
Kidneys	70–260	Settings: Median Region of calculation: 4.00 mm
Aorta	315–445	Settings: Median Region of calculation: 3.00 mm
Skeletal	162–3531	Settings: Median Region of calculation: 5.00 mm

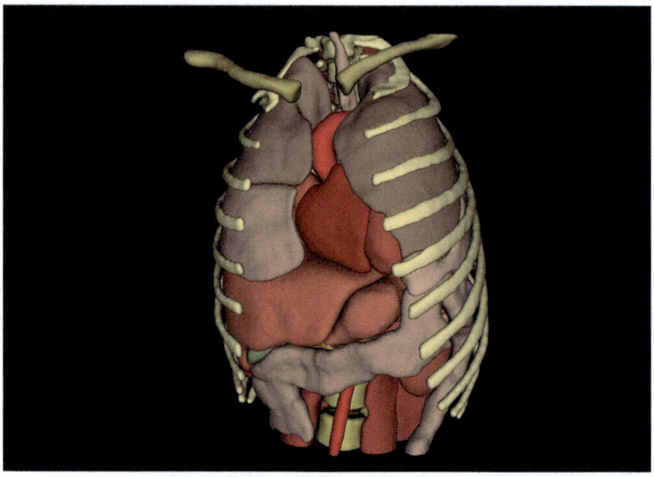

Fig. 4.8 Segmented model

Table 4.5 Polygon count of each structure before and after retopology

Structure	Before retop (polys)	After retop (polys)
Aorta	65,792	2944
Colon	150,592	4853
Oesophagus	23,284	3923
Gallbladder	13,956	958
Heart (atriums and ventricles combined)	170,461	14,228
Kidneys (combined)	105,444	9735
Liver	188,208	1828
Lungs (lobes combined)	599,020	18,715
Pancreas	32,376	4872
Spleen	28,884	1905
Stomach	75,840	5129
Pulmonary artery	27,408	4837
Muscles (combined)	363,492	14,034
Bones (combined)		39,461

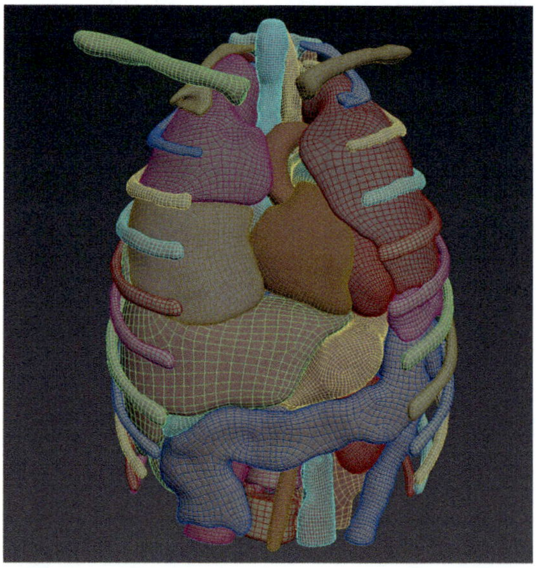

Fig. 4.9 Retopologised model containing 127,422 polygons

4.2.3.2 Model Texturing

Following the completion of the retoplogising process, the models were transitioned into Adobe Substance Painter (Fig. 4.10). Here, the embedded auto-unwrapping functionality within Substance Painter was utilised to efficiently unwrap the models. This process ensured optimal utilisation of the models' surface area for accurate texture mapping. Textures were applied to each model, and a new mesh with a corresponding texture map was exported to be readily available for integration into Unity.

The model mesh exported from Substance Painter was initially re-imported to 3ds Max to overview the poly count and ensure the retopology carried across. It was found that this was successful and aided as an efficient way to swiftly UV unwrap models whilst under time-restricted conditions.

Once the models were imported into Unity, a reconstruction process meant intuitively dragging and associating appropriate textures with their respective material maps, ensuring the

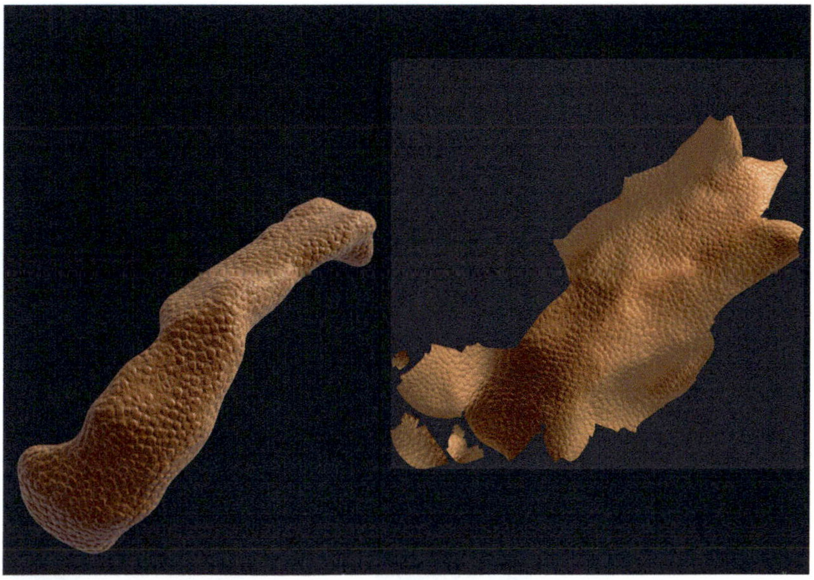

Fig. 4.10 Pancreas textured mesh and texture map containing

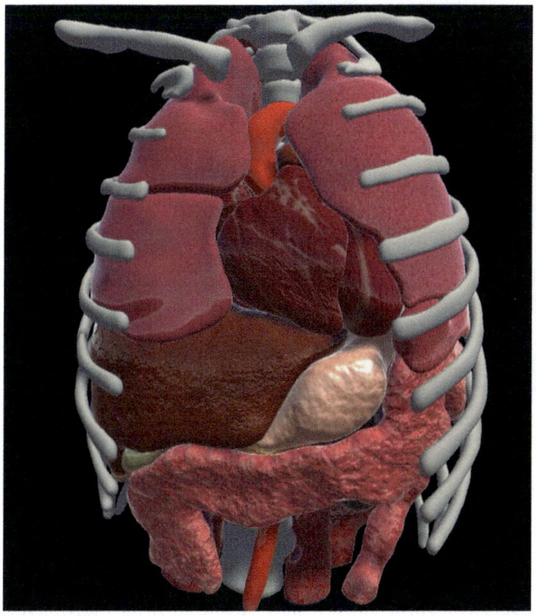

Fig. 4.11 Textured model in Unity game mode

visual attributes corresponded appropriately with the models' geometries.

Finally, the anatomical model was successfully imported into Unity (Fig. 4.11) and a preliminary test was conducted to validate the model with Unity's real-time rendering capabilities for the application development. The models' performance was assessed and approved within the Unity environment to ensure a seamless and responsive visualisation.

4.2.3.3 Application Development

The application was developed to operate on an Android tablet, using Unity's input handling capabilities tailored for touchscreen interactions. Designing the UI involved sizing and placing buttons and panels thoughtfully. Spacing between elements to prevent the cluttering of colliders was crucial to allow the user to navigate through the application without difficulty. Throughout the implementation, continuous functional testing was undertaken to ensure suitable touch interactions.

A bespoke graphics pack (Fig. 4.12) was designed to create a distinctive visual identity throughout the application. The graphics were hand-drawn using Procreate, adhering to the specific colour schemes (Fig. 4.2) initially set out for continuity across the application.

AR interactions within the application were developed using the Unity's AR Foundation package which was downloaded and imported to the Unity project file upon initiation. For this, the ARCore software development kit was set as a subsystem into the project set-up to enable the creation of the AR experiences on Android devices (Fig. 4.13).

Fig. 4.12 Bespoke graphics pack

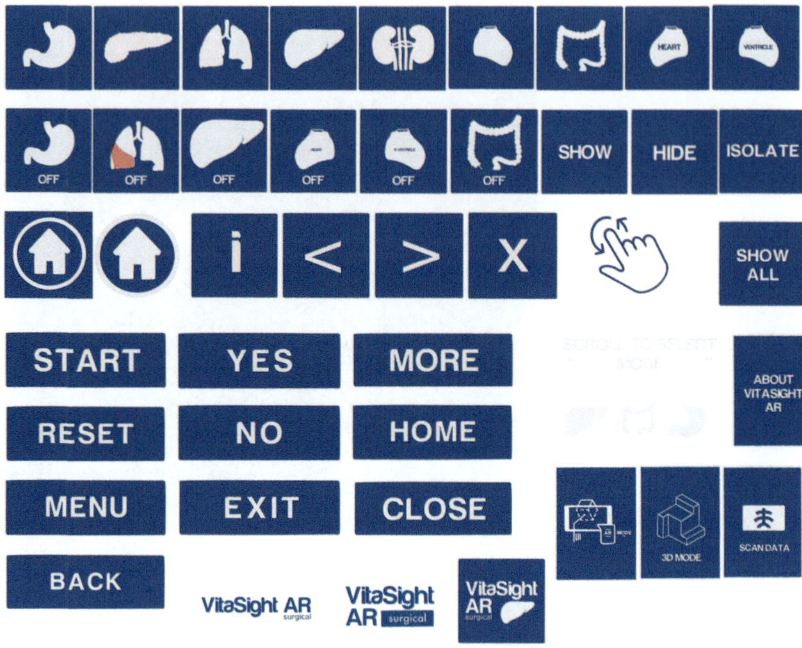

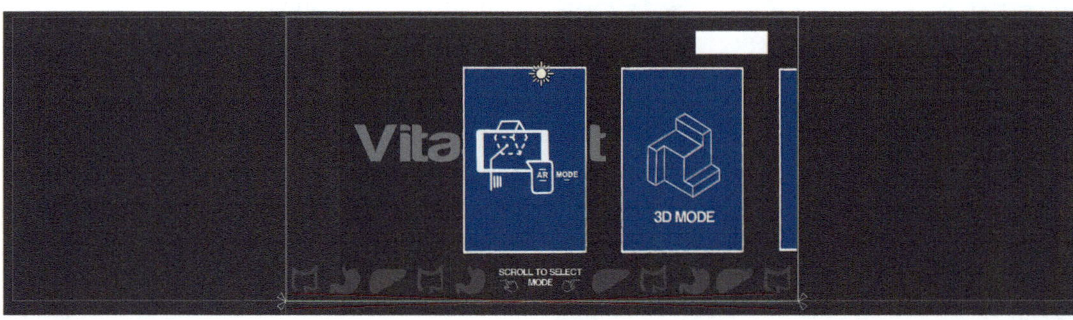

Fig. 4.13 Horizontal scrollbar and sliding area

The development process was conducted using Unity and C# scripting, allowing for a multifaceted application with distinct scenes tailored for various user experiences. The intricacies of touchscreen navigation, model manipulation, and transparency control were paramount in delivering an intuitive and interactive user interface.

The application comprises four distinct scenes. The "AR Mode" would immerse the user into an augmented reality experience, enabling them to explore the inner anatomy of a model through decal tracking. The "3D Mode" was developed to give the user the ability to interact with and customise the anatomical model in real time, offering a dynamic exploration of structures. The "Scan Data Mode" was designed as a prototype to grant the user access to patient-specific data and make notes whilst using the tablet during pre-surgical planning or intraoperatively. Lastly, the "Information Scene" would provide users with contextual knowledge about the application, offering a background overview and intended use cases.

Before generating assets, an initial grey-box prototype (Figs. 4.14 and 4.15) of the application was generated to establish interaction with basic shapes, models, and UI functions. Following the completion of the definitive assets, they were

Fig. 4.14 Prototype scene for UI Menu screen

imported into Unity to replace the primitives of the basic shapes.

The development of the AR mode presented challenges, in marker design and precise anatomical placement within the AR environment. Extensive testing and refinements were undertaken to ensure seamless integration and visualisation of anatomical structures in an augmented reality setting.

The ARObjOverlayImage script, derived from Dr Matthieu Poyade's tutorial, served as a link between AR tracking and digital overlays. It managed AR Markers, detected and tracked the AR Decal Image Marker, and facilitated digital object placement.

Using MarkerPrefabs, it stored marker visuals and object information in a dictionary, allowing instantiation and updating based on marker detection. Integrated into Unity's AR Foundation framework, it connected with the AR Core platform (Android) to enable the AR experience.

A designed box (Fig. 4.15), aligned precisely beneath the AR Marker in the real world, played a vital role in providing depth and realism to the augmented environment. This box, crafted to match the dimensions of a resuscitation doll used for testing, had a calculated depth of 14 centimetres, closely mirroring the actual object's dimensions. The AR system was designed to interact with a physical resuscitation doll used for testing purposes. The Unity-created box served as a platform for AR markers and a visual interface, while the resuscitation doll acted as the physical model for internal anatomy representation and testing.

A mask material was integrated into the AR box's exterior wall, enhancing depth perception through a viewing window aligned with the AR Image Marker (Fig. 4.16). This window provided a distinct perspective into the box's interior, where an anatomical model representing the resuscitation doll's internal structure was strategically positioned.

Given the doll's absence of true internal anatomy, precise placement of the anatomical representation within the doll was a primary focus. While it couldn't achieve perfect anatomical replication, it aimed to closely mirror plausible arrangements based on available CT scan data used to create the model.

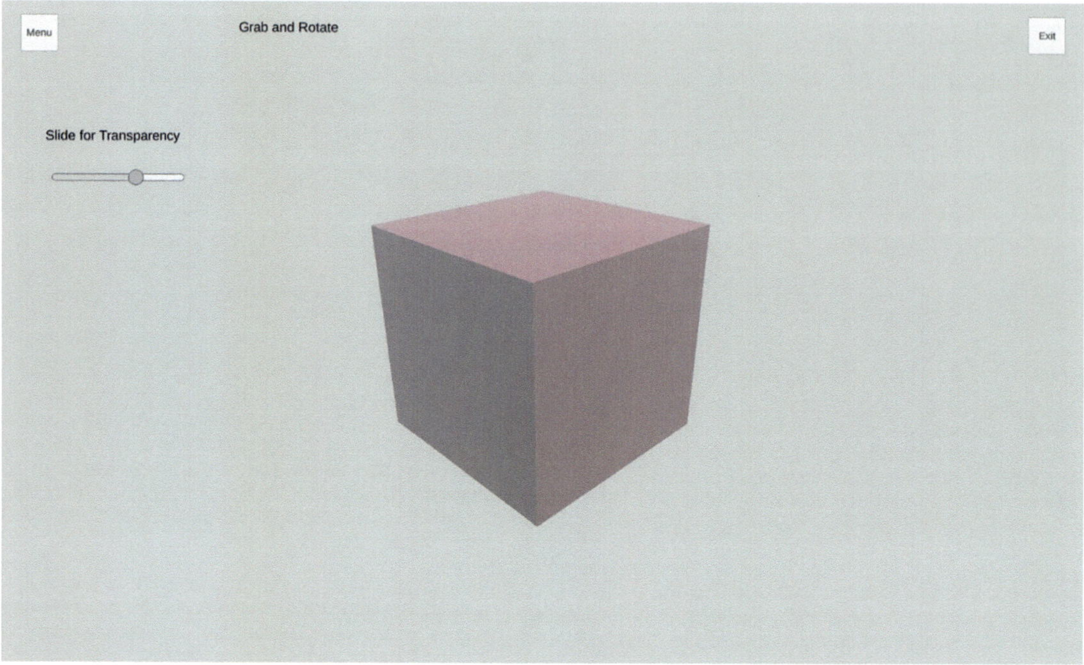

Fig. 4.15 Prototype for 3D model scene—touch and drag to rotate model

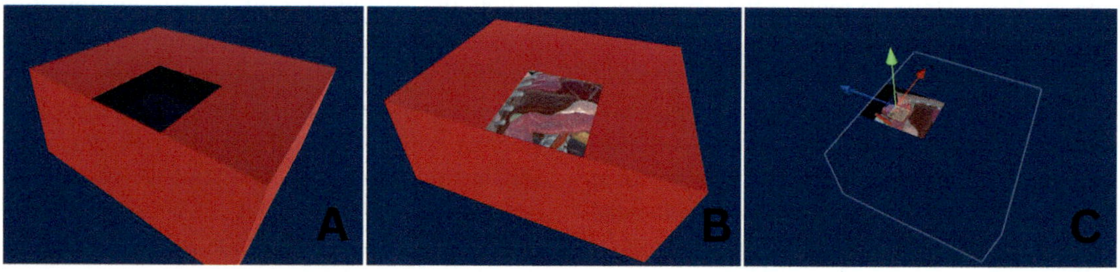

Fig. 4.16 (**a**) Red—Box Exterior Surface Panel. Black—Box Interior Surface Panel. (**b**) Box with model integrated. (**c**) Box with Mask Mesh applied to Exterior Surface panelling to create invisible illusion

For actual patient data, this application would be customised to the individual's unique anatomy, ensuring precise organ and structure placement, resulting in accurate representation based on their specific data.

After testing the initial box set-up with the doll, subsequent phases of testing and refinement were undertaken. Standard cubes were placed inside the box to assess user navigation and interaction within the internal box space in AR. Following this, a skeletal model from the Unity Asset Store was incorporated as a preliminary test to gauge sizing and assess the plausibility of the anatomy within the box boundaries. The final stage involved implementing the final comprehensive model with skin-textured walls (skin model) inside the box (Fig. 4.17).

4.2.3.4 Model Customisation Inside AR

The challenge of enabling and disabling specific anatomical models within the AR environment demanded a sophisticated solution. A refined

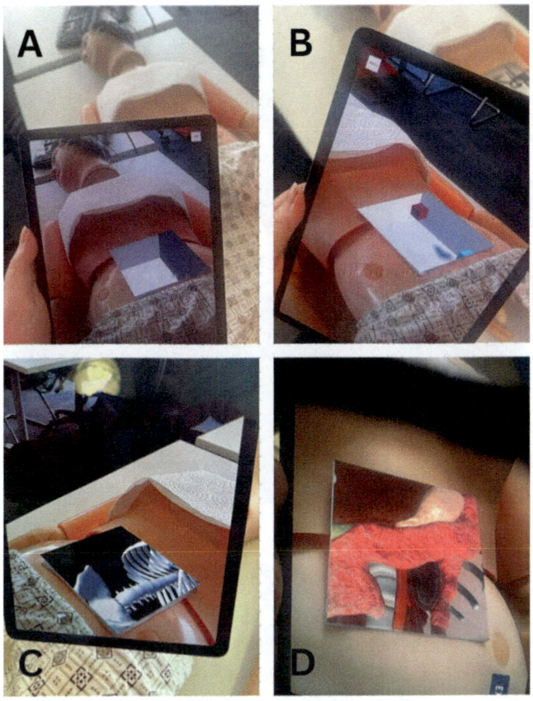

Fig. 4.17 (a) Initial smaller scale box prototype tested on model to test depth perception. (b) Cubes incorporated into the AR scene to test movement. (c) Internal wall colour change and addition of an asset store model. (d) Implementation of final model with skin mode

scripting approach was developed to facilitate a more seamless interaction for users. This involved script modifications that enabled intuitive activation and deactivation of individual organs within the AR environment. The iterations and refinements in this process allowed users to toggle specific models on and off, significantly enhancing exploration and understanding of anatomical structures.

This detailed and iterative development phase ensured that the application not only met functional expectations but also prioritised user experience and interaction in both the 3D and AR modes.

4.2.3.5 AR Tracking Image

Refinements were made to the tracking image, evolving from an interim test image to a bespoke 12 cm × 12 cm AR image decal designed for precise AR tracking. The marker's size and position-

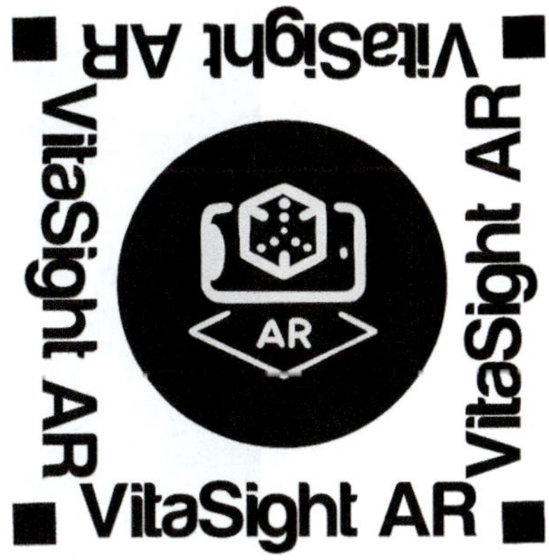

Fig. 4.18 Final AR Image Decal developed for application use during testing

ing were optimised to ensure efficient marker detection and improved visualisation of anatomical structures, enhancing the overall user experience (Pérez-Pachón et al. 2020). Additionally, it is worth considering the possibility of situating the marker outside the confines of the actual AR visualisation area. During testing, the box containing the anatomical representation was deliberately moved from its original position under the reference tracker. This did allow the marker to be scanned, for instance, in the chest area, whilst offering the user a viewing window to the corresponding anatomy of the abdominal region (Fig. 4.18).

In summary, this comprehensive project encompassed stages from 3D model generation to the development of an AR application, emphasising not only usability but also the precision required for paediatric surgical applications.

4.3 Results

4.3.1 Introductory Screen

A custom introductory screen is visible upon start-up of the application following the Unity splash screen. This screen features a "Start" button, which, upon pressing, guides the user into the main menu of the application (Fig. 4.19).

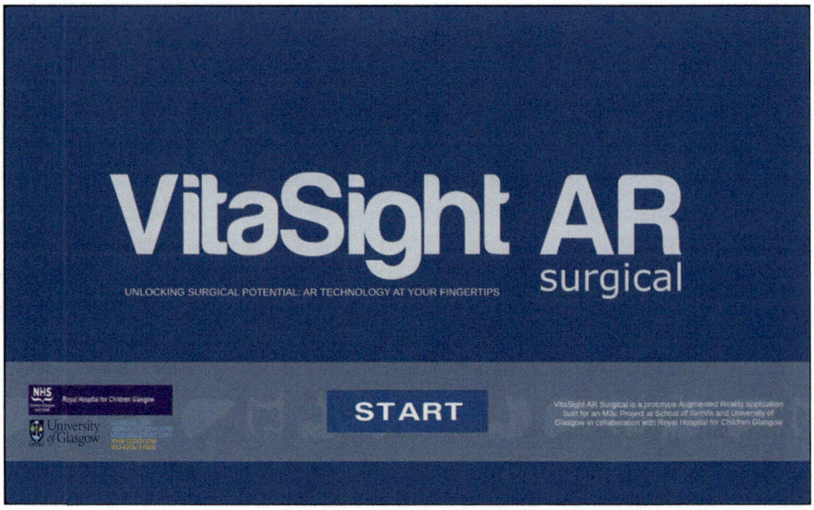

Fig. 4.19 Introductory scene with application logo, slogan, and Start button

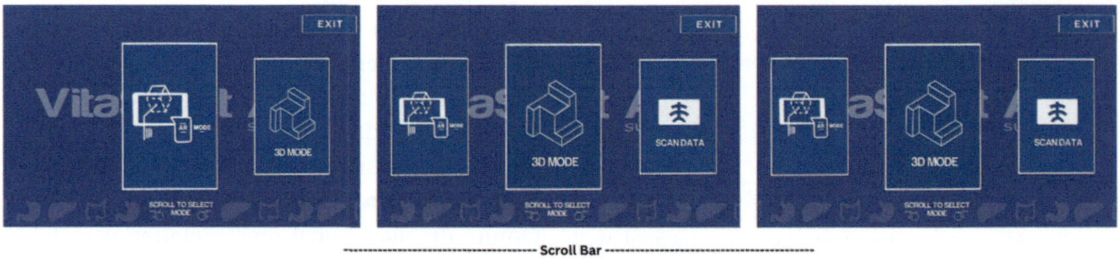

Fig. 4.20 Main menu items along the horizontal scroll bar with enlarged items based on user input along the horizontal scroll

4.3.2 Main Menu

Upon pressing Start, the user is first brought to the main menu, which features an animated swipe-menu feature. Whilst swiping left and right using the touchscreen, "AR Mode," "3D Mode," "Scan Data," and "About" menu items scale according to the user input. Each menu item acts as a button leading to each application scene (Fig. 4.20).

An "Exit" button is present which opens a quit panel, prompting the user to confirm their choice. Selecting "Yes" quits the application, whilst the "No" button closes the panel and returns to the main menu (Fig. 4.21).

4.3.3 AR Mode

When the user presses the AR Mode menu item, the application uses the device's camera to capture the surrounding real-world environment. Live camera feed serves as the foundation for this scene upon which various digital elements are superimposed, such as UI buttons, panels, and interactive components (Fig. 4.22).

An "Info" button is present in the scene, and upon clicking this button, informative panels emerge, offering guidance on how to effectively navigate the AR Mode. These detail instructions on how to manipulate the models within the AR, how to scan the decal, and explanations of typical

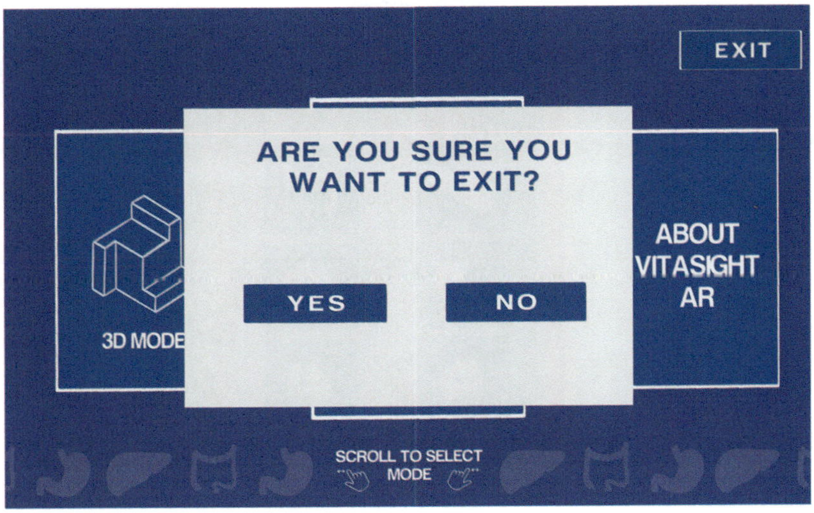

Fig. 4.21 Exit panel

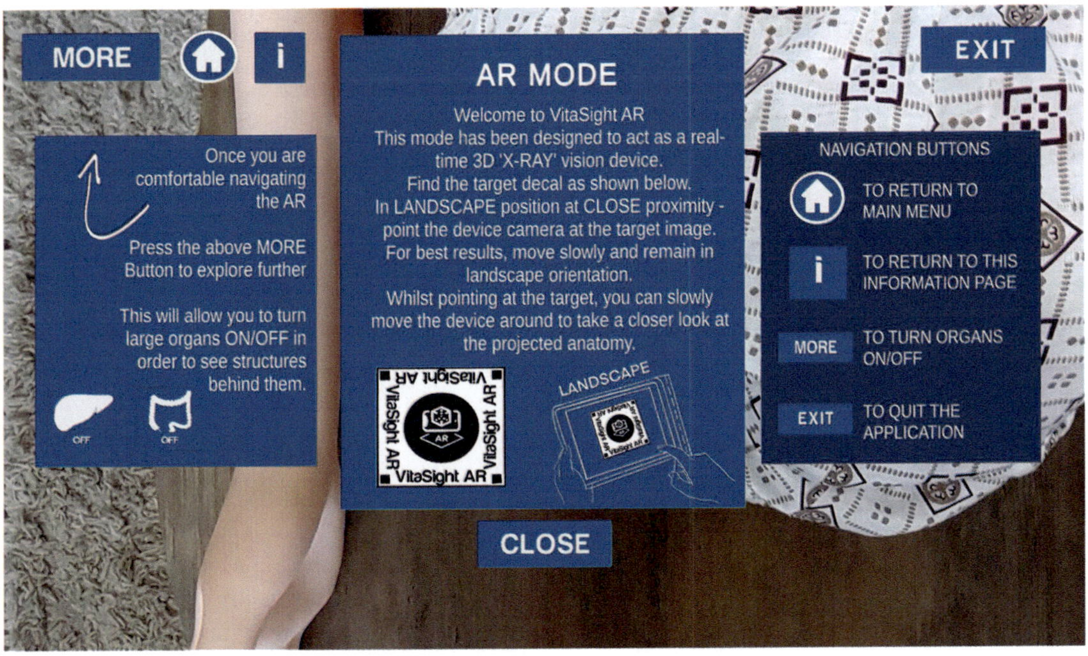

Fig. 4.22 Information shown when pressing the info button

navigation buttons. A "Close" button, or a second click on the info button, allows the user to dismiss these panels when ready.

A home icon is present which leads the user directly to the Main Menu, and an Exit button, with its assigned panel, also allows the user to quit the application at any time (Fig. 4.23).

Once the AR Image Decal is successfully detected and the anatomical model becomes visible within the scene, additional functionality is introduced through the "More" button. This button opens a dedicated panel which features six buttons for the Liver, Colon, Stomach, Right Lung Middle Lobe, Ventricle and Heart. These buttons allow the user to interactively toggle the associated 3D models on and off within the AR space.

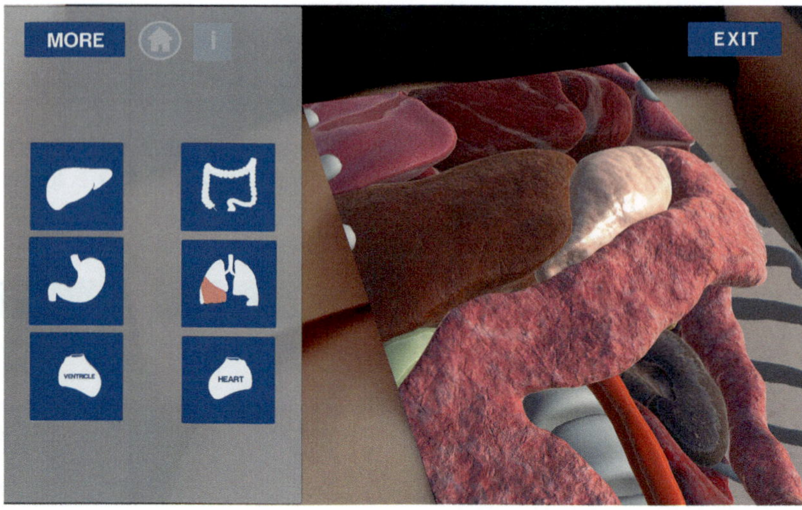

Fig. 4.23 Items inside the "More" button panel

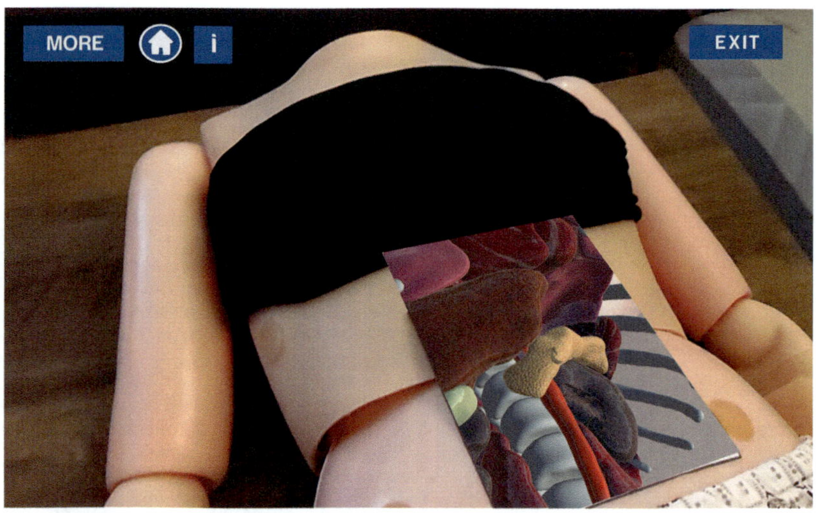

Fig. 4.24 AR Mode in use showing depth of the abdomen with colon and stomach removed

A second click on the More button will close the panel again (Fig. 4.24).

4.4 3D Mode

Upon selecting the 3D Mode menu item, users are transitioned into the 3D model scene. In this environment, the 3D anatomical model is displayed within a 2D application space. Here, the user can engage with the model by touching the screen to rotate and examine it from various viewpoints (Fig. 4.25).

When entering the 3D Mode scene, an informative panel is automatically activated. This provides the user with an overview of how the scene functions. This panel also features an Explore button which leads users to an extended 3D Mode scene where they can further customise the model through specific organ selection. This panel also offers a Hide button which allows the user to conceal the panel at their discretion, collapsing it into an info button which can be reactivated again at any time (Fig. 4.26).

A home icon is present which leads the user directly to the Main Menu, and an Exit button

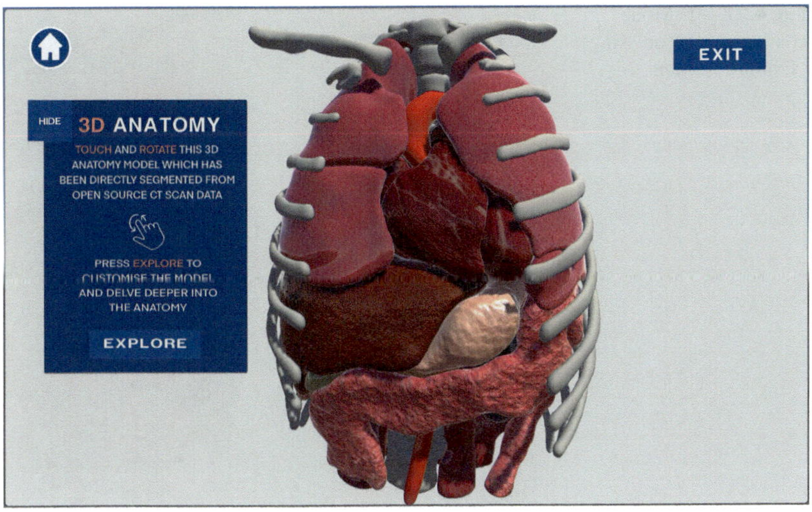

Fig. 4.25 3D Mode directly from Main Menu with info panel automatically activated

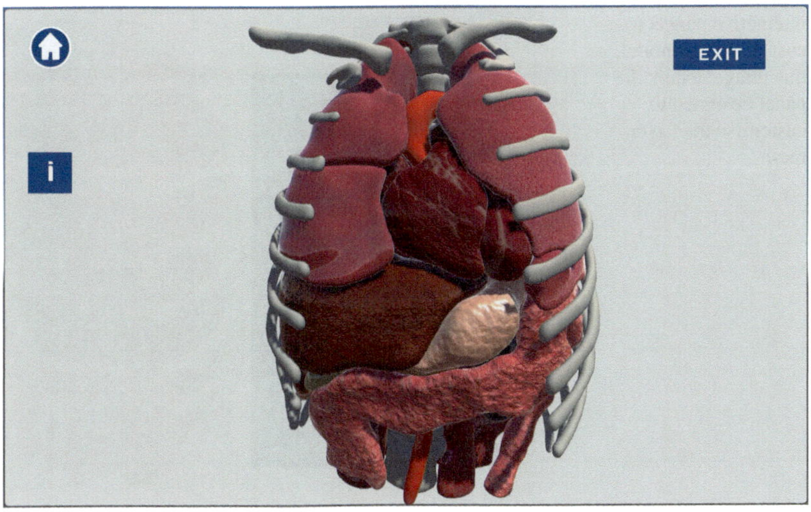

Fig. 4.26 3D Mode when info panel is deactivated using the “Hide” button

with its assigned panel also allows the user to quit the application at any time.

When the users initiate the Explore button, the 3D Mode scene presents a selection of seven buttons, each representing anatomical models within the scene: Liver, Lungs, Colon, Heart, Pancreas, Kidneys, and Stomach. Pressing any of these buttons opens a model-specific panel which allows the user to customise the displayed organ within the 3D viewer according to their preferences (Fig. 4.27). The user can opt to showcase or conceal the model, change its opacity using the UI slider, and isolate the structure completely. Each model-specific panel features an “X” close button which dismisses the panel when adjustments are made (Fig. 4.28).

A home icon is present which leads the user directly to the Main Menu, and an Exit button with its assigned panel also allows the user to quit the application at any time.

A Back button within this scene leads the user directly back into the initial 3D Mode Scene where there was no distraction of UI buttons.

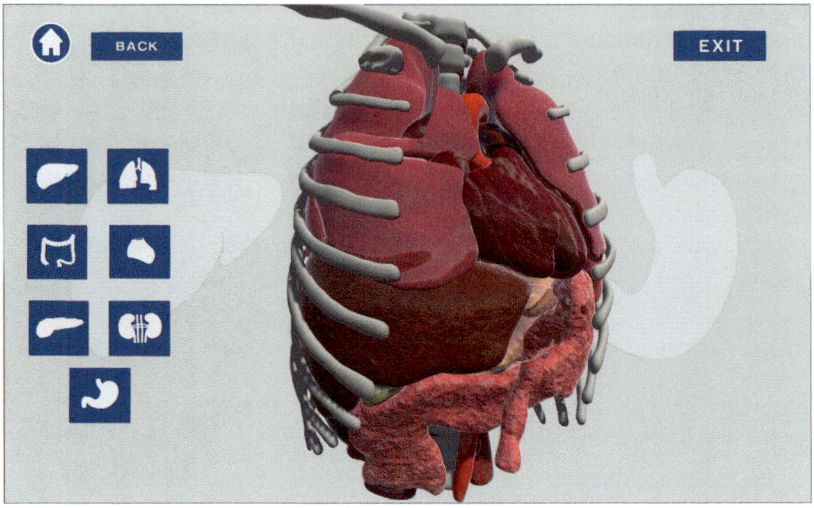

Fig. 4.27 3D Mode continued after pressing "Explore" button

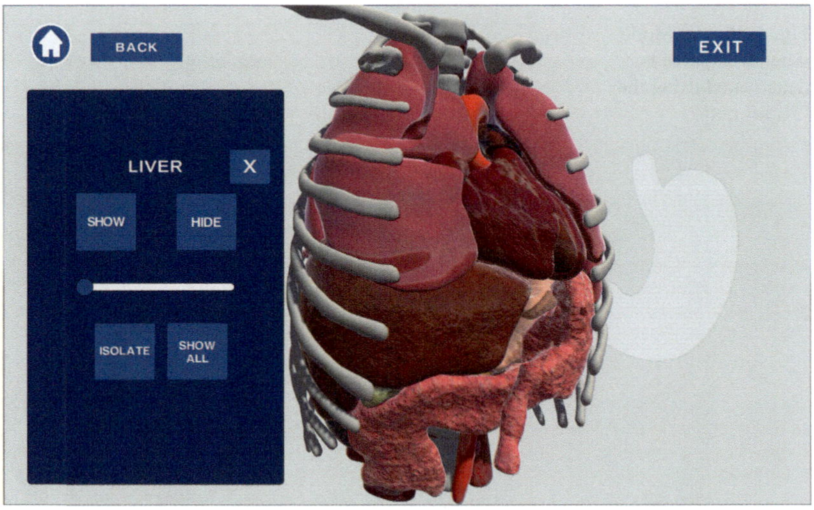

Fig. 4.28 One of seven interactive panels to customise the model, this image details the panel designed to customise the Liver mesh

4.4.1 Scan Mode

Scan Mode allows the user to view medical data whilst note-taking on the tablet device for convenience. The user can interact with the scan data using the "<" previous and ">" next buttons to change the slice displayed in the viewport (Fig. 4.29).

Text boxes with feature prompt placeholders such as "Patient Name," "Date," and "Notes" are featured within the scene. When the user taps on any of these text boxes, the tablet's keyboard is triggered and appears, allowing them to input notes (Fig. 4.30). After typing in the desired content, users can either press the "OK" button on keyboard or tap anywhere outside the keyboard and text box area. This causes the keyboard to deactivate, and the inputted text is visible within the respective box (Fig. 4.31).

A home icon is present which leads the user directly to the Main Menu, and an Exit button with its assigned panel also allows the user to quit the application at any time.

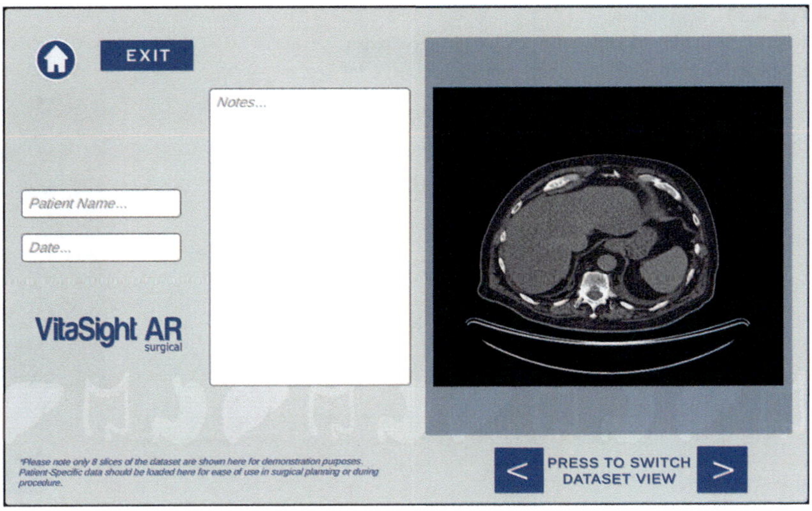

Fig. 4.29 Scan Mode opened directly from the Main Menu

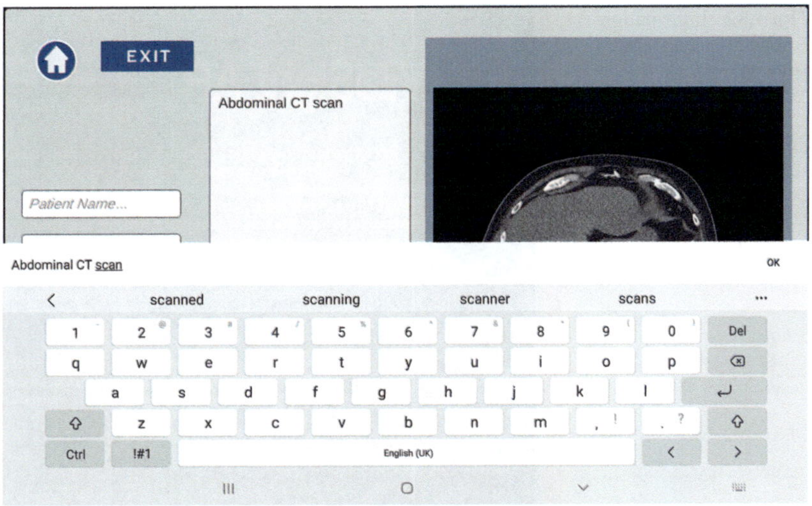

Fig. 4.30 Scan Mode when typing into the provided notes area

4.4.2 Information Scene

This scene offers comprehensive information regarding the application development and its intended purpose. The only interaction features in this scene are the home icon leading the user directly to the Main Menu and an Exit button with its assigned panel also allowing the user to quit the application at any time (Fig. 4.32).

4.5 Evaluation

4.5.1 Participants

The investigation delved into the usability and impact of an augmented reality (AR) application in the medical field, focusing on complex surgical procedures and healthcare protocols. Conducted at the Royal Hospital for Children, Glasgow, the study comprised a diverse group of 21 participants; 15 females (71.43%) and 6 males (28.57%) were recruited by Dr Michael Jacovides and Dr Giuliana Torpiano at the Royal Hospital for Children, Glasgow.

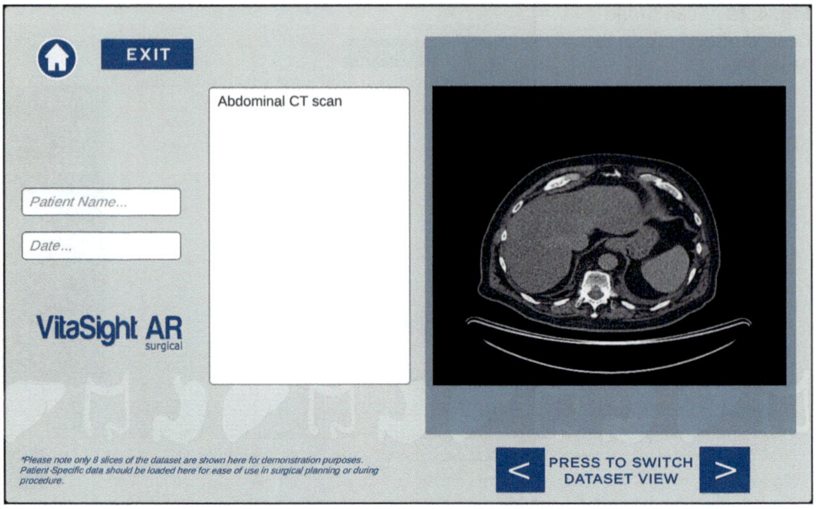

Fig. 4.31 Scan Mode with note displayed and keyboard deactivated

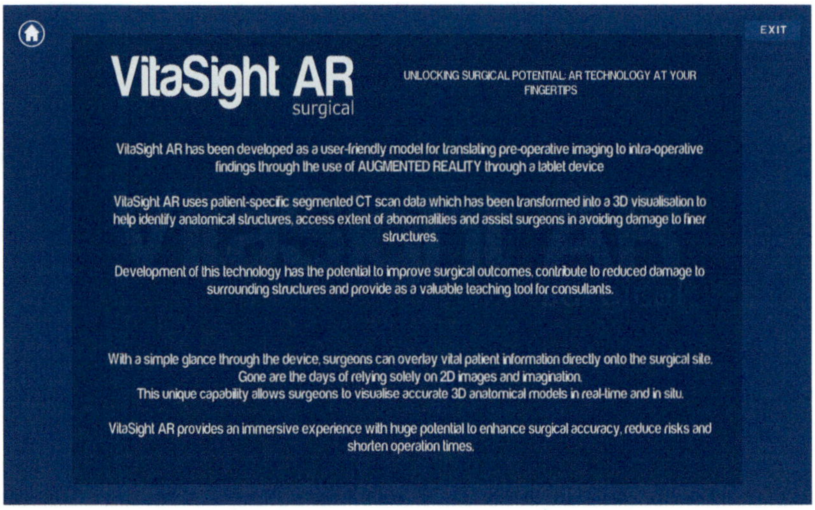

Fig. 4.32 Information Scene opened directly from Main Men

This group encompassed a wide spectrum of positions including foundation doctors, surgical trainees, associate specialists, experienced consultants, and nurse practitioners, collectively contributing to the comprehensive demographic of professionals within the domain of paediatric surgery and related fields.

Participants exhibited varying levels of comfort and familiarity with technology and AR. The majority felt moderately comfortable with technology but were relatively new to AR. This diversity in familiarity provided a comprehensive spectrum of perspectives.

4.5.2 Experimental Set-up and Procedure

The experimental set-up consisted of the AR application running on an Android tablet Samsung Tab S5 adjacent to a resuscitation doll, with an AR tracking decal affixed to the doll's abdomen. This arrangement allowed real-time tracking of AR content, creating an interactive experience for participants.

The procedural framework involved several steps, including initial information dissemination using a personal information sheet, consent acquisition, competence initial assessments, and free exploration of the application. After using the application, participants were asked to answer a series of usability questions.

Participants were invited to the Royal Hospital for Children Seminar Room on Level 3, where they were initially provided with a personal information sheet outlining details of the study. Consent acquisition was then signed by both the researcher and the participant should they decide to proceed and engage in the experimental testing.

Prior to using the application, participants were requested to complete initial competence assessments, outlining their initial familiarity with AR applications and articulating their anticipations of a successful application.

Participants were then given unrestricted time to explore the application, while the researcher remained in close proximity, addressing any inquiries that may arise throughout. After concluding their use of the application, participants were prompted to fulfil a ten-question usability questionnaire, followed by an eight-question survey assessing their user experience.

4.5.3 Data Analysis

A questionnaire structure was devised for the pre-test competence questionnaire, featuring multiple-choice questions with A, B, C, and D answer options. Participants were prompted to select the most applicable responses from these options. The data collected was analysed by tallying the frequency of each response for every question, which enabled a quantitative evaluation of participants' initial knowledge and expectations.

The System Usability Score (SUS) was used to measure the usability of the application and collected data was imported into Microsoft Excel for analysis.

SUS scores were calculated following the methodology outlined by Brooke (1996). Each response was translated into a numerical value ranging from 0 to 4, where 0 represented "strongly disagree" and 4 indicated "strongly agree." Given the contrasting positive and negative phrasing of odd and even-numbered questions, distinct analytical approaches were applied (Table 4.6). The mean SUS score was computed and juxtaposed against an established SUS grading framework, as detailed by Bangor et al. (2009).

Table 4.6 SUS analysis

X	(Sum of all odd-numbered question responses)—5
Y	25—(sum of all even-numbered question responses)
Score out of 40	X + Y
SUS score (out of 100)	(X + Y) × 2.5

A three-point answer questionnaire was implemented, wherein participants were presented with dynamic response options denoted as "A," "B," and "C." These options varied across different sections of the questionnaire to capture a range of user experiences, ensuring a nuanced and comprehensive assessment of the application. This structured questionnaire facilitated participants in providing feedback and insights regarding their interaction with the application. The questionnaire collected both quantitative and qualitative metrics. An added text box gathered participant feedback and suggestions, enhancing the exploration of their perceptions in detail.

The quantitative data was organised and tabulated, categorising the responses based on the number of participants who agreed with each statement. For instance, responses falling under the "A" category, "B" category, and the "C" category were counted and tallied separately using Microsoft Excel for each statement.

Within the evaluation form, participants were presented with a 0–10 scale ranking system to express their assessment of the overall user experience. A score of 0 denoted an evaluation of "extremely unsatisfactory," while a score of 10 indicated a rating of "extremely satisfactory." This provided a standardised and quantifiable measure.

4.6 Results

The application's System Usability Scale (SUS) assessment yielded a mean score of 84.17 (Fig. 4.33), which indicates a substantial margin of 16.17 points above the established benchmark median score of 68.

An evaluation of the overall user experience was conducted through a structured 0–10 scale ranking system, with a score of 0 signifying "extremely unsatisfactory" and a score of 10 corresponding to "extremely satisfactory." Individual scores from the pool of 21 participants were collected. The total sum of these scores yielded a total score, which was subsequently divided by the total number of participants (21), resulting in a mean score of 8.14.

Sixteen out of the 21 participants took the opportunity to provide comments and insights within the designated "specific suggestions or improvements" section of the evaluation questionnaire. Positive comments described the application as "excellent to explain to parents/patients," "overall, very good," and that they "liked the transparency button to fade organs." One participant stated that the application "would be great in our teddy hospital" and another stated that they would "definitely be able to use this with good effect for families." Four participants provided feedback suggesting that further anatomical detail would benefit the application such as having "more information available for smaller complex structures" and to "show blood vessels on individual organs to help explain complications." One participant expressed that they would like the "opportunity to try it out again to practice further." A further suggestion was made to explore "using two (or more) smaller markers instead of one bigger one."

4.7 Discussion

This research explores the user-friendly integration of AR in surgery, aiming to potentially impact on precision and outcomes. Augmented reality overlays digital information onto real-time surgical views, offering 3D visualisation, accurate identification of structures, and improved planning.

4.7.1 Challenges and Methodological Reflections

While a majority found the application's interactive features and guidance to be intuitive and clear, some encountered technical issues or glitches during their interaction with the AR elements of the application. The identification of technical challenges and glitches during the eval-

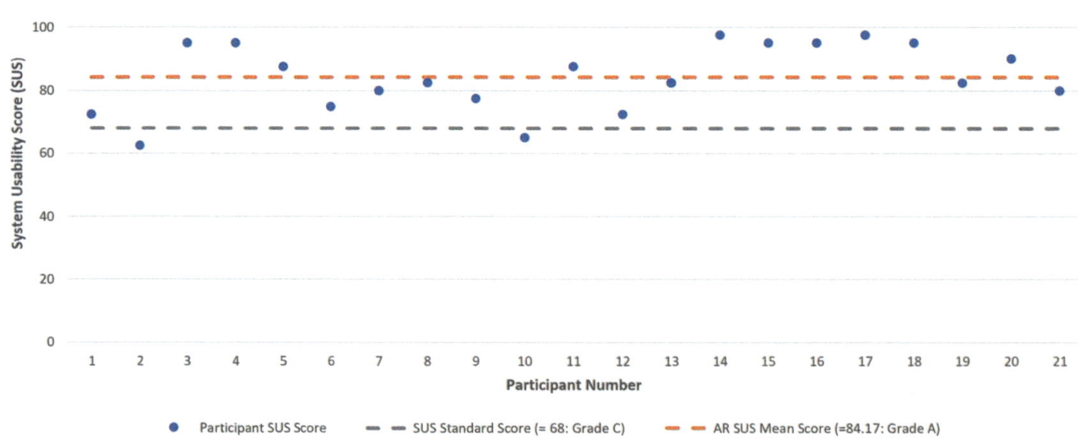

Fig. 4.33 Scatterplot of SUS scores for application

uation process brings attention to the possible influence of the testing set-up to the influence of participant height on the application's performance. It was observed that technical issues tended to arise when participants were positioning the tablet at a lower height, causing them to scan the AR decal from an angle rather than directly overhead. Participants who were taller seemed to experience fewer glitches, indicating a potential correlation between participant height and technical issues. Careful consideration of optimal scanning angles in future should be addressed; however, the height of the table that the resuscitation doll was placed on could have been considered prior to testing.

The choice of a large 12 × 12 cm AR marker for testing presented concerns related to practicality, especially in a surgical context. The apprehension that the marker might be obstructive or prone to damage during surgery was valid. An avenue for improvement could involve exploring the use of smaller AR markers or distributing a few smaller markers strategically outside the surgical field, to project AR anatomy on the surgical field. Testing the application with smaller markers or alternative marker arrangements could have provided further data for insights into enhancing usability.

The development of 3D anatomical models using software like Slicer, Autodesk 3ds Max, and Adobe Substance Painter presented both rewarding and challenging aspects. While segmentation techniques in 3D Slicer were effective for most structures, challenges in precise liver segmentation necessitated a dataset change, emphasising the need for early consideration of exclusion criteria. Notably, the attempted use of the AI tool "Segment CT Liver Plug-In" on Slicer initially proved unsuccessful, adding an additional layer of complexity to the segmentation process. This highlighted the importance of exploring alternative approaches. Additionally, unforeseen complications during the transition to Unity raised issues with mesh rendering, revealing the importance of proactive planning for rendering mode adjustments.

Similar challenges were faced during application development. Unforeseen complexities in AR mode design resulted in delays, particularly regarding opacity adjustments for AR objects. Methodological reflections highlighted the necessity for scenario analysis and earlier planning for unique script requirements, improving efficiency and mitigating unforeseen challenges.

4.7.2 User-Friendly AR Model Development

The developed AR model, specifically designed for paediatric surgery and deployed on a tablet device, underwent extensive testing among a group of 21 participants at different stages of training. Ranging from foundation doctors to experienced consultant surgeons at the Royal Hospital for Children, Glasgow, their feedback proved invaluable. The application's usability, measured by the standard System Usability Score (SUS), significantly surpassed the median benchmark score, indicating a high level of user-friendliness. Participants reported high satisfaction, particularly praising its potential in conveying complex medical concepts to patients and parents, showcasing its potential as a communication tool within the medical context.

However, insights from a subset of participants emphasised the need for specific refinements to facilitate the application's use in an intraoperative setting. A smaller, less invasive decal markers and additional anatomical information for seamless integration into the surgical environment. Optimising AR for use during procedures proved important, particularly focusing on real-time tracking precision and intuitive interface design.

4.7.3 Evaluation and Suggestions for Improvement

Participant feedback suggested the application's potential to improve patient engagement, visualise complex medical concepts, and enhance surgical procedures. The responses to research questions indicated that a significant number of participants perceived this application as having the potential to enhance various aspects of medical practice. Particularly noteworthy was the consensus that the application could contribute to improving patient engagement, visualising medical concepts, and enhancing surgical procedures. These findings suggest that the application aligns with participants' aspirations for AR tools that can facilitate communication and understanding within medical contexts.

A notable observation during the evaluation was that certain icons within the user interface inadvertently led users to exit the application unexpectedly. This could be improved by optimising the user interface to ensure intuitive navigation and minimise similar instances. Ensuring that icons and controls are more logically placed may contribute to a smoother and more seamless interaction. Further, the 3D models, while serving as effective visual aids, could benefit greatly from more anatomical detail to provide a more comprehensive understanding of medical complications and structures. Incorporating details such as blood supply and venous drainage would provide a more holistic representation. This would also enhance the application's ability in a surgical setting.

A distinctive feature of the application is its innovative approach to creating visible depth and internal perspective. Rather than relying on a typical AR overlay set-up, the application was built to emulate the sensation of peering inside the model's abdomen. The result was a compelling illusion of depth, and participants verbalised their appreciation for the design by noting how effective it was to be able to observe the anatomical structures from different angles—downward, upward, and even through the chest from the abdomen. Whilst this was well-received, there is potential for further refinement in the design by changing the shape of the virtual box which holds the model to align more closely with the contours of the human body. A rounded box shape would mimic natural curvature, and the illusion of peering inside could be further enhanced.

4.7.4 Limitations and Ethical Considerations

While time constraints presented a challenge, it is noteworthy that the final application managed to encompass all scenes and significant functionalities originally outlined in the initial storyboard. The project was executed within a condensed timeline of 12 weeks, posing a significant challenge to the comprehensive development and thorough user testing required for a fully functional application of this nature.

Ethical considerations imposed a limitation on the utilisation of patient-specific data, which, on reflection, could have otherwise been used to significantly enhance the application's authenticity. Prior to contemplating this, ethical guidelines and considerations had already been established and agreed upon, and the main focus was on the application's ability to perceive depth, not on the physical models. Subsequently, the choice was made to use open-source data, which, although offering valuable anatomical structure references, fell short of the additional authenticity that patient-specific data could have provided to participants during testing.

4.7.5 Future Research Directions

The comprehensive insights gained from the study highlighted the significance of a more extensive participant pool and the collection of demographic data to gain a more holistic understanding of the application's usability and impact. Additionally, considerations regarding the technical challenges and the application's practicality in surgical settings were highlighted for future development and refinement.

It should be noted that further research should be conducted after further refinement, and a subsequent investigation should involve revisiting the application's use in the intraoperative setting to assess its improved functionality and effectiveness. This should prioritise the integration of patient-specific data, rather than using open-source data. This may aid to shift the application from a prototype-like feel to a clinically relevant tool, and by using real patient data, medical professionals can better connect the application's visualisations to actual cases, improving utilisation in both educational and intraoperative contexts.

Further testing and data collection should be considered to expand the scope of insights. Specifically, evaluating knowledge acquisition both with and without the application could test its impact in surgical contexts, assessing its use as an educational tool.

4.8 Conclusion

The use of AR in medical surgery shows promise for improving precision, safety, and technical outcomes. AR can overlay digital information onto a surgeon's real-time view, enhancing visualisation, accuracy, and planning. It offers 3D visualisation of anatomical structures and patient data and can aid in critical tasks like tumour localisation and instrument placement. However, most research focuses on head-mounted displays (HMDs), which may introduce distractions and ergonomic challenges, potentially affecting surgical performance. Depth perception is an ongoing concern, as distorted perceptions can lead to visibility issues and scene distortions. Further research is needed on user-friendly, cost-effective AR interfaces that minimise distractions and depth perception challenges while maximising benefits.

This project aimed to develop a user-friendly model for translating preoperative imaging to intraoperative findings using augmented reality on a commercially available tablet device for paediatric surgery. Initial user testing showed promising results for the implementation of this application into the healthcare system, with the potential to improve patient engagement and understanding. While additional refinement and user testing would be advantageous, this endeavour showcases the potential of an AR application on a tablet device to convert pre-operative imaging into intraoperative findings by utilising segmented 3D anatomical models. Notably, this approach involves using depth cues to accurately position the models within anatomical context, departing from the conventional projected AR overlay method. The successful implementation of AR in this context could extend its utility across various healthcare applications within the hospital setting and encompass a wide array of functions, enhancing patient care, surgical precision, and ultimately medical outcomes.

References

Barcali E et al (2022) Augmented reality in surgery: a scoping review. Appl Sci 12(14):6890. https://doi.org/10.3390/app12146890

Bangor A et al (2009) Determining what individual SUS scores mean: Adding an adjective rating scale. J Usability Stud 4(3):114–123

Borovanska Z et al (2020) Engaging with children using augmented reality on clothing to prevent them from smoking. Adv Exp Med Biol:59–94. https://doi.org/10.1007/978-3-030-43961-3_4

Brecevich AT et al (2019) 121. Machine-vision image guided surgery (mvigs): an intraoperative and radiation-free spine navigation system workflow analysis. Spine J 19(9). https://doi.org/10.1016/j.spinee.2019.05.135

Brooke J (1996) Sus: a "quick and dirty" usability scale, Usability evaluation in industry, pp 207–212. https://doi.org/10.1201/9781498710411-35

Carmigniani J, Furht B (2011) Augmented reality: an overview, Handbook of augmented reality, pp 3–46. https://doi.org/10.1007/978-1-4614-0064-6_1
Carswell V et al (2022) Is it time to Fona friend? A novel mixed reality front of neck access simulator. Med Vis Appl Technol:3–25. https://doi.org/10.1007/978-3-031-06735-8_1
Choi H et al (2015) An effective visualization technique for depth perception in augmented reality-based surgical navigation. Int J Med Robot Comput Assist Surg 12(1):62–72. https://doi.org/10.1002/rcs.1657
Cutolo F (2019) Letter to the editor on "Augmented reality based navigation for computer assisted hip resurfacing: a proof of concept study". Ann Biomed Eng 47(11):2151–2153. https://doi.org/10.1007/s10439-019-02299-w
Deng W et al (2013) Easy-to-use augmented reality neuronavigation using a wireless tablet PC. Stereotact Funct Neurosurg 92(1):17–24. https://doi.org/10.1159/000354816
El Jamiy F, Marsh R (2019) Survey on depth perception in head mounted displays: distance estimation in virtual reality, augmented reality, and mixed reality. IET Image Process 13(5):707–712. https://doi.org/10.1049/iet-ipr.2018.5920
Ieiri S et al (2011) Augmented reality navigation system for laparoscopic splenectomy in children based on preoperative CT image using optical tracking device. Pediatr Surg Int 28(4):341–346. https://doi.org/10.1007/s00383-011-3034-x
Kruijff E et al (2010) Perceptual issues in augmented reality revisited, 2010 IEEE international symposium on mixed and augmented reality [preprint]. https://doi.org/10.1109/ismar.2010.5643530
Léger É et al (2020) Marin: an open-source mobile augmented reality interactive neuronavigation system. Int J Comput Assist Radiol Surg 15(6):1013–1021. https://doi.org/10.1007/s11548-020-02155-6
Lex JR et al (2022) Clinical applications of augmented reality in orthopaedic surgery: a comprehensive narrative review. Int Orthop 47(2):375–391. https://doi.org/10.1007/s00264-022-05507-w
Mahadevan V (2018) Anatomy of the vertebral column. Surgery (Oxford) 36(7):327–332. https://doi.org/10.1016/j.mpsur.2018.05.006
Mamone V et al (2020) Projected augmented reality to drive osteotomy surgery: implementation and comparison with video see-through technology. IEEE Access 8:169024–169035. https://doi.org/10.1109/access.2020.3021940
Marescaux J, Diana M (2015) Next step in minimally invasive surgery: hybrid image-guided surgery. J Pediatr Surg 50(1):30–36. https://doi.org/10.1016/j.jpedsurg.2014.10.022
Meulstee JW et al (2018) Toward holographic-guided surgery. Surg Innov 26(1):86–94. https://doi.org/10.1177/1553350618799552
Miner RC (2017) Image-guided neurosurgery. J Med Imaging Radiat Sci 48(4):328–335. https://doi.org/10.1016/j.jmir.2017.06.005
Mondal SB et al (2020) Head-mounted devices for non-invasive cancer imaging and intraoperative image-guided surgery. Adv Funct Mater 30(37). https://doi.org/10.1002/adfm.202000185
Pérez-Pachón L et al (2020) Image overlay surgery based on augmented reality: a systematic review. Adv Exp Med Biol:175–195. https://doi.org/10.1007/978-3-030-47483-6_10
Pérez-Pachón L et al (2021) Effect of marker position and size on the registration accuracy of Hololens in a non-clinical setting with implications for high-precision surgical tasks. Int J Comput Assist Radiol Surg 16(6):955–966. https://doi.org/10.1007/s11548-021-02354-9
Prevost GA et al (2019) Efficiency, accuracy and clinical applicability of a new image-guided surgery system in 3D laparoscopic liver surgery. J Gastrointest Surg 24(10):2251–2258. https://doi.org/10.1007/s11605-019-04395-7
Princle A et al (2018) [poster] using an industry-ready AR HMD on a real maintenance task: AR benefits performance on certain task steps more than others, 2018 IEEE international symposium on mixed and augmented reality adjunct (ISMAR-adjunct) [preprint]. https://doi.org/10.1109/ismar-adjunct.2018.00075
Puladi B et al (2022) Augmented reality-based surgery on the human cadaver using a new generation of optical head-mounted displays: development and feasibility study. JMIR Serious Games 10(2). https://doi.org/10.2196/34781
Sielhorst T et al (2006) Depth perception—a major issue in medical AR: evaluation study by twenty surgeons. Med Image Comput Comput Assist Inter 2006:364–372. https://doi.org/10.1007/11866565_45
Souzaki R et al (2013) An augmented reality navigation system for pediatric oncologic surgery based on preoperative CT and MRI images. J Pediatr Surg 48(12):2479–2483. https://doi.org/10.1016/j.jpedsurg.2013.08.025
Wasserthal J et al. (2023) TotalSegmentator: robust segmentation of 104 anatomical structures in CT images, arXiv.org. Available at: https://arxiv.org/abs/2208.05868.
Wen R et al (2017) Augmented reality guidance with multimodality imaging data and depth-perceived interaction for robot-assisted surgery. Robotics 6(2):13. https://doi.org/10.3390/robotics6020013
Zhao Z et al (2021) Augmented reality technology in image-guided therapy: state-of-the-art review. Proc Inst Mech Eng H J Eng Med 235(12):1386–1398. https://doi.org/10.1177/09544119211034357

Controllerless Control: A Review of Peripheral Technologies for VR Veterinary Spinal Tap Training

5

Liam Pearce, Matthieu Poyade, Rodrigo Gutierrez Quintana, and Julien Guevar

Abstract

Across veterinary education, students are required to develop complex clinical skills and in-depth knowledge of diagnostic techniques to achieve the best possible outcome for patient care. One of which is the process of cerebrospinal fluid (CSF) collection, vital for the diagnosis of disease progression of animal neurological disease and degeneration. Ethical and educational barriers across this industry such as access to ethically sourced specimens and a lack of education resources have neglected clinical skill development across the veterinary curriculum, resulting in fatal consequences for animal welfare. The use of virtual reality (VR) has been researched as a supplementary educational tool, providing a platform to visualise abstract concepts in knowledge acquisition, however, little empirical data regarding the use of fully immersive technology in psychomotor training for clinical skills and the parameters that impact this acquisition process currently exists. This study developed a simulation development pipeline for providing insights regarding interaction paradigms and associated factors that improve or hinder technical skill acquisition across virtual skill training. This was achieved via the design and assessment of a VR CSF sampling training simulator. Despite the current consensus of hand tracking presenting a sense of dissonance in immersive environments, findings from this study found that hand tracking was objectively perceived to be the most immersive paradigm compared to controller-based interactions, providing a more valid experience for transferable psychomotor skills Findings from this study propose a potentially safe and ethical solution for repeated practice and refinement of veterinary skills, however, more research should be conducted to understand the impact of high versus low fidelity of VE's and their contribution to skill development, independent of the interaction paradigm.

L. Pearce (✉)
School of Medicine, Dentistry and Nursing, College of Medical, Dentistry and Nursing, University of Glasgow, Glasgow, UK

School of Simulation and Visualisation, The Glasgow School of Art, Glasgow, UK

M. Poyade
School of Simulation and Visualisation, The Glasgow School of Art, Glasgow, UK
e-mail: M.Poyade@gsa.ac.uk

R. G. Quintana
School of Biodiversity, One Health and Veterinary Medicine, University of Glasgow, Glasgow, UK
e-mail: Rodrigo.GutierrezQuintana@glasgow.ac.uk

J. Guevar
College of Veterinary Medicine, University of Bern, Bern, Switzerland

J. Clancy, M. Poyade (eds.), *Medical Visualization and Applications of Technology – Volume 2*, Biomedical Visualization 5, https://doi.org/10.1007/978-3-031-63463-5_5

Keywords

Virtual reality · Veterinary education · Interactive education · Training simulation development · Cerebrospinal fluid sampling

5.1 Introduction

Diagnostic investigation within veterinary medicine necessitates an array of highly specialised procedures for the identification of diseases and pathologies across varying animal species. In cases where radio imaging cannot sufficiently identify causation or progression of disease and disorders with confidence (Lowrie and Anderson, 2011), cerebrospinal fluid (CSF) sampling may be employed to provide improved diagnostic accuracy for neurodegenerative diseases, critical indicators for establishing patients care plans (Chandler, 2008).

Although presenting minimal risks of long-term complications (Fentem et al., 2023), the growing strain on the veterinary curricula, and access to ethically sourced specimens, present significant barriers to students' development of essential clinical skills (Martinsen and Jukes, 2005; Patronek and Rauch, 2007; Bernigau et al., 2021; Karkera, 2021). This presents an inherent danger to animal welfare from failed punctures (Luján Feliu-Pascual et al., 2008).

5.1.1 Research Rational

The use of immersive technologies has been witnessed across research as an educational tool for veterinary sciences to combat limitations, by developing foundational knowledge of animal anatomy and clinical skills through digital interactivity (Bot et al., 2005; Avdic et al., 2014). For CSF collection, current simulations utilise semi-immersive environments through stereoscopic virtualisation devices to visualise 3-dimensional environments to assist with cognitive knowledge acquisition associated with the learning environment (Mossel et al., 2021; Cipresso et al., 2018). Research covering the use of immersive technologies in the context of veterinary education remains limited (Xu et al., 2022), offering little empirical evidence regarding the efficacy of fully immersive peripherals on veterinary students' development of psychomotor skills and knowledge acquisition. An increased focus on building frameworks for how we use virtual reality (VR), and its potential peripherals, to create environments that allow for knowledge acquisition whilst also building essential clinical skills is required.

5.1.2 Theoretical Background

Veterinary students and clinicians are required to repeatedly practice and train physical clinical skills for procedures such as CSF sampling for adaptiveness towards changes in patient care (Baillie et al., 2015). Where modern educational systems lack the resources to provide this training, immersive paradigms have shown potential as a learning apparatus to supplement physically based learning in areas where resources are scarce (Balogh, 2014; Xu et al., 2022).

5.1.2.1 Process of CSF Collection

Cerebrospinal fluid (CSF) is a clear fluid produced in the leptomeninges and ventricular choroid plexus through the filtration of blood plasma, providing chemical and physical protection for the central nervous system (Thomson et al., 2012). This fluid typically is found entering the subarachnoid spaces, allowing clinicians to access CSF through the Cerebellomedullary cistern via needle insertion above the first cervical vertebrae. Flexion of the animals' head distally beyond a 90 angle whilst placed in a lateral recumbent position, exposes the position of the cistern in which a needle may be advanced to access CSF in the subarachnoid space (Fig. 5.1) (Terlizzi and Platt, 2006; Platt and Di, 2009; Kenny, 2015; De Lorenzi and Mandara, 2016). Neurodegenerative diseases and inflammation may alter the characteristics of CSF, therefore analysis of the proteins and inflammatory markers within the sample provides insight into animal health (Lowrie and Anderson, 2011; Chandler, 2008). CSF sampling technique

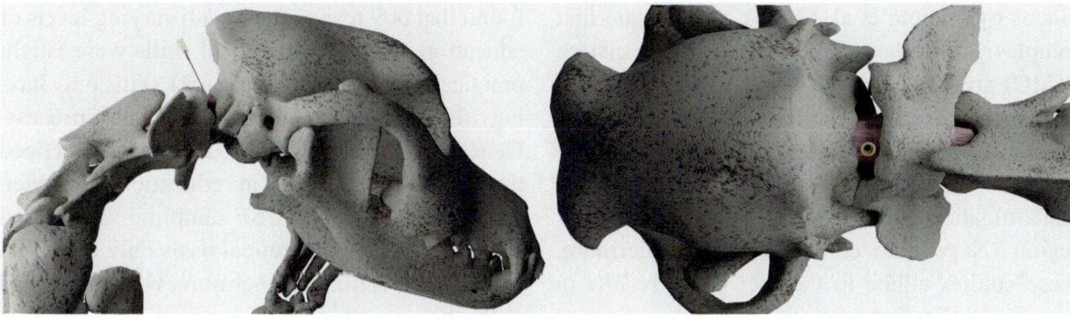

Fig. 5.1 Lateral view (left) and superior view (right) of needle advancement into the cistern using the mandible as a reference point state the animal. Image by Liam Pearce

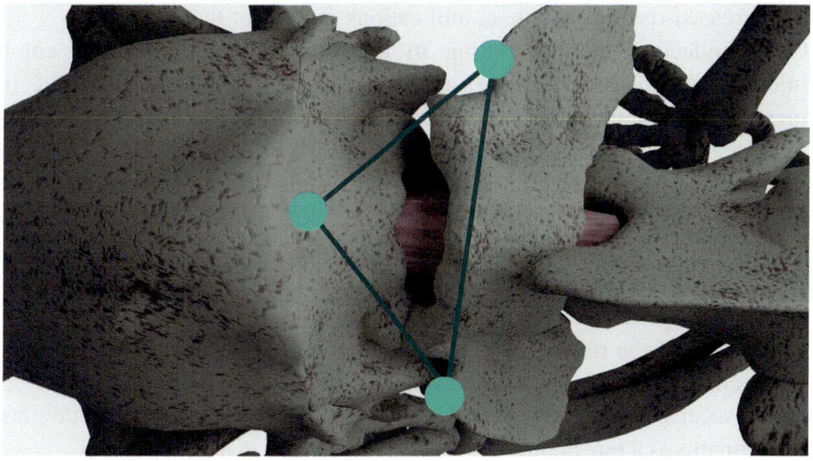

Fig. 5.2 Lateral view of triangulation of Cerebellomedullary cistern position using occipital bone and atlas wings as reference markers. Image by Liam Pearce

requires a level of technical skill and trained dexterity to mitigate the risk of potential damage from improper needle placement (Fentem et al., 2023). To train this skill, veterinary students and clinicians are required to perform this task repetitively to confirm accurate Cerebellomedullary cistern and lumbar cistern identification and proper insertion technique (Fig. 5.2), however, barriers to accessibility surrounding training for this procedure continue to hinder potential learning opportunities in modern teaching (Karkera, 2021; Bernigau et al., 2021) to the detriment of animal welfare from structural damage relating to the spinal cord (Luján Feliu-Pascual et al., 2008). Factors attributing to a lack of educational opportunities can be primarily identified as; a lack of provisional access to practical learning opportunities across veterinary curricula, and the inconsistencies in the presentation of proper procedures of needle placement and cistern identification across medical literature regarding the proper procedure (Platt and Olby, 2013; Kenny, 2015; Dewey and Da Costa, 2016; Platt and Olby, 2013; Bernigau et al., 2021; Karkera, 2021).

Physical training of clinical skills is highly regarded as the most efficient way to develop the motor skills necessary for performing high-risk clinical procedures and preparing students to face scenarios closer to that which they will experience across real clinical settings (Bot et al., 2005; Avdic et al., 2014). However, from the current climate surrounding medical education across veterinary sciences, access to physical training becomes increasingly difficult for students enrolled in veterinary sciences, often being presented with inconsistent information on what skills they should be developing, and what skills need supplementing with physical educational opportunities. Examples of this can be witnessed in studies detailing other CSF sampling techniques by Fentem et al. (2023), which state that samples from the Cerebellomedullary cistern (CMC) are an objectively easier process, with a 95.8% success rate collection, compared to 86.1% of lumbar samples. The percentage of samples that do fail is often attributed to blood contamination of collected CSF from the lumbar region (Nagendran et al., 2020). Furthermore, these studies allude to the fact CMC results in fewer complications due to this higher success rate.

However, reviews of the CMC sampling process by Luján Feliu-Pascual et al. (2008) found an increased risk of adverse complications from CMC collection failure relating to brainstem injury. Where the authors agree with current findings that CMC collection is considered an easier practice, this is attributed to a decreased likelihood of blood contamination. Authors within this research area do not claim CMC sampling as a safer practice, the risk associated with this procedure stems from long-term complications due to the proximity of the collection needle to vital structures and the risk of striking the brainstem, when compared to the lumbar sampling. (Luján Feliu-Pascual et al., 2008) Where the authors mention this as a rare complication, it is indicated this is also due to the experience of professionals conducting the process and the necessity for expert training to mitigate neurological damage during the procedures.

5.1.2.2 Barriers to Accessible Clinical Training

A lack of opportunities for practical clinical skills development for veterinary students is often cited as a factor for the lack of overall quality training (Rösch et al., 2014), problems such as shifts in the curriculum to accommodate strained resources across educational establishments (Bernigau et al., 2021; Karkera, 2021) and access to ethically sourced specimens are key contributors in the drop of practical learning opportunities within the veterinary curricula (Martinsen and Jukes, 2005; Patronek and Rauch, 2007). A review by Rösch et al. (2014) regarding practical training for 49 clinical skills taught to veterinary students through their educational establishment found that 609 respondents with varying levels of education, showed 28 clinical skills were taught practically, with the remaining 21 skills only having theoretical knowledge of their process. General skills were found to have been practiced throughout their time in education, however, techniques specific to CSF sampling were found to be taught on a theoretical basis only across all levels of education. Furthermore, when presented with the opportunity to learn these skills via interactive modalities, students consistently stated they would be willing to supplement their education via simulation-based training for many of these skills.

These findings emphasise the need for clinical skills training and information that presents opportunities to build competency for clinical practice (Ericsson, 2008; Gummery et al., 2018), in a manner that presents prospects for applied skills development whilst maintaining access to theoretical knowledge acquisition to re-enforce practical learning. Though universal techniques are generally not seen across literature, existing evidence supports a digital-focused learning platform for veterinary education using immersive technologies to combat challenges in the veterinary curriculum.

5.1.2.3 Immersive Technology in Veterinary Medical Education

Multiple facets of the education sphere have adapted both theory and physical practices towards digitally assisted learning, offering a blended approach utilising virtual environments (VE's) (de Bie and Lipman, 2012; Routh et al., 2021). VR is often cited as being the most immersive technology in the Extended Reality (XR) spectrum, capable of placing users within computer-generated virtual worlds via multiple channels of sensory input, e.g. sight and sound, to increase the feeling of physical presence (Cipresso et al., 2018). Through varying degrees of movement, the user can move in their real-world space, whilst the VR system responds to kinetic movement by adjusting the 3D space in accordance with user motions to improve feelings of presence, allowing users to experience multi-sensory environments to assist in the interpretation of abstract concepts in context to their use in medicine and developing motor skills through physical learning (Chen et al., 2020; Langebæk et al., 2021). Many authors in this field have stated the importance of VE's in offering a "learning-by-doing" method of education utilising acquired knowledge and skills to develop practical solutions to situations that mirror real-life scenarios helps to reinforce learning, particularly in medical education (Bot et al., 2005; Avdic et al., 2014). VR from a practical perspective accommodates the construction of virtual training to circumvent physical and environmental barriers in a safe and controlled environment (Nagendran et al., 2020; Poyade et al., 2021) and promote reduced rates of future incidents via encouraging mistakes as a learning experience.

In the veterinary education sector, this allows institutions to respond to barriers surrounding animal welfare, whilst still allowing users to experience real-time feedback from their actions (Balogh, 2014). However, parameters such as the requirement for pre-requisite knowledge and guidance for these simulations and hardware affordance, present current barriers to accessibility in education (Lean et al., 2006; Warburton, 2009).

Much of the current literature supporting XR-aided learning, however, is centralised on assessing training simulators from the perspective of knowledge acquisition. However, there is currently little empirical evidence stating the improvement of physical skill development from clinical training simulations. This requires an increased focus on valid simulations to successfully transfer motor skills to real-world environments. Dede et al. (2017) state that, unlike the findings of similar studies such as that of Won et al. (2023) where factors such as sensory and action immersion may impact a user's sense of presence (Dede et al., 2017), this is perceived as beneficial in the process of knowledge acquisition, presenting little impact on skill development in VR, which utilises a model of action and reflection where on participants reflect on the steps taken within the environment.

By analysing VE's in their entirety, much of the current literature neglects the analysis of individual parameters of a simulation and its success in skill attainment and knowledge encoding through learner engagement. Studies following this shift in the digital paradigm present data regarding the impact of interaction methods on validity and learning. A review by McMahan et al. (2016) found that many users will experience dissonance from interacting with VE's if the method of interaction is of mid-fidelity due to inconsistencies from biomechanical and kinematic symmetry with inputted physical movement. However, high-fidelity interactions, such as that of 1:1 recreation of natural movement or fidelity such as controller-based interactions did not result in the same effect. However, the inverse effect could also be witnessed in the finding by Hameed et al. (2021); stating the failure to meet preconceived expectations across hand-tracking paradigms, resulted in controller paradigms outperforming hand-tracking simulations when measuring factors of performance efficiency and usability, despite immersive properties such as haptics providing multi-channel feedback to improve immersion (Maran and Glavin, 2003; Cipresso et al., 2018).

Failure to acknowledge these limitations, results in interaction paradigms failing to meet pre-established expectations of the simulation, increasing cognitive load, and information uptake. The importance of an increased focus on high-fidelity interactivity and validity within VE's cannot be ignored when considering user experience and this technology as a vector for education (Slater, 2009).

Within surgical training, this limiting factor becomes significant due to the necessity of high fidelity within these environments for refining motor skills, However, there is currently a limited amount of empirical evidence detailing the efficacy of fully immersive peripherals specific to veterinary students' psychomotor development and knowledge acquisition. Preliminary study by Xu et al. (2022), for example use hand-tracking for equine anatomy and safety techniques for large animals, however, these are currently model studies with authors acknowledging that research needs to be conducted to gather data about its effectiveness. From the literature, evidence suggests teaching methods present in veterinary curricula cannot keep up with the demands of a strained education system (Rösch et al., 2014). Furthermore, neglecting skills training for a theory-based curriculum has fatal consequences, particularly when performing CSF collection (Luján Feliu-Pascual et al., 2008).

Results from these findings would require the analysis of parameters of varying interaction paradigms and associate impact across transferable skills and theoretical training from VE's to offer the most optimal resource for training clinical procedures. Within veterinary training, there may be an opportunity to analyse the use of these peripherals when the focus is placed on high-fidelity environments and interactions to produce a near 1:1 scaled representation of CSF collection.

Where some evidence suggests the positive impact of VE's as a potential solution to a lack of theoretical education (de Bie and Lipman 2012; Routh et al. 2021), the lack of existing empirical data surrounding this paradigm for the supplementation of physical learning opportunities necessitates the analysis of parameters impacting transferable skills and knowledge from VE's to offer the most optimal resource for training clinical procedures in veterinary education.

5.1.3 Aims and Objectives

This study aimed to investigate the process of motor skill refinement and knowledge acquisition from VE's and discuss the impact of interaction paradigms through empirical evidence.

This was achieved through the segmentation and development of anatomically accurate models of canine anatomy into 3D models suitable for real-time simulations for standalone virtualisation hardware, wherein users completed skills-based training using interaction paradigms involving either controller or hand-tracking interactions for CSF collection. This was achieved using kinematic motion, as well as auditory and haptic feedback to establish natural physical interactions, invoking feelings of immersion and presence.

To measure this, veterinary students evaluated the simulated environment and assessed how interaction paradigms impacted their perceived ability to refine clinical skills and improve their learning experience. This data was recorded and presented as a comparison study to understand the individual facets of immersion and usability, and their overall impact on interaction paradigms as vectors of mimicking physical clinical training.

5.2 Methods and Materials

The creation of the VE saw the development of a production pipeline, synchronising the digital reconstruction of multiple anatomical structures, and the development of interactive functions to produce the final training simulator.

5.2.1 Apparatus

5.2.1.1 Data

To ensure the development of clinical skills in VE's, anatomical accuracy was the key focus throughout the preliminary developmental stages. DICOM datasets, provided by Dr. Rodrigo Gutierrez Quintana and Julien Guevar, would be employed to generate segmentations of canine anatomical structures (Table 5.1).

5.2.1.2 Hardware

The following hardware was utilised in the creation and deployment of the veterinary simulation (Table 5.2). The Meta Quest 2, a fully immersive standalone head-mounted display (HMD) capable of running Android-compatible VR applications natively within the device, was used to run the developed training simulator. The project would target this device due to the versatility of the hardware as a standalone system, and the array of available XR development packages suitable for simulation deployment (Fig. 5.3) (Meta, 2023).

Table 5.1 DICOM Dataset Output meshes

Case number	Series number	Anatomical region	Segmentation	Export use	Provided by
1	*4*	Head and neck	• C-1-5 Spinal vertebrae • Occipital bone • Maxilla • Mandible • Soft Tissue	Rigging of head and neck bones for exposing CMC	Rodrigo Gutierrez Quintana
2	*101* *102* *108*	Brain and CSF	• Atlanto-occipital cistern • CSF • Spinal cord • Dura	Dura, CSF, and spine colliders	Matthieu Poyade
3	6: Neck and paws 7: Thorax	Caudal region of the neck, paws, scapula, and thorax	• Thorax • Scapula • Ulnar • Radius • Metacarpals • Digits • Humerus	Providing anatomical context for neck region for X-ray in the simulation	Matthieu Poyade

Table 5.2 Device specifications

PC specifications	
Desktop	PC Tornado R3
Processor	AMD Ryzen 3 4100 Processor 3.8 GHz/4.0 GHz
GPU	NVIDIA GeForce GTX 1650 4 GB
RAM	8 Gb
HMD specifications	
Headset	Meta (Oculus) Quest 2:
Display	LCD 1832 x 1920 resolution per eye
Refresh rate	72 Hz
Tracking	6 Degrees of freedom, inside out
RAM	6Gb
Input modality	Controllers and hand-tracking

5.2.1.3 Software

The development of the simulation requires individual software packages capable of synchronising created assets from one stage of the pipeline to the next. The anatomical accuracy of organic models required the provision of specialist segmentation software (Table 5.3) for the generation and refinement of 3D anatomical structures. For the simulation aspect, the use of real-time engines was used to build the constructed environment environments for the training to take place, audio feedback was used at various points of the simulation to provide indicators of clinical error, needle position in relation to the spinal cord, and penetration of the dura (Table 5.4).

5.2.2 Design and Development

High-fidelity environments and variations in interaction modalities were identified as essential factors in the transfer of motor skills and knowledge within virtual spaces (McMahan et al., 2016; Dede et al., 2017). In the context of veterinary science, this takes the form of a high-fidelity simulation that, through controller and controller-less modalities, allows users to explore CSF sampling in a safe environment. By eliciting consistent feelings of face validity across all aspects of the simulation, veterinary students would potentially see the development of motor function akin to that of physical clinical practice. Supplying evidence to support this, the environment necessitated the methodologies to assess what parameters affect this validity, understanding specific interaction paradigms and their factors that hinder or supply immersive properties. A waterfall development pipeline was generated to assess the necessary activities that would be undertaken following these parameters for success (Fig. 5.4) and identify the key milestones (Fig. 5.5) throughout the research.

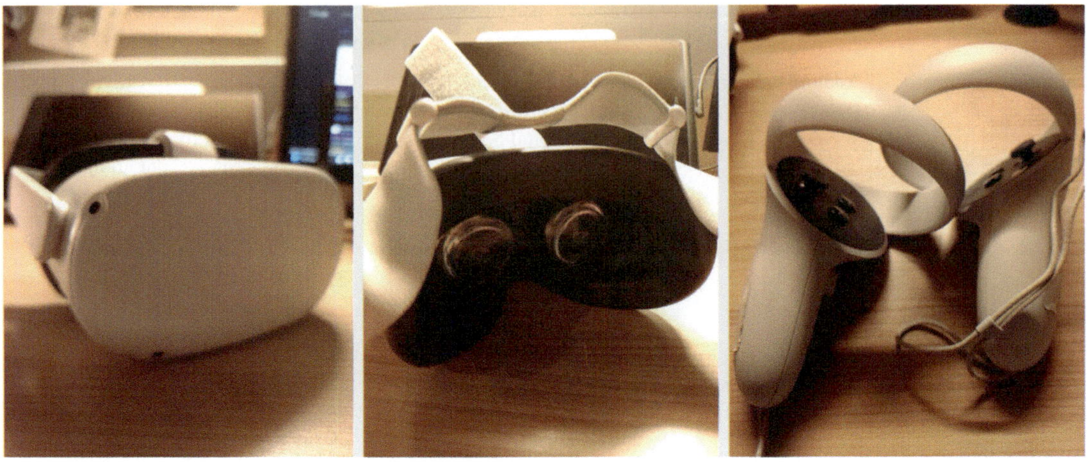

Fig. 5.3 Meta Quest headset (left and centre) and touch controllers (right)

5.2.2.1 Storyboarding

A storyboard was proposed to describe the narrative structure and interactions for a simulated VR experience, detailing potential diversion routes for individual interaction modalities. Figures 5.6, 5.7, and 5.8 show the initial simulation structure and diverging interaction processes.

5.2.2.2 3D Anatomical Segmentation

Segmentation in Slicer3D, a volumetric visualisation platform, is a critical aspect of the process of digital reconstruction of anatomical structures. Producing 3D anatomical assets with this method prioritises the anatomical accuracy of outputted graphics.

DICOM datasets were utilised to attain anatomical structures required for the simulation of CMC sampling. The proposed methodology for the production of viable mesh generation for real-time engines utilised a production pipeline where datasets were refined using imaging filters before necessary anatomical structures in each dataset were identified and segmented to produce a polygonal mesh (Fig. 5.9).

5.2.2.2.1 Case Number 1: Head and Neck Segmentation

Case 1 provided landmark skeletal structures vital in performing a CMC sampling including the occipital bone, cervical vertebrae 1 through 5, and the foramen magnum. Due to the importance of these structures for the identification of the CMC via physical palpation, this dataset was a primary focus for segmentation accuracy for physical interactions within the simulator. Key structures were marked with the mark-up tool throughout the segmentation process to maintain visual on necessary structures to be output. Noise identified within the dataset presented potential issues for segmentation tools utilising isodensity range selection and automatic boundary detection. This noise distortion was corrected via median imaging filtering to add a controlled blur whilst maintaining the edge boundaries of the dataset (Fig. 5.10).

A threshold filter was applied in the slicer segmentation module to generate a base mesh, which would then be refined by shrinking the output segment by 1 mm to conform to the structure's edges more accurately. Minor fusion of segment structures was manually separated. This was exported as label maps to generate exportable mesh data. The surface toolbox was used with Laplacian smoothing and decimation, allowing for boundary edges between bones to be maintained (Fig. 5.11) and maintain accuracy for later physics calculations. This process would then be repeated to attain the soft tissue layer from this segmentation, with the addition of the hollow segmentation tool to hollow the skin layer ready for positioning over the skull (Fig. 5.12).

Table 5.3 List of applications used throughout the generation and implementation of the simulation

Application	Version number	Application use	Accessible from
3D Mesh generation			
3DSlicer 3D Slicer blender	*5.0.3*	• Segmentation of DICOM datasets to create base models • Direct volume rendering to create multi-plane reference material for 3D sculpting	https://download.slicer.org/
Blender	*3.3.1*	• Box-modelling of larger organic structures and hard surface structures • Procedural generation of textures • Exportation of texture maps • UV unwrapping of models • Sculpting and refinement of organic structures • Rigging and animation for real-time engine	https://www.blender.org
Instant meshes	n.a.	• Remeshing sculpted meshes	https://github.com/wjakob/instant-meshes
Simulation development			
Visual Studio Code	*1.78.0*	• C# Programming for simulation interactions and core functionality	https://code.visualstudio.com/

(continued)

Table 5.3 (continued)

Application	Version number	Application use	Accessible from
Adobe Illustrator	*27.7*	• Creation of UI assets	
Unity	*2021.3.11*	• Creation of a simulated environment and core engine • Conversion and exportation to standalone devices	https://unity.com/

Table 5.4 Audio files and their use within the simulation

SFX name	Producer	Use case	Available from
Beep	Qubodup	Menu pop-in sound	https://opengameart.org/content/beep-tone-sound-sfx
Interface	p0ss	For Hand grab SFX	https://opengameart.org/content/interface-sounds-starter-pack
Electric Hum	SoundsForYou	Error Buzz	https://pixabay.com/sound-effects/electric-hum-141075/
Paisaje-sonoro-uem-maquina04	Pixabay	For Distance Detector SFX	https://pixabay.com/sound-effects/paisaje-sonoro-uem-maquina04-98111/
Body Fall On Carpet	Pixabay	For Palpation SFX	https://pixabay.com/sound-effects/bodyfall-on-carpetwav-14747/
Pillow Hit	Sound reality	Dura Puncture SFX	https://pixabay.com/sound-effects/pillow-hit-154187/

5.2.2.2.2 Case Number 2: Brain and Brainstem Segmentation

The goal of this dataset was to produce a mesh capable of inheriting mesh colliders within the simulation program for the needle puncture interactions. It is important to note at this stage, that this segmentation did not aim to replicate complete anatomical accuracy of the brain tissue but to define the dura, subarachnoid space, and spinal cord, to produce the physical sensation of CSF sampling within the simulation. Case 2 provides the shape and size of the spinal cord and cistern, and areas of CSF from the T2 weighted MRI data, using threshold filtering and manual segmentation to conform to the shape of the required anatomical structures. Finally, a Boolean operation was set to subtract between all three segmentation layers to ensure no gaps were present between these layers (Fig. 5.13).

5.2.2.2.3 Case Number 3: Skeleton Segmentation

This segmentation was utilised to improve validity by providing positional context to the head and neck skeleton isolating C5 to T13 vertebrae following the same segmentation methodology as case 1. This produced a lot of artefacts on the model (Fig. 5.14), a combination of removing islands and closing holes to fill any gaps in the mesh produced by removing islands (Fig. 5.15)

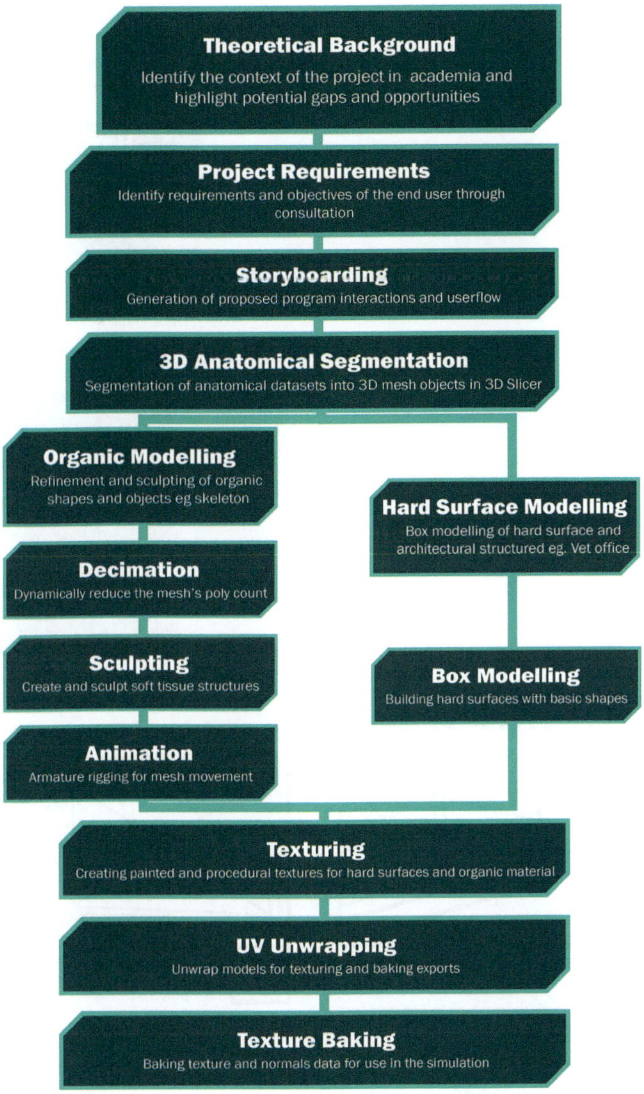

Fig. 5.4 Waterfall diagram detailing the activities to be undertaken throughout the research

this would be refined further in the next stage of the pipeline. Output from Cases 1–3 would be imported into the 3D modelling software blender for refinement.

5.2.2.3 3D Modelling and Sculpting

Mesh outputs from segmentation software are unsuitable for deployment across real-time engines when unrefined, due to high polygon density and mesh distortion becoming difficult to process on low-end hardware, such as that of standalone HMDs. Output models go through a process of mesh decimation, retopologising, and texture mapping to allow mobile processors to rapidly render real-time changes to the mesh data. The modelling and animation software, Blender, was chosen as the ideal program to fit this workflow, due to its multi-faceted capabilities of completing many steps within a synchronous environment through its powerful editing tools and geometry filters. This accommodated both organic modelling and the hard surface modelling of the simulated environment.

5.2.2.3.1 Collation and Decimation of the Skeleton

Wavefront Object (.OBJ) meshes from 3DSlicer were imported into Blender to create the CMC

Fig. 5.5 Waterfall diagram detailing the key milestones throughout the research

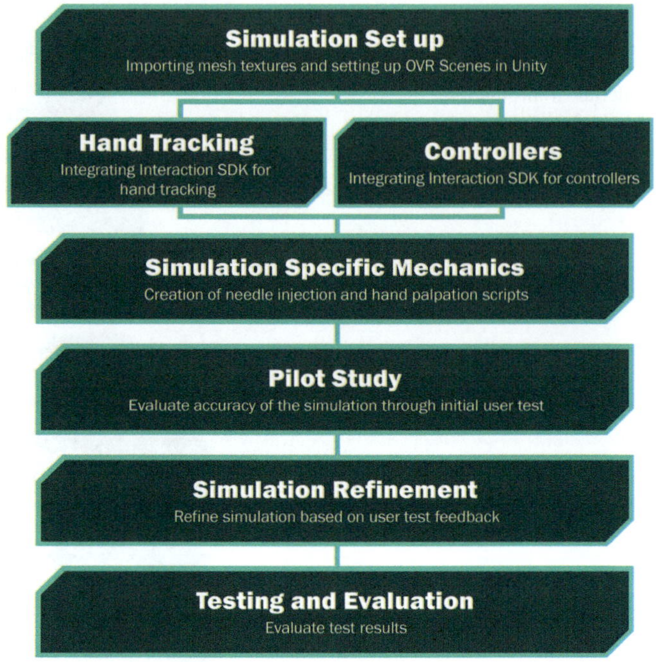

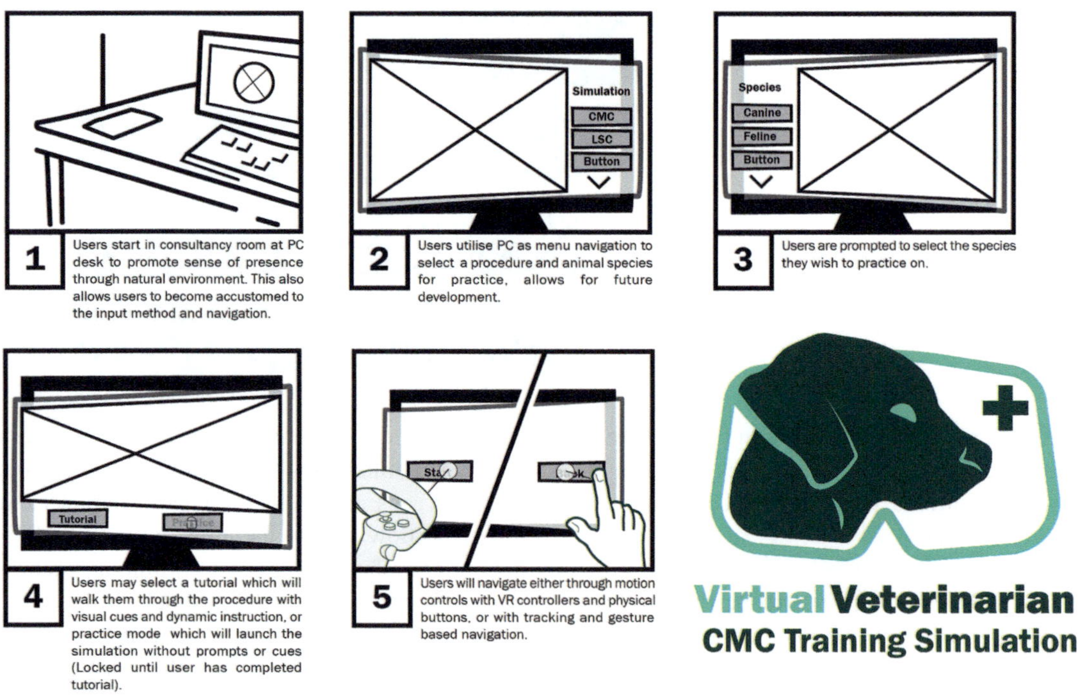

Fig. 5.6 Proposed application structure for onboarding users into the simulation

and underlying spinal structures. The head, neck, and thorax mesh were positioned in context to their neighbouring structures, using anatomical landmarks from the segmentation process as reference points. Finally, the layered brain and cistern mesh were placed in between the occipital

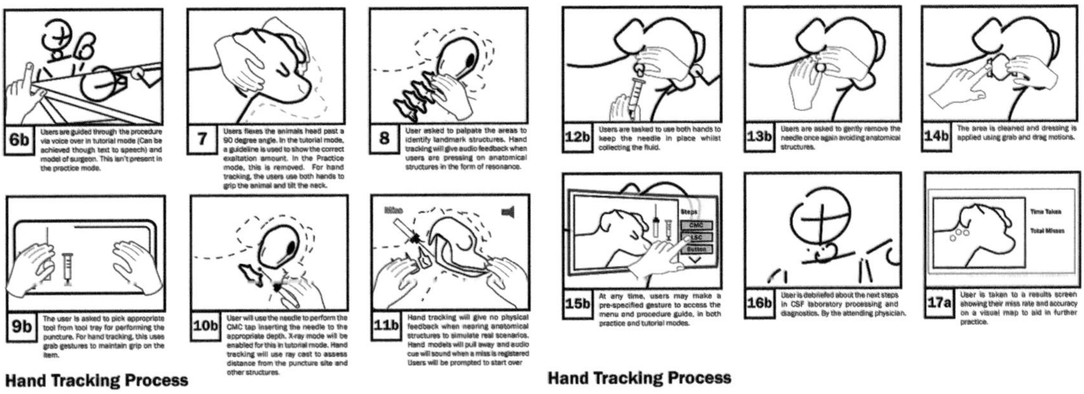

Fig. 5.7 Diverging program structure detailing modality of hand-tracking-based interactions

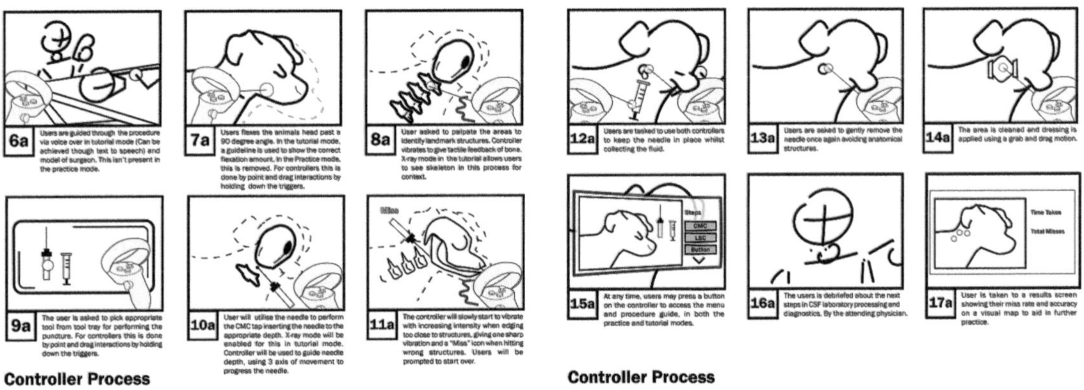

Fig. 5.8 Diverging program structure detailing modality of controller-based interactions

bone and through C1 (Fig. 5.16). Overlapping segmentations such as C5 from the thorax and paws mesh, were unified using a union Boolean operation to combine the separated mesh (Fig. 5.17). A full explanation of this modifier and all 3D tools used can be found in Table 5.5 with explanations from (Blender, 2023).

Finally, to prepare the skeleton models for real-time engines, the polygon counts of these elements required reduction to a level that maintained the structure's anatomical accuracy, whilst reducing the polygon count to its lowest possible factor. Using decimation tools, a range of values was assessed (Table 5.6) to bring each element to its lowest suitable mesh density (Fig. 5.18). C1 and the occipital bone received the least amount of decimation due to the necessity of higher poly values for physics calculations within the simulation.

5.2.2.3.2 Organic Sculpting

Soft tissue data was required to cover the CMC and provide opportunities to develop landmark palpation skills. Case 1 was used to form the soft tissue layer of the head, however, other datasets failed to supply adequate soft tissue for the thorax and appendicular skeleton, due to the variation in canine species. Therefore, to improve the accuracy of the rigged dog object, it was decided to sculpt a body mesh to encapsulate the skeleton. To maintain some level of accuracy, indirect volume rendering of case 2 would create reference images for the sculpt (Fig. 5.19).

The base sculpts used a primitive box mesh, to provide a base shape for sculpting (Fig. 5.20). The head and the body mesh were added into sculpt mode and remeshed to generate an even mesh density between the two objects.

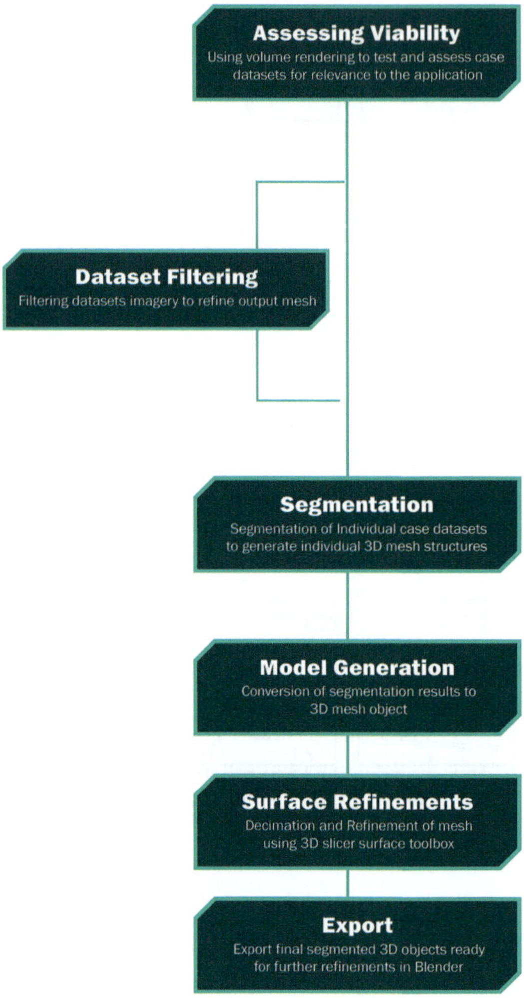

Fig. 5.9 Segmentation pipeline, from input DICOM to export mesh

It was decided to further add elements of validity by sculpting fur on the soft tissue mesh, to circumvent texturing limitations of stereoscopic devices, and hardware limitations of hair particles. Brush packs from GameDev (2022) were used to sculpt fur detailing which could later be baked to surface normal to limit the number of polygons on the mesh whilst maintaining detail. Table 5.7 details the brushes used within this process and their use cases (Fig. 5.21).

The skin mesh would then be re-topologised using Instant Meshes (Bokun and Jakob, 2019). This allowed for a quick automatic retopology algorithm to dynamically reduce an object's vertex count, by marking areas critical for maintaining edge flow and anatomical structure boundaries. Figure 5.22 shows the final output from Instant Meshes; this was remeshed to quads once more to maintain consistent edge flow.

The box-modelling technique was repeated to create hard surface objects such as the room and collection needles (Fig. 5.23).

5.2.2.3.3 Texturing and Baking

An initial limitation consideration involved stereoscopic-focused environments and an inability to utilise common texturing methods, often making textures appear washed out and larger height variations emitting harsh shadows. As an alternative solution, baked normal maps would be generated from the sculpted mesh to give the illusion of a higher detailed mesh. For the hard surface models, procedural textures were generated using the shader pipeline.

This approach would allow for textures to conform to the room layout with minimal distortion, whilst also allowing for procedural height data generation.

To apply 2D image data to a 3D object, mesh faces are required to be flattened and ripped into mesh religions to conform to a 2D plane in a process deemed UV unwrapping. This is performed via marking mesh seams where faces are separated and unfolded on the texture map. These are then scaled and positioned, with detailed areas taking scale priority on the map. For the soft tissue, these edges were marked as loops around the neck, legs, and tail (Fig. 5.24). This would allow for the accurate generation of textures in the VE.

5.2.2.3.4 Rigging and Animation

Mesh Animation would be vital in displaying the accurate positioning of the animal for CSF collection. For this, armature deformation was utilised to deform and position the organic structures to display lateral recumbency and angle of flexion for collection. To begin this process, an armature was constructed using the skeletal mesh as a reference, and armature bones were assigned a percentage of influence over mesh vertices to mimic the elasticity and muscle of soft tissue using the weight painting module (Fig. 5.25).

Finally, the armature was posed using the newly rigged armature, and animated using key-

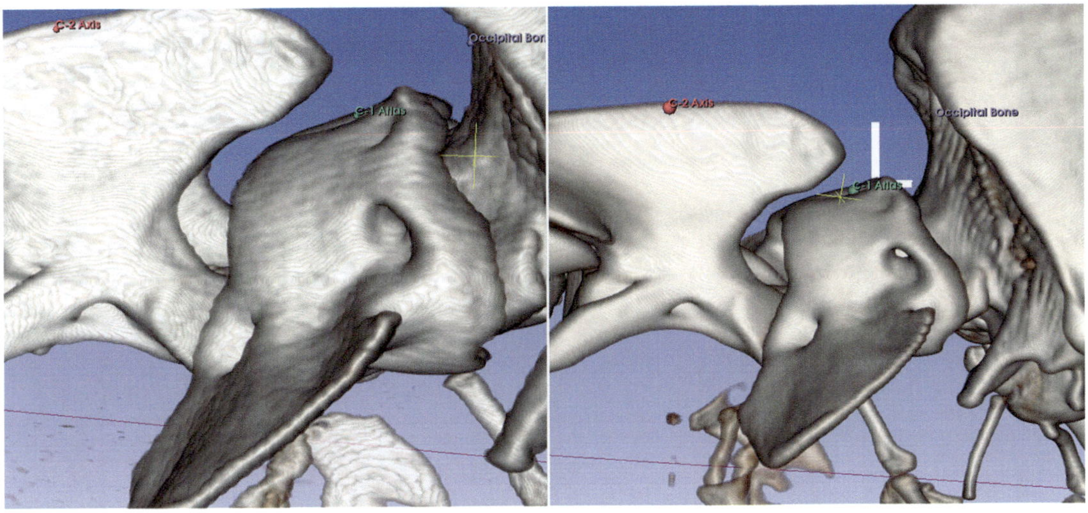

Fig. 5.10 Noisy dataset with soft structure boundaries (left) and dataset Series median image filter applied (right)

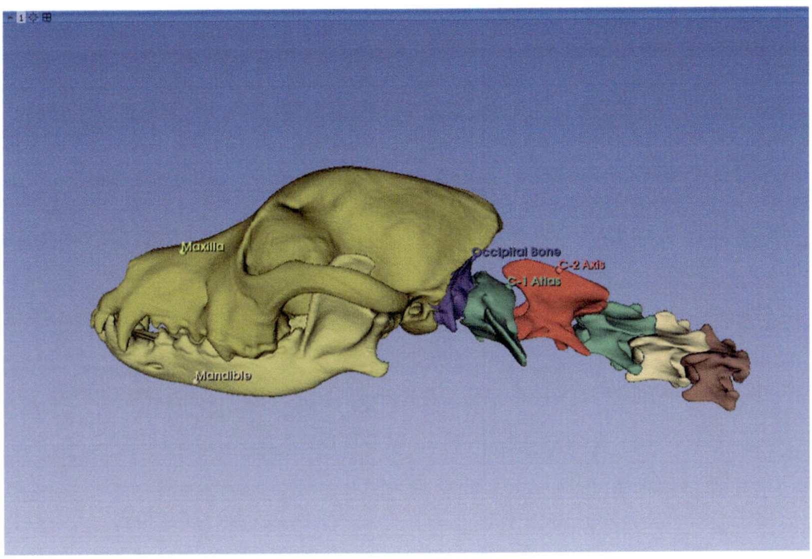

Fig. 5.11 Lateral view of final output segmentation from Case 1

frames to a lateral recumbent position with neck flexion with inverse kinematics to control child bone rotation (Unity 2023a, b, c) (Fig. 5.26). These assets would be imported into unity for the creation of the VE.

5.2.2.4 Unity

Unity within this project, in combination with the Oculus Interaction SDK, accommodates fully immersive environments to be generated across multiple scales of immersive interaction paradigms. These processes utilised organic and hard surface assets, augmented with scripting using the programming language C#, to produce bespoke interactions specific to the context of surgical simulations. The following sections detail the method used for the generation of this high-fidelity VE.

5.2.2.4.1 Setting Up the Simulated Environment

The interaction paradigm needed to remain consistent across both hand-tracking and controller interactions, to ensure equal opportunity for the

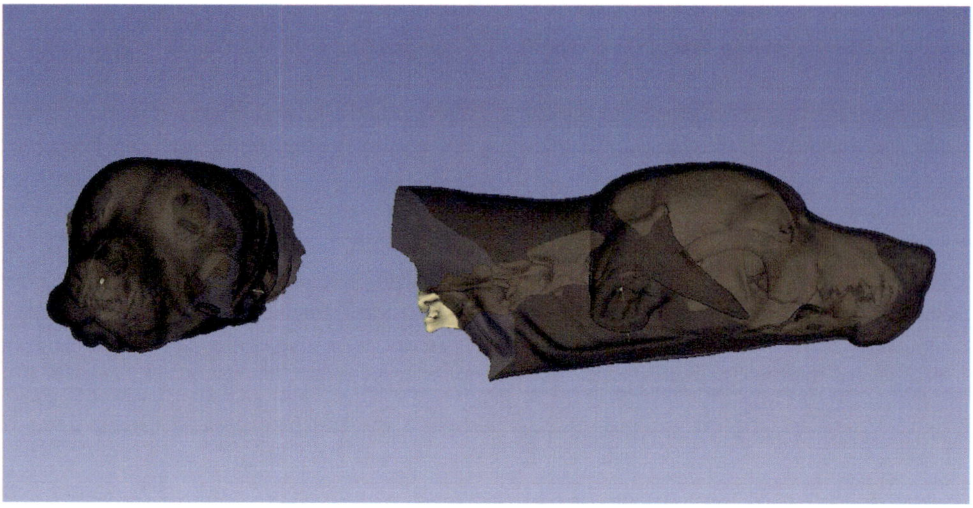

Fig. 5.12 Oblique view (left) and lateral view (right) of final skin segmentation from Case 1

Fig. 5.13 CMC segmentation output mesh

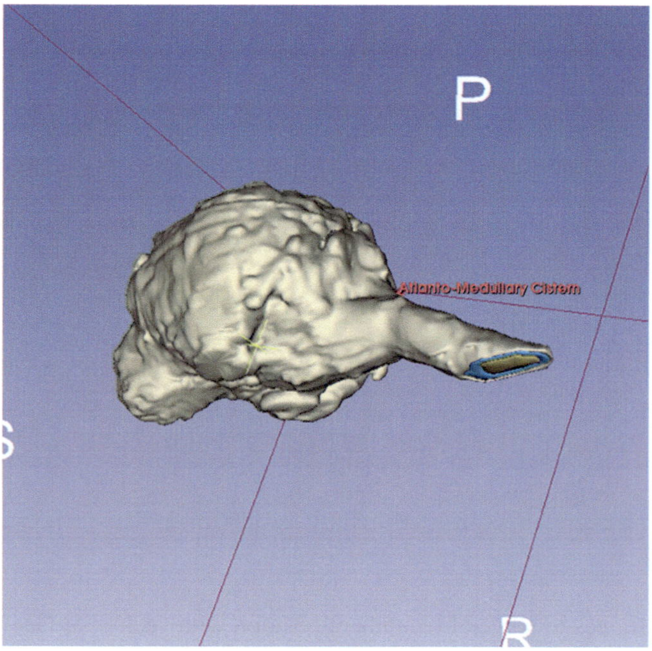

same level of knowledge and transferable skills attainment from both.

The Oculus Interaction SDK was utilised to implement base VR functionality into the simulation for interactions such as grabbing, locomotion, and UI interaction. To function, each interaction paradigm must be referenced in the interactions table found in the OVR interactions prefab, and interactable objects featuring matching component scripts. Table 5.8 below details each OVR interaction element feature in the simulation and their purpose for interaction.

5.2.2.4.2 CSF Sampling Interactions

The use of haptics, auditory and visual feedback as a conduit for realism, and feedback from the simulation across between interaction paradigms, played a key role in directing this interactivity for

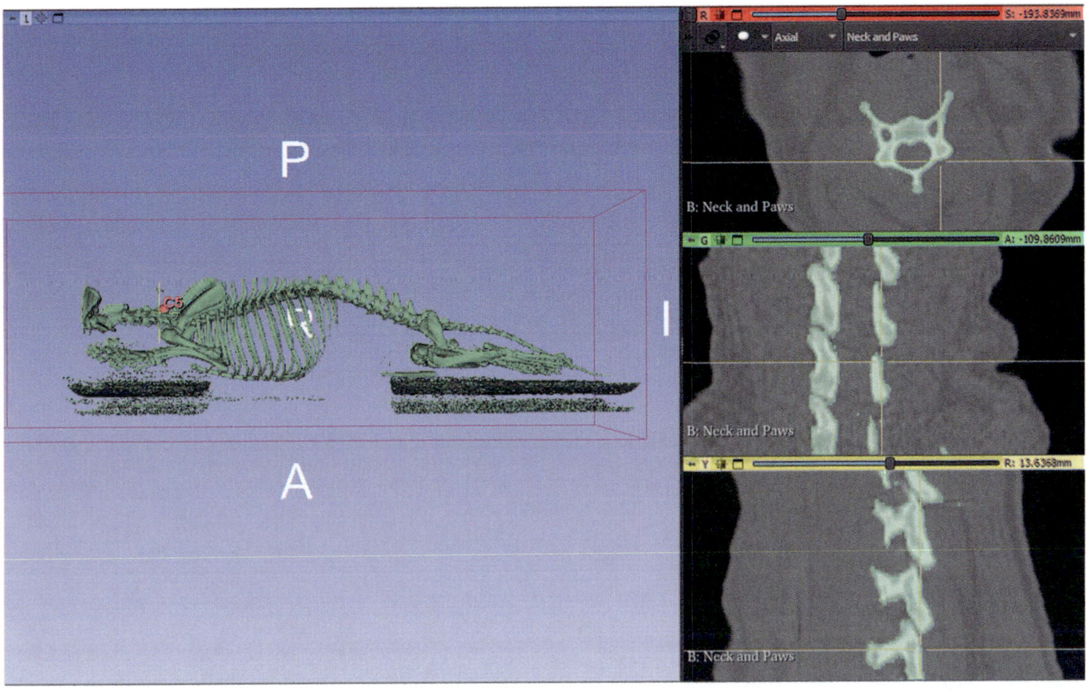

Fig. 5.14 Base mesh produced by threshold filter

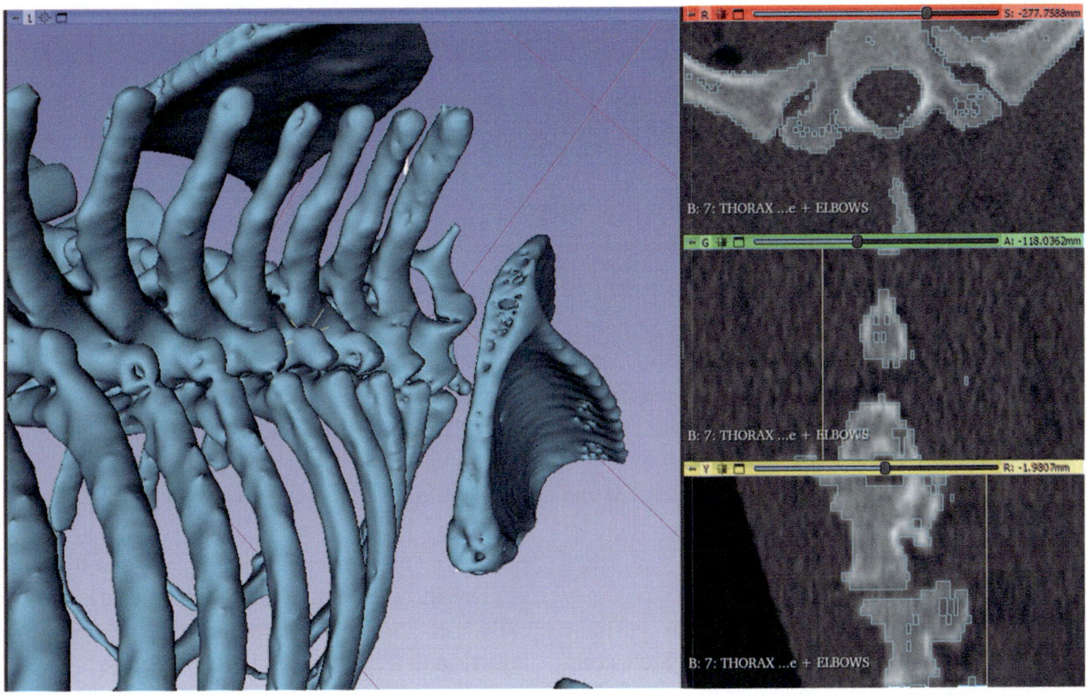

Fig. 5.15 Mesh holes produced by threshold settings

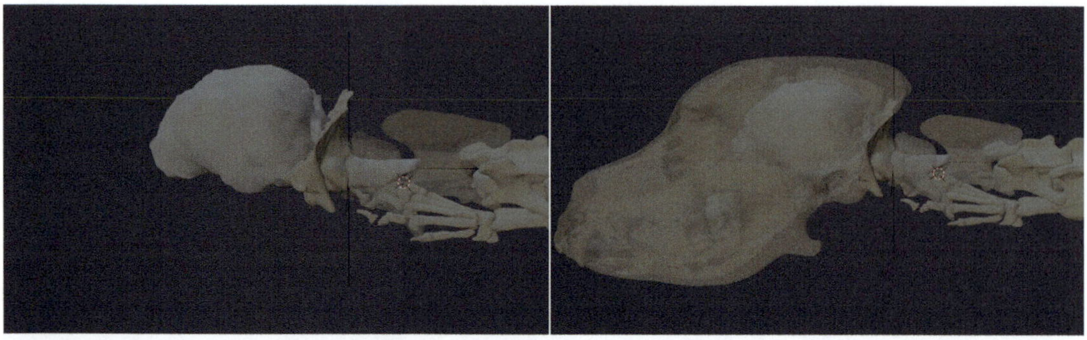

Fig. 5.16 Placement the dura, CSF, and spinal cord caudal to the foramen magnum

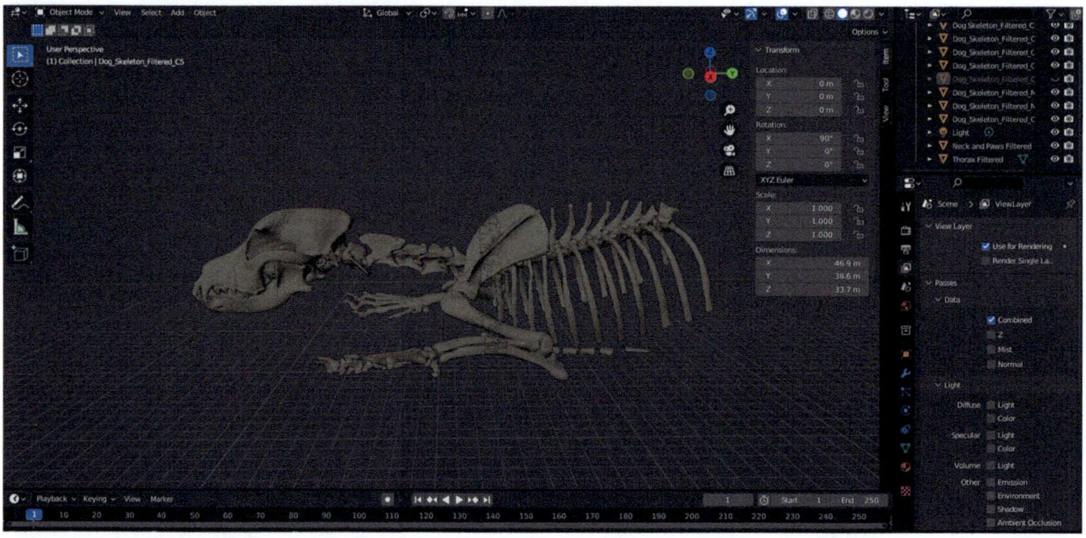

Fig. 5.17 Overlapping Skeleton mesh pre-Boolean modification

mimicking the physicality involved in CSF collection. The placement of the fingertips and articulation of finger joints when grabbing the virtual objects were recorded in the simulated space, using the pose recorder function available within the Oculus Interaction SDK. This accommodated the consistent replication of finger placement and natural grabbing motions to mirror what the user expects to experience with the object's physical counterparts (Fig. 5.27).

The interaction method utilises a bespoke "Needle Puncture Manager" script, which communicates with the game manager to record when the sampling needle made contact with the spinal cord or the surrounding bone. The goal was to relay to the user via the interaction paradigm when the procedure was successful, or when a clinical error was made.

Where collision detection was a consideration for this application, for collision data to register one of the colliding objects must contain a non-kinematic rigid body (Unity 2023a, b, c). Grabbable objects in accordance with the Oculus SDK must be kinematic, as well as non-kinematic elements are restricted to 255 polygons on convex mesh colliders (Unity 2023a, b, c), drastically reducing the potential for accuracy in injection detection (Fig. 5.28).

Trigger functions were found to provide more reliable detection error by comparison, whilst maintaining core functionality, however, still may trigger false errors. An offset in mesh detec-

Table 5.5 Explanation of geometry modifiers used throughout the project (Blender, 2023)

Modifier	Explanation	Input parameters
Sub-division surface	*Procedurally divides mesh geometry by a specified factor, increasing polygon count whilst maintaining edge flow, and smoothing the appearance of the mesh*	Catmull-Clark: A formula of sub-division primarily focusing on mesh appearance and face smoothing
Mirror	Mirrors a mesh across its object's origin across a specified local axis	X-axis mirror: Mirrors mesh geometry in accordance with the object's origin point on the X-axis Clipping: Combines mesh geometry at the mirror's intersection point preventing geometry from moving past the mirror plane Merge: Combines verts where they intersect the mirror plane
Remesh	Generates new quad topology based on the edge flow of the input mesh	Voxel: Creates a new manifold mesh whilst maintaining the original input geometries volume Voxel size: Input parameter for the output mesh's resolution Adaptivity: Input parameter for the threshold of triangulated faces where detail is not needed
Decimation	Dynamically reduce the vertex count of a selected mesh whilst maintaining the original shape	Collapse: the collapse and merge of neighbouring vertexes whilst taking the original mesh shape into account Ratio: Input parameter for the number of verts to be removed (0.0–1.0)
Boolean	Uses the intersection points of two meshes to produce a single combined mesh	Union: Adds the target mesh to the selected mesh by removing interior and overlapping polygons, producing a whole combined mesh
Armature	Deform the mesh based on the bone's area of influence set via weight painting	N.A

Table 5.6 Decimation values and output polygon count of the canine skeleton

Model	Decimation ratio	Original face count	Decimated face count
Mandible	0.04	134,170	2682
Skull	0.02	461,225	9223
Occipital bone	0.1	41,507	4149
C1	0.1	37,913	3791
C2	0.045	33,890	1524
C3	0.035	30,366	1062
C4	0.035	31,623	1105
Shoulder, legs, and paws	0.02	738,792	29,315

tion was added to accommodate incongruities in error registration.

When the sampling needle made contact with the spinal cord or the surrounding occipital bone or vertebrae, the simulation would trigger an audio, or a haptic pulse from controllers, to inform the user that a clinical error was made or when the dura was punctured using collision functions and audio source components.

Controller interactions were generated utilising a similar development process, whilst still using hand models as a general representation of natural interactions, posable grabbing was not utilised due to the inability to determine accurate finger position via controller modalities. Finally, controllers would send haptic pulses to the user via the controller to mimic physical sensation.

5.2.2.4.3 Palpation and X-Ray Mechanics

The palpation of anatomical landmarks was replicated in the simulation using ray casting functions, initially achieved via casting from joints of the OVR hands. However, due to the refresh rate of hand-tracking, the ray would often miss the bone due to jittering. Instead, an empty game object's transform was positioned around the left and right index fingers to use as a stable reference point for the ray.

Upon collision, the application would emit a sound to indicate when users interact with the occipital bone or cervical vertebrae, with control-

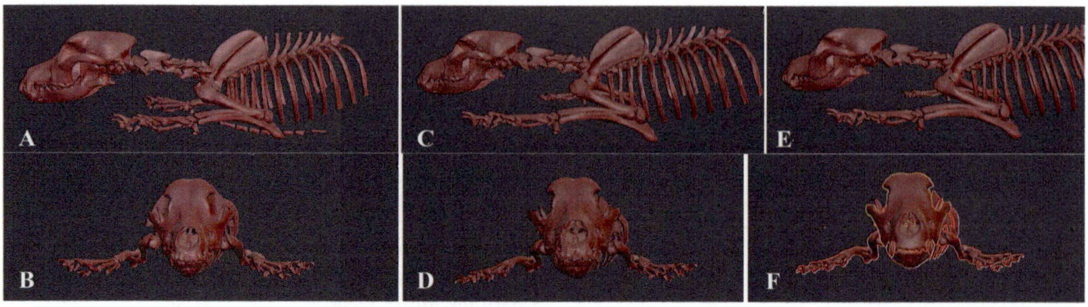

Fig. 5.18 Side profile and front of the decimation process, showing pre-decimation (**a** and **b**), post-decimation (**c** and **d**), and post-decimation with smooth shading (**e** and **f**)

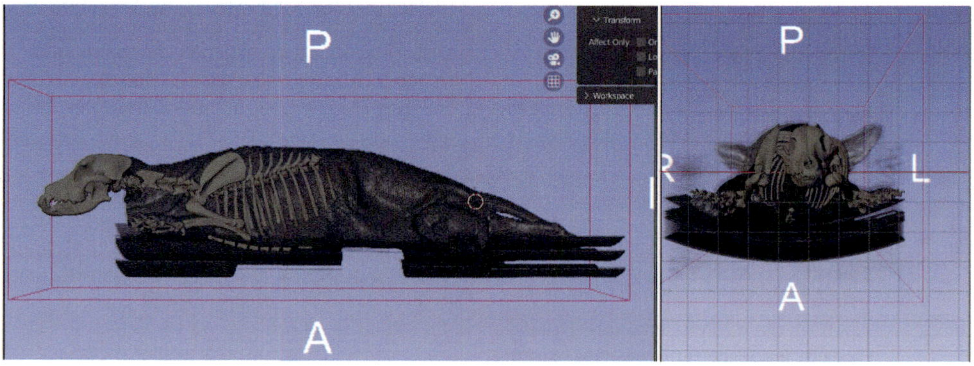

Fig. 5.19 Using DICOM imaging to set up sculpt reference for soft tissues using anatomical structures as placement reference

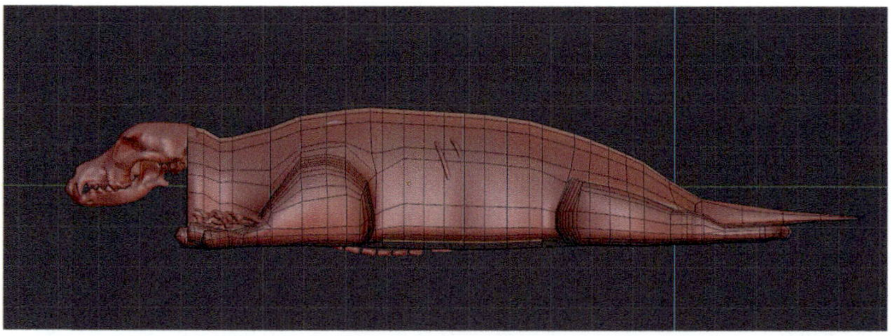

Fig. 5.20 Box modelling to attain the general shape of the canine soft tissue

lers also emitting a haptic pulsing to mimic physical touch. To circumvent an inability to deform soft tissue when palpating, decal markers from the UPR decal component were used to inform the user of an approximate location for landmark structures. Finally, to see the full skeleton for an educational context, an X-ray mode was added, using transparent shaders created using the URP shader graph.

5.2.2.4.4 Refinements

Upon initial testing with nine veterinary participants (3 veterinary students, 2 veterinary graduates, 2 veterinary neurologists, and 2 veterinary

Table 5.7 Blender sculpting tools and their uses

Tool	Definition	Use case
Dynamic retopology	Dynamically add extra geometry around the cursor whilst sculpting	Add geometry to the mesh whilst sculpting the definition
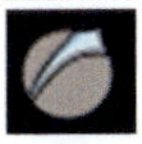 Crease	Create crevasses and valleys in the mesh	Create muscle definition and crease areas where the legs meet the body
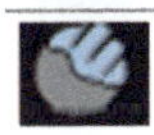 Clay strips	Add strips of extra geometry on top of the mesh surface	Add extra geometry around specific areas to define muscular structures
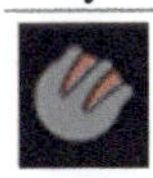 Fill	Bridge creases in the geometry	Bridge gaps between paws and bridge remnants between the head and body meshes
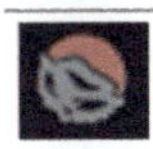 Smooth	Smooth peaks in the mesh	Smooth out mesh after remesh
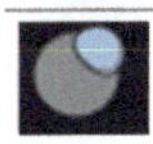 Inflate	Expand the geometry and pull it away from the mesh	Define whole body shape
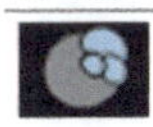 Blob	*Spherize geometry at the location of the cursor*	Refine back leg shape
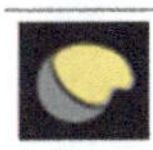 Elastic deform	*Dynamically pull/push the mesh at the point of the cursor*	Conform the mesh to the underlying skeleton
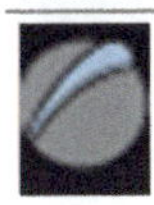 Draw	Create small detailing on the mesh	Fur detailing and mouth definition

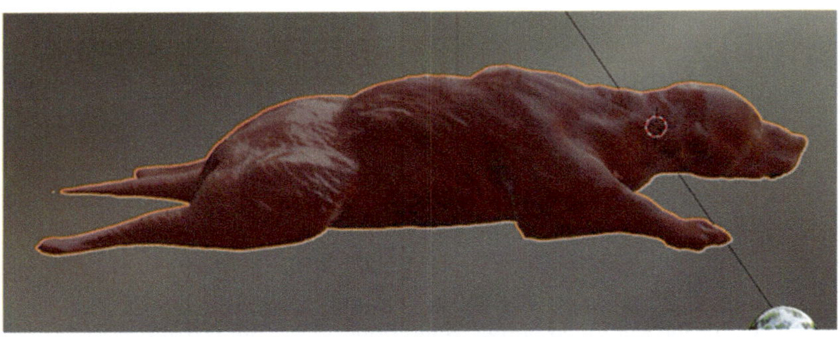

Fig. 5.21 Canine mesh with sculpted fur detailing

surgeons), the program would be further refined based on user feedback relating to difficulty. The false triggering of clinical errors was found to be a consistent issue and therefore changes to the size of the cistern and the needle detection offset were implemented to accommodate for a wider grace period of error detection. This would mark the end of the development pipeline, producing a complete skills training simulation.

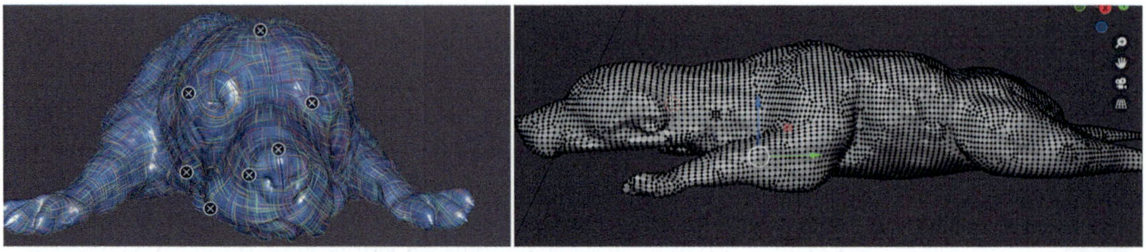

Fig. 5.22 Marked edge flow and final output mesh

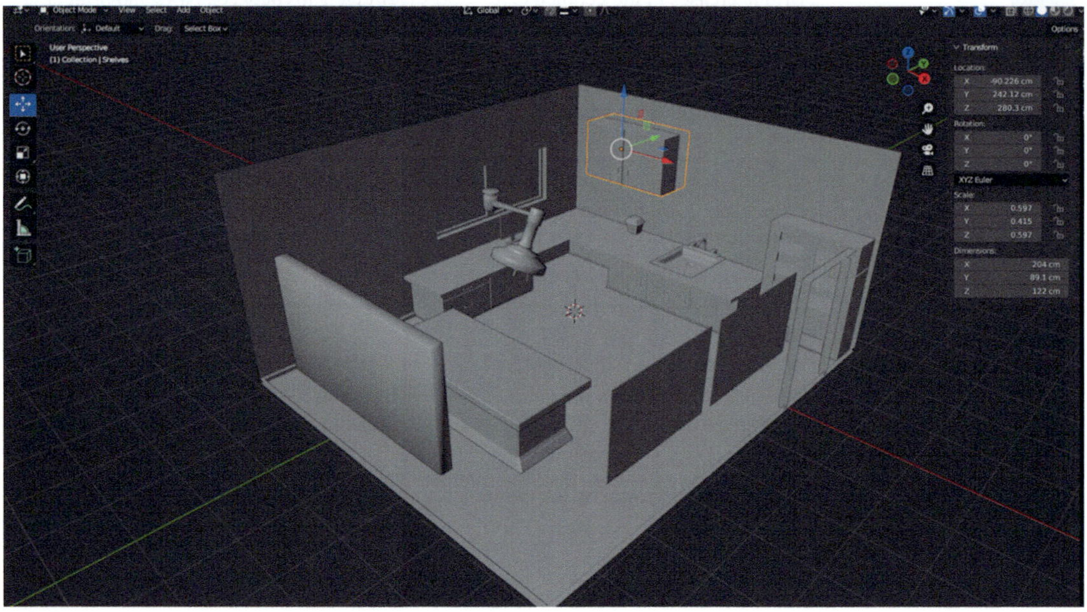

Fig. 5.23 Populating simulation room using hard surface modelling techniques

5.3 Development Outcomes

The following section documents the outcome assets for the environment and the final VR simulation. Outcomes from the proposed methodology produced an interactive spinal tap VR simulation within the real-time engine unity, which would be deployed across standalone virtualisation hardware. This simulation would allow users to repeatedly practice CMC sampling of CSF in canine species to further refine clinical and motor skills in a safe environment using both controller and hand-tracking paradigms of interaction.

5.3.1 Organic Modelling Assets

5.3.1.1 Canine Model

Figure 5.29 shows the fully rendered skeleton including the legs and thorax. This was rigged and animated to expose the cistern upon flexion of the neck. The final soft tissue mesh was generated from a mix of segmentation models and sculpting seen in Fig. 5.30.

5.3.1.2 Cerebellomedullary Cistern

The final cistern model was segmented into dura, CSF, and spinal cord meshes from the case 2 dataset. The final layered model can be seen in Fig. 5.31.

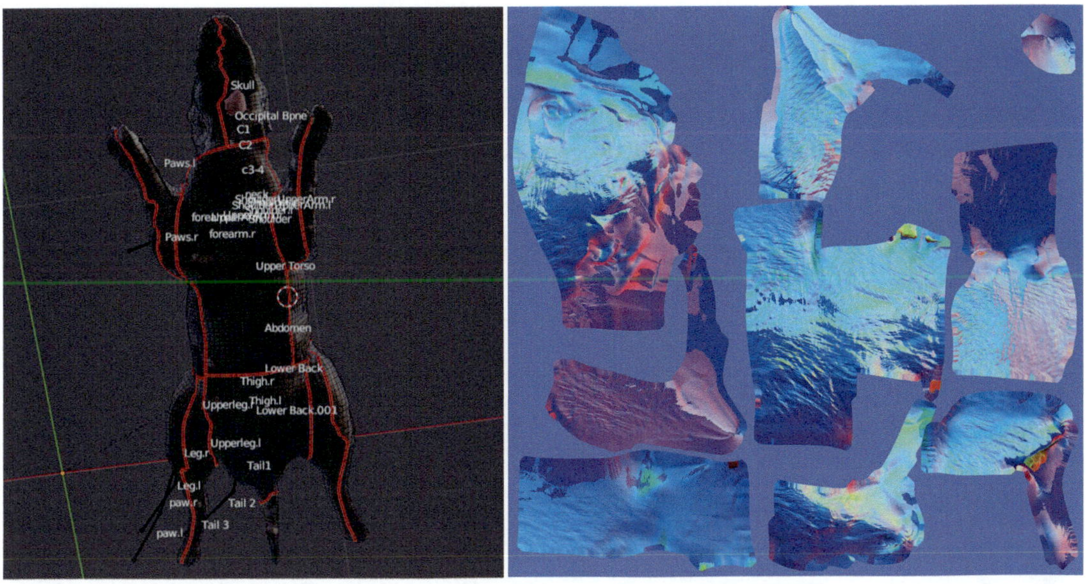

Fig. 5.24 Marking seams to unwrap organic mesh (left) for texture map baking (right)

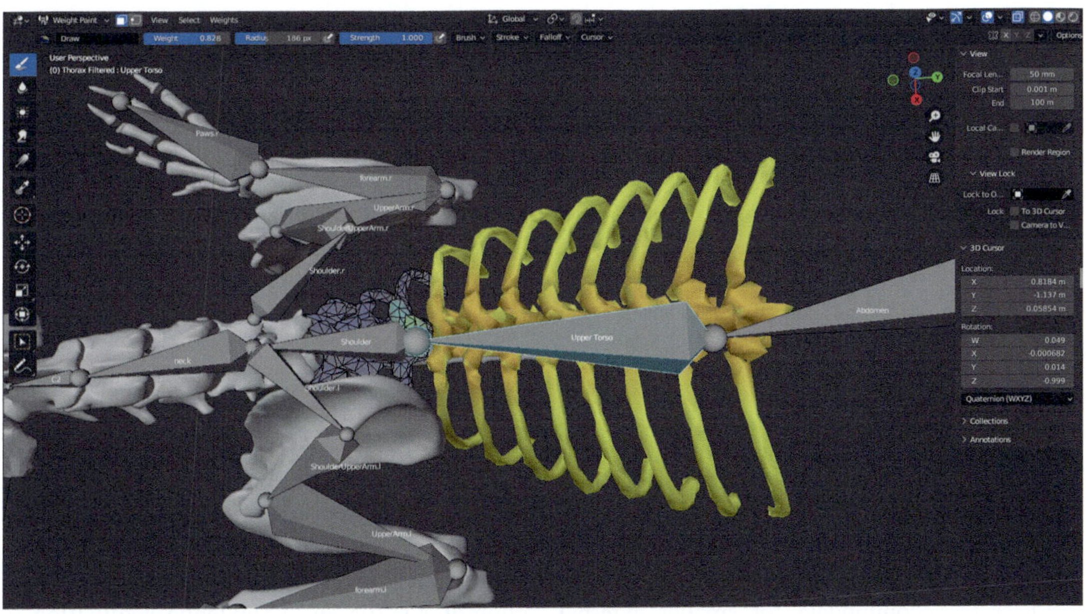

Fig. 5.25 Process showing weight painting, assigning vertex weights to the selected bone

5.3.2 Simulation

The final simulation was deployable across android comparable HMDs where interaction paradigms for both controllers and hand-tracking were supported. Users would be presented with the canine for practice sampling techniques and an information panel explaining paradigm-specific instructions.

Users could use physical grab or poke actions to interact with the environment (Fig. 5.32) or utilise distance grabbing whereby by reaching

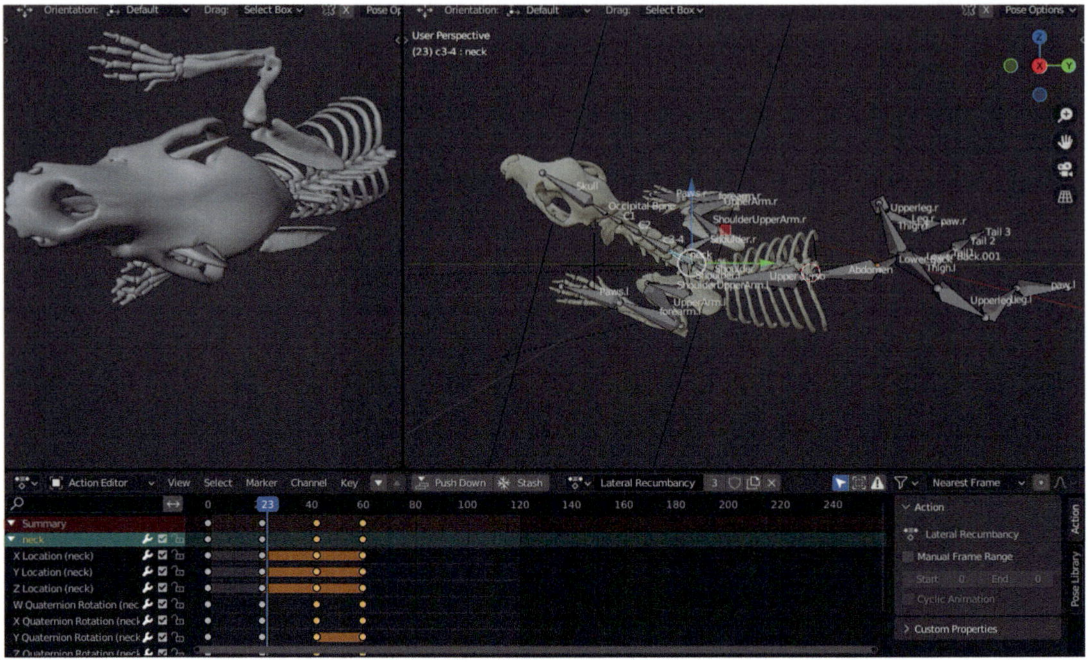

Fig. 5.26 Using keyframe animation to control pose position and rotation

Table 5.8 OVR Interactions and their use

Description	Description
Grabbable	Allows objects to be grabbed in any form
Hand grab interactable	Allows objects to be physically grabbed using pinch or button inputs
Distance hand grab interactable	Allows objects to be grabbed from a distance, moving them towards the user
Ray interactable	Allows elements to be ray cast from hands (used for distance UI)
Poke interactable	Allows canvas UI to be physically pressed

out and pinching, objects would move towards the user to accommodate for smaller external environments.

Users would be able to palpate the area and listen to or feel for auditory and haptic feedback for confirmation of landmark and CMC location, users could then advance the needle into this cistern and once again listen for an audible pop to confirm entering the dura. Finally, users would maintain the needle in the CSF until CSF drainage from the hub is present. Clinical errors would be registered whenever the user made contact with the spinal cord or surrounding cervical vertebrae and occipital bone with the sampling needle. Upon making a clinical error, users would hear a warning buzzer indicating they would need to start over.

5.4 Evaluation

To evaluate the interaction paradigms a mixed method modality aims to answer questions regarding if interaction modality would have a significant impact on the development of psychomotor skills and knowledge acquisition in veterinary skills training. Participants would be presented with the ITC Sense of Presence Inventory (Lessiter et al., 2001) for assessing presence and immersion, promoting participants to score statements regarding the simulation on a 5-point Likert scale where 1 meant strongly disagree, 2 meant disagree, 3 meant neutral, 4 meant agree, and 5 meant strongly

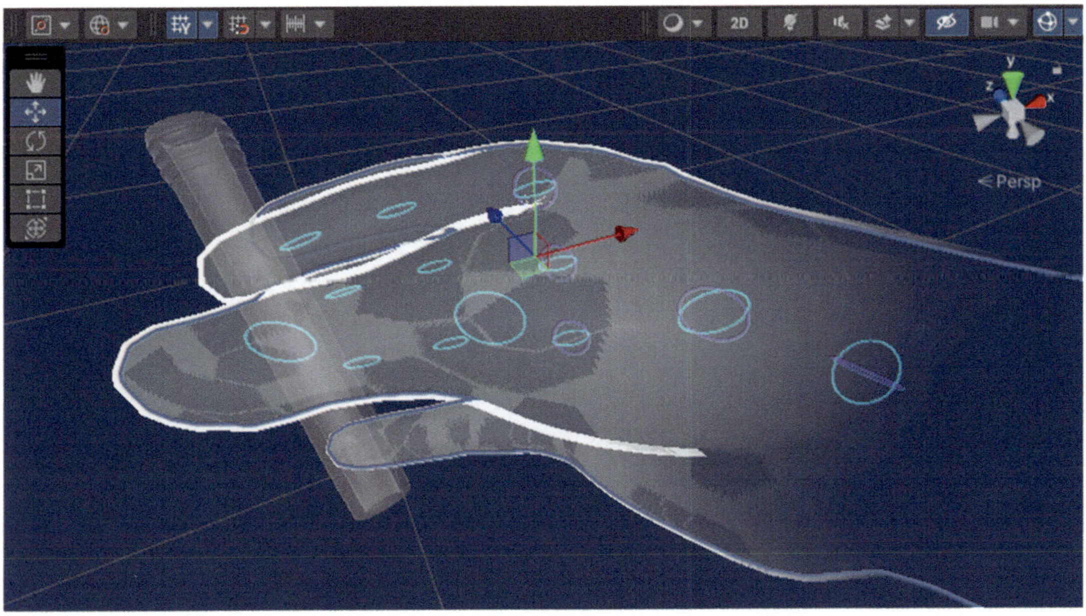

Fig. 5.27 Adjusting hand poses to create realistic grab motions for needle puncture instruments

Fig. 5.28 Convex mesh limitations create collider inaccuracies

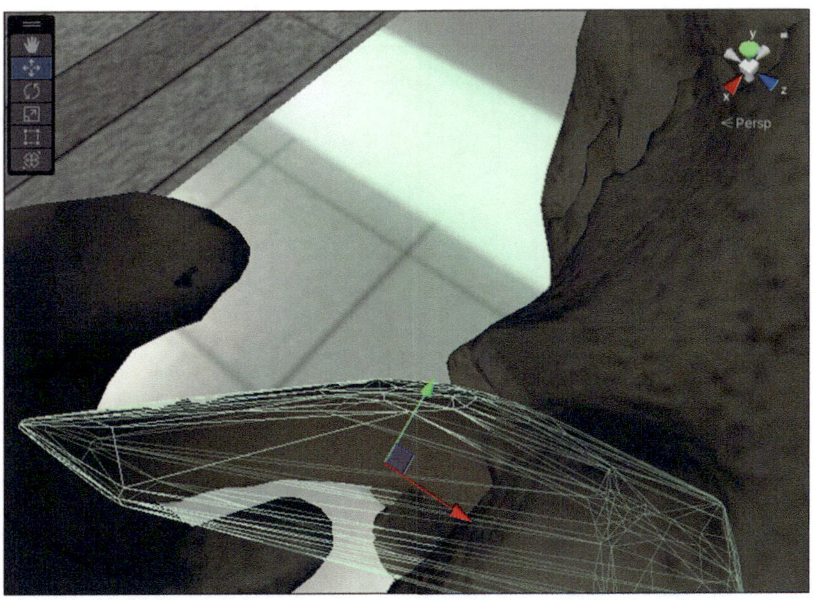

agree. Participants were also asked to complete a qualitative questionnaire, prompting users to assess what they considered positive and negative aspects of the simulation, perspective improvements they wished to see, and the potential of the technology within their education.

5.4.1 Methods

5.4.1.1 Participants

Fourteen participants were recruited from a cohort of veterinarians, from a range of experience levels, from the University of Glasgow's Small Animal Hospital in Glasgow. Participants

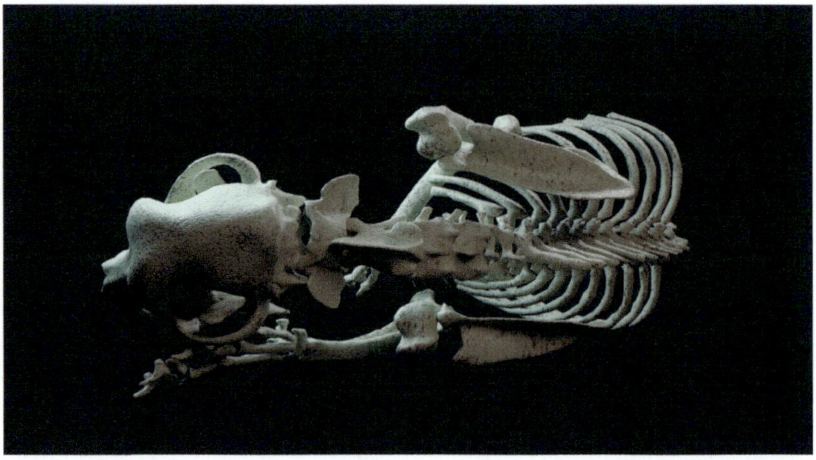

Fig. 5.29 Segmented, textured, and rigged canine skeleton in lateral recumbency with flexed head

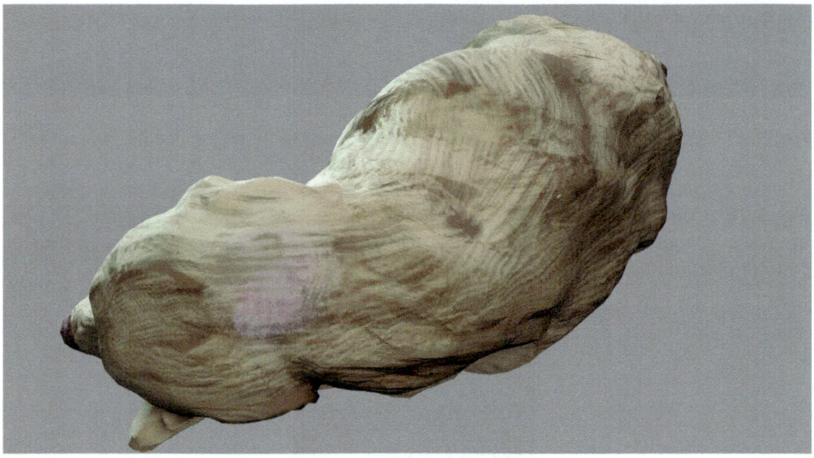

Fig. 5.30 Sculpted, textured, and rigged canine mesh in lateral recumbency with flexed head

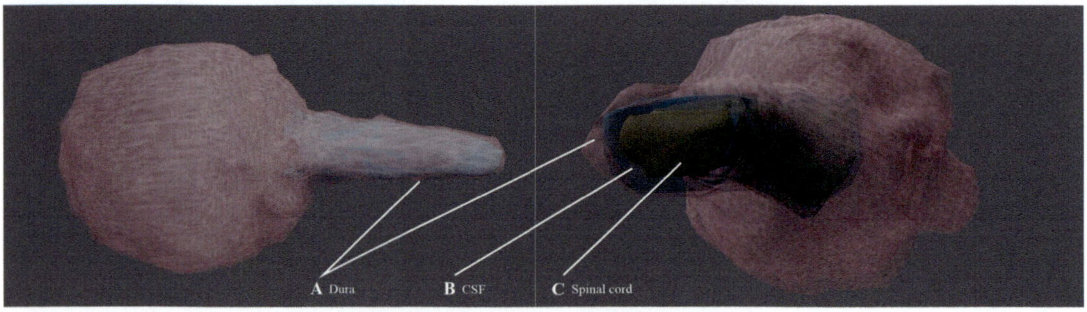

Fig. 5.31 Final Layered Cistern showing dura (**a**), CSF (**b**), and spinal cord (**c**)

were presented with an information sheet and consent form, detailing the apparatus, purpose, procedure, and associated risks of the study prior to their participation. This research was granted ethical approval by the Glasgow School of Art Learning and Teaching office.

From the 14 participants (4 Males, 10 Females), veterinary science qualifications

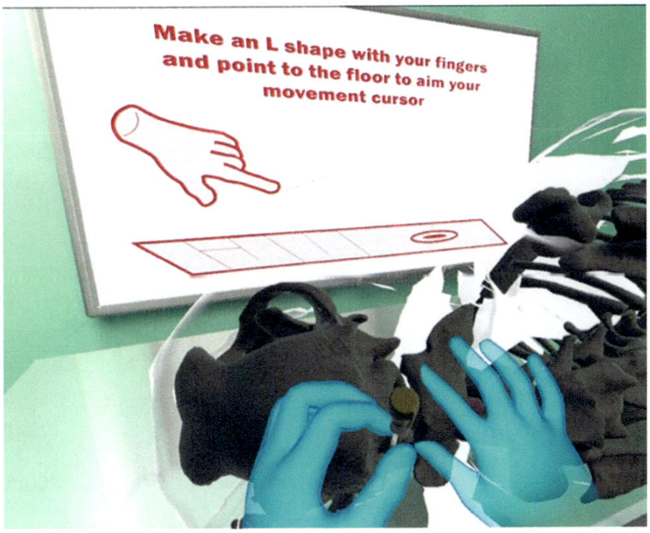

Fig. 5.32 Needle puncture process using grab interactable needle

equated to 6 veterinary students, 5 graduate veterinarians, and 1 veterinary surgeon 1 veterinary nurse. The age of participants ranged from 23 to 44 ($\sigma = 6.13$) years, and an average age of 30 years($\overline{x} = 30$).

5.4.1.2 Procedure

This study took place in the Small Animal Hospital in Glasgow using 2 Meta Quest HMDs to deploy the simulated environment, using controllers and hand-tracking (Fig. 3.1). From the participant pool, 8 participants completed the controller simulation, and 6 completed the hand-tracking simulation.

Participants were briefed on their task to collect the CSF sample from the CMC using their chosen interaction paradigm.

Participants started in front of the injection site, with an instructional panel to their immediate left. Users were asked to read these instructions and collect their tools either via hand grabbing and locomotion or through stationary movement and distance grabbing.

Participants would be asked to perform palpation using markers as a guide, listening for auditory feedback for landmark identification and CMC location. Controller participants would also note haptic feedback when palpating. Participants would advance the needle through the CMC to collect CSF after holding for 1.5 s. Puncturing the dura would produce a pop sound, with controllers also emitting haptic vibrations. If the participant made contact with the spinal cord, or surrounding bone structures such as the cervical vertebrae and occipital bone with the sampling needle, an auditory buzzer would sound, informing the user of a clinical error being made, and must re-attempt collection.

Upon completion of the task, users would then be asked to fill out the post-test survey an ITC-SOPI questionnaire (Lessiter et al., 2001) was presented to participants post-simulation. The four factors of presence presented in this survey would aim to measure a participant's spatial presence in the simulation, their engagement rate, the ecological validity, and potential negative effects.

5.4.1.3 Data Analysis

The mean values ($\overline{x}$) and standard deviation (σ) of participant responses for each section of ITC-SOPI were calculated. Results compared controller groups to those using hand tracking, to measure facets of spatial presence, engagement, ecological validity, adverse effects, and perceived ease of the interaction paradigm to understand users' sense of presence and immersion within the simulation across both paradigms.

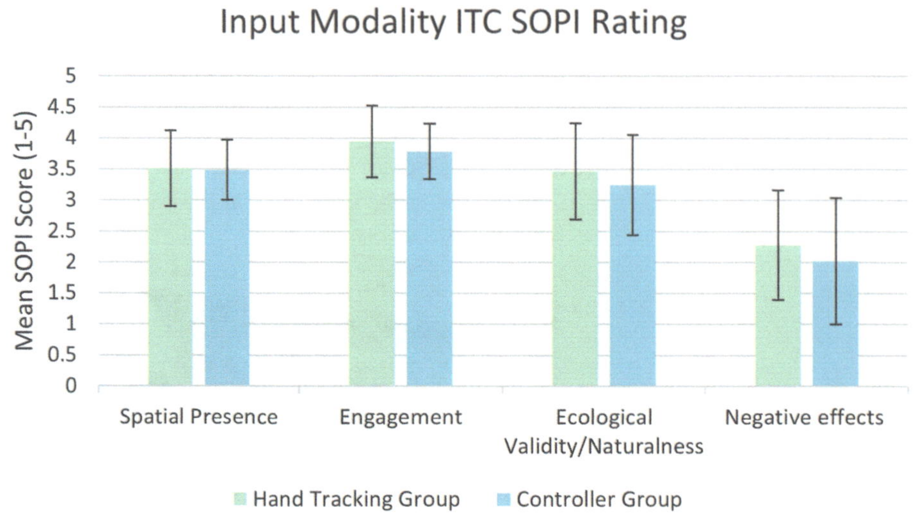

Fig. 5.33 ITC-SOPI comparison detailing immersion and presence across modalities

5.4.2 Results

Results from the ITC-SOPI presented hand-tracking results as a marginally higher perceived sense of presence versus the controller paradigm. Spatial remained in relative consistency across hand-tracking ($\overline{x}$ = 3.51) when compared against the controller paradigm ($\overline{x}$ = 3.48), however, hand-tracking presented a wider response variation ($\sigma = 0.61$) compared to controllers ($\sigma = 0.47$).

Engagement and ecological validity were much higher for hand-tracking (engagement $\overline{x}$ = 3.95 ± 0.58, ecological validity $\overline{x}$ = 3.47 ± 0.78) versus controllers (engagement $\overline{x}$ = 3.78 ± 0.45, ecological validity $\overline{x}$ = 3.25 ± 0.81).

Participants were more likely to experience negative effects such as difficulty using the interaction paradigm and dissonance in movement within the VE whilst utilising hand-tracking ($\overline{x}$ =2.28) compared to controllers ($\overline{x}$ =2.02). However, participant responses varied significantly across this facet, with controllers presenting a wider variance in the score (σ = 1.02) compared to hand-tracking modalities ($\sigma = 0.89$). Figure 5.33 details this comparison in graph format. Out of 14 participants, 13 fully completed the qualitative answer section (Table 5.9). Across both hand tracking and controller groups, participants were in consensus that the simulation both felt realistic and could visually relate the scenario to real-world scenarios. Where improvements were prompted, controller participant responses varied in comparison to hand tracking, with the general trend showing controller participants feeding back on the environment and overall navigation, whereas hand-tracking participants wished to see the interaction accuracy improved. When asked if they perceived this as a useful tool as part of their education, all participants responded positively, stating they would want to see similar simulations in some form in their curriculum.

5.5 Discussion

Collating results there is evidence to support hand-tracking as a superior modality of interaction, presenting heightened levels of immersion and presence. Evaluation findings suggest hand-tracking has a significant impact on a user's ecological validity in drawing connections between the virtual environment and their physical environment in that participants would be capable of immersing themselves consistently in this environment. Furthermore, hand-tracking consistently results in more positive engagement, whilst lower limits remain consistent across both groups. From this, neither modality can be considered detrimental to a user's engagement.

Table 5.9 Participant survey responses

Participant number	What did you like the most about the simulation?	What did you like the least about the simulation?	What would you like to see changed about the simulation?	Do you believe this approach would improve education within veterinary science? Why/Why not?
1	The details, landmarks etc.	N/A	More animal variety (possibly after successful with dog, move on to cat etc.)	Yes, it allows a more realistic visualisation
2	Experience for me was new	Didn't work as it should and a lot of repreogramming was necessary	More realism	Yes, as a first hand experience before clinical work
3	That it is not real and you can actually try as many times as you like because you cannot kill your patient comparing to real life	The graphic needs improvement	I would love to use the gloves in thinking about, however, i do not know whether is technologically possible	Definitely. I think would be amazing to be able to try small procedures or even surgeries in this way before you are actually exposed to that
4	The reaction if you put the needle in wrongly	Picking things up	Possibly an easier way to pick things up	Yes definitely to immerse yourself in a real-world environment to practice and know the steps before trying in real life
5	The ability to practice such a technical skill in a safe environment	The difficulty in navigating the system and the unrealistic animal	Easier to use	Yes, technical skills that are important do not necessarily have the space to practice in a safe environment
6	I did feel like I was in a room	I could not reach out and touch anything	Better hand–eye coordination	Yes but it needs finer tuning
7	Practicing the motions of a skill	Not understanding what the buzzes meant, which button to use	If hands could work, it allows for more realistic hand placement	100% yes, practice is the key to improving
8	Is really interacting and it feels that you are in the simulation	Maybe a little bit more of motion when you touch some of the objects	More approaches	Yes. It makes it more enjoyable
9	The novelty and the option to display X-ray vision	I was initially unfamiliar with the controls	More realistic looking environment	Yes absolutely—the ability to see positioning and switch on/off X-ray vision was so informative
10	Very interactive	I would like to be able to do more things	Put more procedures	I think it will allow to teach in a very enjoyable manner
11	Real application, included X-rays for landmarks	Some functions were inconsistent (reaching objects)	Different sizes of animals/lumbar CSF instead of cisternal	Yes, could be very helpful
12	Being immersed in the environment	Not having anything solid to lean on	Have something to lean on and steady the hand	Yes for understanding approach. No for actually doing the procedure

(continued)

Table 5.9 (continued)

Participant number	What did you like the most about the simulation?	What did you like the least about the simulation?	What would you like to see changed about the simulation?	Do you believe this approach would improve education within veterinary science? Why/Why not?
13	Much smoother with controllers than my own hands	Unable to palpate anatomy, so need to use X-ray setting	Ability to palpate somehow with hands	Yes, I feel it would be very helpful for students to appreciate the anatomy and procedure for spinal taps
14	n.a.	n.a.	n.a.	n.a.

Although controllers share a consistent difficulty and lower rates of immersion and presence through a narrower range of deviation, negative effects were found to be consistently lower compared to hand-tracking. Users reported that controller-based modalities would require more guidance in learning the system than hand-tracking, suggesting a level of complexity associated with controller-based interactions that impact engagement. Much of this contests with what is currently understood in literature, instead displaying the use of hand tracking as a highly immersive paradigm of interaction with a positive rate of engagement despite participants' feedback of kinematic dissonance and findings from previous studies (Hameed et al., 2021; Maran and Glavin, 2003).

Overall, across both modalities, users reported they would see the integration of similar tools implemented in veterinary education, with user feedback presenting an overwhelmingly positive response when questioned about the potential future of this technology in education. Many participants attested this to the ability to attain transferable skills from realism aspects presented through the simulation, and the ability to practice these skills in a repeatable and safe manner suggesting the potential of VR veterinary simulations as a plausible alternative to physical workshops, concurrent with previous findings (Balogh, 2014; Chen et al., 2020; Nagendran et al., 2020).

Where participants made improvement comments, many lay with environmental fidelity for controllers, and interaction fidelity for hand tracking, citing comments such as issues with kinematic motion, coordination of hand movements, and a lack of physical sensation associated with the program. Many of the SOPI results would reflect this, showing a range of negative effects associated with these individual tracking modalities. However, relating the findings to comments made by participants and the lower ecological and spatial validity, much of the negative feedback measured in this facet can be attributed to fidelity for the environment controller groups, despite the digital environment being the same across both groups. This was not as prevalent in the hand-tracking group, potentially because of increased feelings of naturalness present in the increased ecological validity. This remains consistent with fidelity studies regarding VE's, displaying a mid-level of fidelity often detrimental to engagement and a sense of presence (Slater, 2009; Won et al., 2023).

Finally, common traits of controller-based input such as haptic feedback showed little impact on immersion and presence, despite prior literature suggesting this would be beneficial.

5.5.1 Critical Reflection on Methodologies

This study proposed a development pipeline for high-fidelity environments and VE rendering which could be used across hand-tracking and controller modalities, utilising anatomical segmentation of DICOM datasets. This was beneficial in creating the anatomical accuracy necessary for the validity of the simulation; however, it is important to acknowledge that the decimation process to reduce model vertex count to improve overall simulation performance, the anatomical accuracy of the initial output from segmentation to a suitable real-time engine asset will be proportional to the amount of mesh decimation applied to the mesh. Detail mapping was an ideal equilibrium to bridge validity whilst reducing mesh density, however, this cannot impact larger elements of geometry, thus still requiring some sacrifice of accuracy for optimisation, and therefore may not account for complete 1:1 accuracy. An increase in accuracy could potentially account for an increase in ecological validity through higher fidelity and therefore improve the transfer of information (Slater, 2009), however, current hardware limitations of standalone HMDs present a challenge for high-fidelity virtualisation.

As outlined by McMahan et al. (2016) and Hameed et al. (2021), the emphasis on face validity through of high-fidelity digital environments is of the utmost importance for valid simulations, a facet of particular importance in surgical simulation training to maintain accurate skill transfer, where methods presented in this paper found a workable pipeline for low-end hardware, more research is needed to present alternative methodologies for working across HMD's with higher computational loads to produce increased anatomical accuracy and account for improved face validity.

The use of procedural generation of textures for hard surfaces was found to be an ideal process for creating adaptive and dynamic textures that may conform to the object surface with more control over parameters of diffuse and height maps compared to image texturing, at a much lower processing cost on already overstretched hardware for high-fidelity interactions.

Where a similar procedural approach may be implemented across organic structures, the mesh complexity often results in texture distortion, potentially impacting a user's face validity. Future works using procedural generation for organic materials could potentially accommodate these limitations during mesh generation phases, aiming to mitigate texture distortion through a considered placement of UV seams in areas of high geometry density, and across hidden areas of geometry to obscure texture wrapping. This could potentially produce a more adaptive approach to lower-end hardware by reducing the number of required texture maps within the simulation, however, it is unknown if repeating textures on organic materials would impact immersion or presence.

Furthermore, accommodations must be considered when simulating complex veterinary anatomy on low-powered virtualisation hardware. Complex particle systems (such as those used to generate hair or fur) continue to be inaccessible for real-time rendering without high-power computational hardware due to increased mesh density and physics calculations needed for dynamic movement. For standalone virtualisation devices, a similar effect may be achieved through a combination of normal mapping and diffuse textures to replicate the presence of fur without a significant increase in computational processing time or mesh density.

Finally, the Oculus Interaction SDK was found to be invaluable for constructing interactive VE's with accessible interactions across paradigms, however, this did sacrifice some bespoke elements of interactivity relating to the ability to physically interact with meshes over a 255-triangle count, hindering the potential anatomical accuracy. Where this limitation is an inherent issue for Unity and mesh colliders, the functionality of the Oculus SDK grabbable components is dependent on kinematic elements resulting in sacrifices to potential interaction and construct validity. Further development surrounding virtual interactions may wish to be approached from a completely bespoke perspective aiming to mitigate prerequisites present in the Oculus Interactions SDK to avoid polygonal limitation and impact of anatomical accuracy of these simulations.

5.5.2 Further Development

Furthering this study, it may be beneficial to analyse varying levels of simulator fidelity, potentially assessing environmental fidelity as an independent factor to understand its relation and impact on interaction paradigms. This could strengthen potential relationships on motor skill transfer in high-fidelity virtual environments akin to real surgical settings, versus the lower fidelity of a gamified environment.

Furthermore, assessing usability, using for instance the System Usability Scale (SUS) (Brooke, 1996), possibly involving a wider cohort of participants, would allow obtaining further insights about the user experience, ease of use, and learning of the simulation. This could potentially strengthen the validity of the proposed simulation to support transferable skills and knowledge into the real world, whilst also gaining further insight into potential problem areas for individual interaction paradigms.

Finally, the potential for more qualitative questioning may be employed to find targeted data about user perceptions of controller and hand-tracking usage in these training simulators to further reinforce previously obtained experimental results. This may be beneficial in providing targeted aid in increasing the overall user experience for digital novices and improving accessibility across interaction paradigms.

5.6 Conclusion

The development process constructed throughout this study, founded and structured a replicable high-fidelity simulation developmental pipeline using anatomical segmentation and real-time game engines, capable of deployment across a variety of clinical skills, allowing for the development of motor skills suited towards clinical skills training. Experimental deployment across veterinary education found positive feedback from both student and professional veterinarians; further re-enforcing evidence of high-fidelity interaction paradigms and their positive effect across transferable skill assertation in clinical training.

Though future research necessitates the analysis of differing interaction modalities towards specific clinical skill sets, preliminary findings support that transferable skills may be attained from VE's, through heightened feelings of engagement and naturalness, when against standardised user input from controllers-oriented training tools. This leads to suggest that VR-based clinical training could be a modern clinical training asset, essential to combating current barriers facing veterinary education curricula in a post-pandemic era.

References

Avdic D, Lundborg P, Vikström J (2014) Learning-by-doing in a highly skilled profession when stakes are high: evidence from advanced cancer surgery. IZA Discussion Paper No 8099. https://doi.org/10.2139/ssrn.2426853

Baillie S, Booth N, Catterall A, Coombes N, Crowther E, Dilly M, … Read E (2015) Veterinary clinical skills laboratories (1st edn). Retrieved 17 June 2023, from https://www.researchgate.net/publication/254738658_Collection_and_interpretation_of_cerebrospinal_fluid_in_cats_and_dogs

Balogh M (2014) Applying games technology to veterinary teaching. Vet Rec 174(3):63–64. https://doi.org/10.1136/vr.g151

Bernigau D, Bahramsoltani M, Corte GM, Reese S, Pfarrer C, Fietz D (2021) Task force veterinary anatomy: joint efforts of the five German veterinary schools to ensure education during the COVID-19 pandemic. GMS J Med Educ 38(5):Doc87. https://doi.org/10.3205/zma001483

Blender (2023) Blender 3.6 manual. Retrieved 30 July 2023, from https://docs.blender.org/manual/en/latest/index.html

Bokun D, Jakob W (2019) Instant meshes. Retrieved 8 Aug 2023, from https://github.com/wjakob/instant-meshes

Bot L, Gossiaux P-B, Rauch C-P, Tabiou S (2005) 'Learning by doing': a teaching method for active learning in scientific graduate education. Eur J Eng Educ 30(1):105–119. https://doi.org/10.1080/03043790512331313868

Brooke J (1996) SUS-A quick and dirty usability scale. In: Jordan PW, Thomas B, Weerdmeester B, McClelland IL (eds) Usability evaluation in industry. Taylor and Francis, London, pp 189–194. Retrieved 14 July 2023

Chandler K (2008) CSF sampling: when, how and why? British small animal veterinary congress. Veterinary Information Network, Hertfordshire. https://www.vin.com/doc/?id=3862902

Chen J-C, Huang Y, Lin K-Y, Chang Y-S, Lin H-C, Lin C-Y, Hsiao H-S (2020) Developing a hands-on activity using virtual reality to help students learn by doing. J Comput Assist Learn 36(1):46–60. https://doi.org/10.1111/jcal.12389

Cipresso P, Giglioli IA, Raya MA, Riva G (2018) The past, present, and future of virtual and augmented reality research: a network and cluster analysis of the literature. Front Psychol 9. https://doi.org/10.3389/fpsyg.2018.02086

de Bie M, Lipman L (2012) The use of digital games and simulators in. J Vet Med Educ 39(1):13–20. https://doi.org/10.3138/jvme.0511.055R

De Lorenzi D, Mandara MT (2016) Chapter 14—the central nervous system. In: Canine and feline cytology, 2rd edn. W.B. Saunders, St. Louis, pp 369–407. https://doi.org/10.1016/B978-1-4557-4083-3.00014-0

Dede CJ, Jacobson J, Richards J (2017) Introduction: virtual, augmented, and mixed realities in education. In: Liu D, Dede C, Huang R, Richards J (eds) Virtual, augmented, and mixed realities in education. Springer, Singapore, pp 1–16. https://doi.org/10.1007/978-981-10-5490-7_1

Dewey CW, Da Costa RC (2016) Practical guide to canine and feline neurology, 3rd edn. Wiley, Chichester. Retrieved 5 June 2023, from https://eleanor.lib.gla.ac.uk/record=b3143560

Ericsson KA (2008) Deliberate practice and acquisition of expert performance: a general overview. Acad Emerg Med 15(11):988–994. https://doi.org/10.1111/j.1553-2712.2008.00227.x

Fentem RS, Nagendran AS, Marioni-Henry KS, Madden MS, Phillipps SS, Cooper CS, Gonçalves RS (2023, February 17) Complications associated with cerebrospinal fluid collection in dogs. Vet Rec. https://doi.org/10.1002/vetr.2787

GameDev V (2022) Sculpting fur and hair brushes for blender, vol 2. Retrieved 8 Aug 2023, from https://blendermarket.com/products/blender-fur-hair-brushes

Gummery E, Cobb KA, Mossop LH, Cobb MA (2018) Student perceptions of veterinary anatomy practical classes: a longitudinal study. J Vet Med Educ 45(2):163–176. https://doi.org/10.3138/jvme.0816-132r1

Hameed A, Perkis A, Möller S (2021) Evaluating hand-tracking interaction for performing motor-tasks in VR learning environments. 2021 13th international conference on quality of multimedia experience (QoMEX). Institute of Electrical and Electronics Engineers, Montreal, pp 219–224, https://doi.org/10.1109/QoMEX51781.2021.9465407

Karkera S (2021) Impact of COVID-19 on the future of cadaveric dissection and anatomy teaching. Int J Res Med Sci 9(3):908–913. https://doi.org/10.18203/2320-6012.ijrms20210901

Kenny P (2015) How to take a cisternal CSF sample. In: BSAVA congress 2015: scientific proceedings. British Small Animal Veterinary Association, Birmingham, pp 168–168. https://doi.org/10.22233/9781910443521.16.7

Langebæk RS, Berendt M, Tipold A, Engelskirchen S, Dilly M (2021) Evaluation of the impact of using a simulator for teaching veterinary students cerebrospinal fluid collection: a mixed-methods study. J Vet Med Educ 48(2):217–227. https://doi.org/10.3138/jvme.2019-0006

Lean J, Moizer J, Abbey C, Towler M (2006) Simulations and games: use and barriers in higher education. Act Learn High Educ 7(3):227–242. https://doi.org/10.1177/1469787406069

Lessiter J, Freeman J, Keogh ED (2001) A cross-media presence questionnaire: the ITC sense of presence inventory. Presence Teleop Virt 10(3):289–297. Retrieved 14 July 2023

Lowrie M, Anderson J (2011) Cerebrospinal fluid: analysis and interpretation in small animals. In Pract 33:75–85. https://doi.org/10.1136/inp.d455

Luján Feliu-Pascual A, Garosi L, Dennis R, Platt S (2008) Iatrogenic brainstem injury during cerebellomedullary cistern puncture. Vet Radiol Ultrasound 49(5):467–471. https://doi.org/10.1111/j.1740-8261.2008.00410.x

Maran NJ, Glavin R (2003) Low- to high-fidelity simulation—a continuum of medical education? Med Educ 27:22–28. https://doi.org/10.1046/j.1365-2923.37.s1.9.x

Martinsen S, Jukes N (2005) Towards a humane veterinary education. J Vet Med Educ 32(4):454–460. https://doi.org/10.3138/jvme.32.4.454

McMahan RP, Lai C, Pal SK (2016) Interaction Fidelity: the Uncanny Valley of virtual reality interactions. In: Virtual, augmented and mixed reality. VAMR 2016. 9740. Springer, Cham, pp 59–70. https://doi.org/10.1007/978-3-319-39907-2_6

Meta (2023) Meta quest. Retrieved 8 Aug 2023, from https://developer.oculus.com/resources/oculus-device-specs/

Mossel A, Schönauer C, Froeschl M, Peer A, Goellner J, Kaufmann H (2021) Immersive training of first responder squad leaders in untethered virtual reality. Virtual Reality 25:1–15. https://doi.org/10.1007/s10055-020-00487-x

Nagendran AS, Sanchez-Masian DS, Bersan ES, Cooper CJ, Gonçalves RS (2020, May 16) Risk factors for blood-contaminated cerebrospinal fluid collection in dogs. Vet Rec 186:e8. https://doi.org/10.1136/vr.105192

Patronek GJ, Rauch A (2007) Systematic review of comparative studies examining alternatives to the harmful use of animals in biomedical education. J Am Vet Med Assoc 230(1):37–43. https://doi.org/10.2460/javma.230.1.37

Platt S, Di T (2009) The function, composition and analysis of cerebrospinal fluid in companion animals: part II—function and composition. Vet J 180(1):15–32. https://doi.org/10.1016/j.tvjl.2007.11.024

Platt S, Olby NO (2013) BSAVA manual of canine and feline neurology, 4th edn. British Small Animal Veterinary Association, Gloucester. Retrieved 18 June 2023, from https://ebookcentral.proquest.com/lib/gla/detail.action?docID=4806820

Poyade M, Eaglesham C, Trench J, Reid M (2021) A transferable psychological evaluation of virtual reality applied to safety training in chemical manufacturing. ACS Chem Health Saf 28(1):55–65. https://doi.org/10.1021/acs.chas.0c00105

Rösch T, Schaper E, Tipold A, Fischer MR, Dilly M, Ehlers JP (2014) Clinical skills of veterinary students—a cross-sectional study of the self-concept and exposure to skills training in Hannover, Germany. BMC Vet Res 10(1):969. https://doi.org/10.1186/s12917-014-0302-8

Routh J, Paramasivam SJ, Cockcroft P, Nadarajah VD, Jeevaratnam K (2021) Veterinary education during Covid-19 and beyond—challenges and mitigating approaches. Animals 11(6):1818. https://doi.org/10.3390/ani11061818

Slater M (2009) Place illusion and plausibility can lead to realistic behaviour in immersive virtual environments. Philos Trans R Soc Lond B Biol Sci 364(1535):3549–3557. https://doi.org/10.1098/rstb.2009.0138

Terlizzi RD, Platt S (2006) The function, composition and analysis of cerebrospinal fluid in companion animals: part I—function and composition. Vet J 172(3):422–431. https://doi.org/10.1016/j.tvjl.2005.07.021

Thomson C, Hahn C, Johnson C, Roper Q (2012) Veterinary neuroanatomy: a clinical approach, 4th edn. Saunders Elsevier, Edinburgh. Retrieved 6 June 2023, from https://go.exlibris.link/wVR9VDw5

Unity (2023a) Unity documentation: Mesh Collider component reference. Retrieved 2 Aug 2023, from https://docs.unity3d.com/Manual/class-MeshCollider.html

Unity (2023b) Unity documentation: collider on collision enter(collision). Retrieved 2 Aug 2023, from https://docs.unity3d.com/ScriptReference/Collider.OnCollisionEnter.html

Unity (2023c) Unity documentation: inverse kinematics. Retrieved 6 Aug 2023, from https://docs.unity3d.com/Manual/InverseKinematics.html

Warburton S (2009) Second life in higher education: assessing the potential. Br J Educ Technol 40(3):414–426. https://doi.org/10.1111/j.1467-8535.2009.00952.x

Won M, Ungu DA, Matovu H, Treagust DF, Tsai C-C, Park J et al (2023) Diverse approaches to learning with immersive virtual reality identified from a systematic review. Comput Educ 195:104701. https://doi.org/10.1016/j.compedu.2022.104701

Xu X, Kilroy D, Puggioni A, Campbell AG (2022) Co-located mixed reality for teaching equine radiology techniques to veterinary students. Institute of Electrical and Electronic Engineers, St. Michael, Barbados. Retrieved 19 June 2023 https://doi.org/10.1109/GEM56474.2022.10017893

The Effectiveness of a 3D Virtual Reality Model of a Paediatric Abdominal Neuroblastoma for Surgical Planning and Junior Doctor Education

6

Karen Lacey, Giuliana Torpiano, Michael Jacovides, and Matthieu Poyade

Abstract

Neuroblastoma (NB) is a rare embryonic cancer that presents surgical challenges, particularly in high-risk cases. High-risk cases are those stratified according to image-defined risk factors (IDRFs) in medical imaging. In abdominal NB, common IDRFs include encasement of major vessels: the abdominal aorta and inferior vena cava (IVC) among others, which poses an increased surgical risk. With a surgical resection goal of over 90% for optimal survival, three-dimensional (3D) models derived from patient datasets have proven beneficial for pre-surgical planning.

This chapter presents the framework used to create a prototype 3D neuroblastoma model within a virtual reality (VR) application for surgical planning and junior doctor education. The 3D VR model displays a large abdominal neuroblastoma with encasement of the IVC and inferior mesenteric artery (IMA), spatial relationship to the abdominal aorta, tributary vessels and abdominal organs. Key features of the VR development include (1) tumour transparency, (2) a customisable interactive toggle display, (3) CT dataset overlay, (4) 360-degree rotation of the model, (5) medical information relating to neuroblastoma, including tumour volume and (6) notation.

User testing was conducted at the Royal Hospital for Children, Glasgow (RHCG) with 20 medical professionals participating. Results demonstrate the application had a good usability rating (SUS 79.75) and sense of presence (ITC-SOPI) rating, with resulting scores in each category: sense of presence (mean 3.75 ± 0.55 SD), engagement (mean 4.08 ± 0.4 SD), ecological validity (mean 3.72 ± 0.83 SD) and negative effect (mean 1.77 ± 0.78 SD).

A counterbalanced anatomical identification experiment comparing the 2D dataset to the 3D VR model showed a significant difference ($p < 0.05$) in errors committed between the control and VR groups, demonstrating that participants performed better in VR ($M_{VR} = 0.35$, $\sigma = 0.59$) compared to 2D ($M_{control} = 0.85$, $\sigma = 0.93$). A significant dif-

K. Lacey (✉)
School of Innovation & Technology, The Glasgow School of Art, Glasgow, UK

School of Medicine, Dentistry and Nursing, College of Medical, Veterinary and Life Sciences, University of Glasgow, Glasgow, UK

G. Torpiano · M. Jacovides
Royal Hospital for Children, Glasgow, UK

University of Glasgow, Glasgow, UK

M. Poyade
School of Innovation & Technology, The Glasgow School of Art, Glasgow, UK

J. Clancy, M. Poyade (eds.), *Medical Visualization and Applications of Technology – Volume 2*, Biomedical Visualization 5, https://doi.org/10.1007/978-3-031-63463-5_6

ference ($p < 0.05$) was also noted in the evolution of error between groups, suggesting that group 1 participants who have first undertaken the control condition and then VR have seen the number of errors decreasing indicating that the VR condition promotes greater accuracy for anatomical identification.

Limitations to this study include a small participant number ($n = 20$) and a broad spectrum of knowledge among participants. Future research could address such limitations by increasing participant numbers and narrowing the education-level demographic, focusing on one cohort of participants.

Keywords

3D surgical planning · Virtual reality · Paediatric tumour · Neuroblastoma · Junior doctor education · Surgical education

6.1 Introduction

6.1.1 Neuroblastoma Aetiology

Neuroblastoma (NB) is a complex paediatric cancer, being the most common extracranial solid tumour in children that derives from early neural tissue (Newman et al. 2019). NB is primarily diagnosed in young children, typically before the age of 5 years, with around 100 children diagnosed with neuroblastoma yearly in the UK (Cancer Research UK 2022).

Neuroblastoma is characterised by the abnormal growth of neuroblasts, which derive from neural crest cells, a transient cell population that arises during embryonic development and gives rise to various cell types, including neurons and glial cells (Maris 2010). Diagnosis usually occurs in very young children, sometimes in infancy, given that neuroblasts are most commonly found in the foetal stages or the very early stages of childhood (Lundberg et al. 2022). This development period involves the differentiation of neuroblast cells into normal neural tissue and when the cancer-predisposing neuroblast cells are most often found.

The process of neurogenesis involves the migration of neuroblasts to their final destinations within the developing nervous system and establishing connections with other neurons, forming neural circuits. Neuroblastomas can arise anywhere along the sympathetic nervous chain, with vast areas populated by neural crest cells (Matthay et al. 2016; Park et al. 2010). The most common location for neuroblastoma development is in the adrenal glands in the abdomen, but they can occur in other parts of the body such as the neck, chest and pelvis.

Genetic abnormalities can result in a significant predisposition for neuroblastoma, resulting in rapid proliferation of abnormal cells rather than differentiation into normal tissue (Barr and Applebaum 2018). One such factor includes dysregulated expression and amplification of the transcription factor MYCN, which strongly predicts prognosis (Otte et al. 2021).

Neuroblastoma can present interesting phenotypic heterogeneity, with a range of clinical outcomes, from spontaneous regression to treatment-resistant progression (Lundberg et al. 2022).

6.1.1.1 Treatment for Neuroblastoma

Treatment for NB often requires surgical intervention as part of a multimodal treatment approach alongside chemotherapy, radiation therapy and stem cell transplantation. Treatment is patient-specific and determined by which risk group a patient falls under: low risk, intermediate risk and high risk. In the low-risk category, observation or surgery alone may be required, while intermediate risk may receive chemotherapy presurgical excision, and high-risk patients receive surgery in combination with intensive multimodal therapy (Sokol and Desai 2019). Treatment for NB generally follows the expert guidelines recommended by the Children's Cancer and Leukemia Group (CCLG) Neuroblastoma Special Interest Group (CCLG 2020).

6.1.1.2 Staging and Risk Stratification of Neuroblastoma

The course of action and operative approach largely depend on both the location and extent of the tumour. Currently, the International Neuroblastoma Risk Group Staging System (INRGSS) is used to classify stages of disease (Table 6.1), with patients being stratified at diagnosis according to the presence and number of image-defined risk factors (IDRFs) (Cohn et al. 2009; Monclair et al. 2009).

Table 6.1 INRGSS staging system for neuroblastoma (Sokol and Desai 2019)

INRG stage	Description
L1	Localised tumour with no image-defined risk factors
L2	Localised tumour with one or more image-defined risk factors
M	Distant metastatic disease
MS	Metastatic disease in children under 18 months with metastases limited to skin, liver and/or bone marrow (<10% involvement)

IDRFs are imaging features that are classified at the point of NB diagnosis, which exhibit a greater risk of surgical complications as presented in Table 6.2. In the abdomen, IDRFs include encasement of the primary vessels: the aorta and/or tributary branches, the inferior vena cava (IVC), the iliac vessels, tumour invading one/both renal pedicles, tumour infiltrating the porta hepatis and/or hepatoduodenal ligament (Cohn et al. 2009). In the case of abdominal neuroblastoma, encasement and compression of the abdominal vessels are commonplace, especially the inferior vena cava due to a thinner, less muscular wall (Uehara et al. 2013; Li et al. 2014).

Table 6.2 IDRFs for neuroblastoma

	Image-defined risk factors (IDRFs)
Ipsilateral tumour extension within two-body compartments	Neck-chest, chest-abdomen, abdomen-pelvis
Neck	Tumour encasing carotid and/or vertebral artery and/or internal jugular vein
	Tumour extending to the base of the skull
	Tumour compressing the trachea
Cervico-thoracic junction	Tumour encasing brachial plexus roots
	Tumour encasing subclavian vessels and/or vertebral and/or carotid artery
	Tumour compressing the trachea
Thorax	Tumour encasing the aorta and/or major branches
	Tumour compressing the trachea and/or principal bronchi
	Lower mediastinal tumour, infiltrating the costo-vertebral junction between T9 and T12
Thoracoabdominal	Tumour encasing the aorta and/or vena cava
Abdomen/pelvis	Tumour infiltrating the porta hepatis and/or hepatoduodenal ligament
	Tumour encasing branches of the superior mesenteric artery at the mesenteric root
	Tumour encasing the origin of the coeliac axis, and/or of the superior mesenteric artery
	Tumour invading one or both renal pedicles
	Tumour encasing the aorta and/or vena cava
	Tumour encasing the iliac vessels
	Pelvic tumour crossing the sciatic notch
Intraspinal tumour extension whatever the location provided that	More than one-third of the spinal canal in the axial plane is invaded and/or the perimedullary leptomeningeal spaces are not visible and/or the spinal cord is abnormal
Infiltration of adjacent organs/structures	Pericardium, diaphragm, kidney, liver, duodeno-pancreatic block and mesentery
Conditions to be recorded, but not considered IDRFs	Multifocal primary tumours, pleural effusion, with or without malignant cells, ascites with/without malignant cells

Adapted from Sokol and Desai (2019)

6.1.1.3 Surgical Intervention

The current surgical approach for neuroblastoma aims to achieve gross tumour resection >90% while avoiding damage to surrounding structures (Fischer et al. 2017; Fati et al. 2021). With surgical procedures carrying a high degree of complexity, especially in high-risk cases, research into the use of patient-specific 3D-printed and virtual models for pre-surgical planning has grown rapidly. With gross total resection being a prognostic factor, the use of a 3D virtual model may help to improve surgical management in complex cases.

6.1.2 3D-Printed Models for Surgical Planning

The application of 3D technology is advancing in planning complex surgical interventions. This technology aids in the 3D conceptualization of spatial relationships among anatomical structures and delineates the geometry of tumour masses. This utilisation enhances surgical precision and contributes to a more thorough understanding of the intricate anatomical details involved in challenging procedures. 3D printing in medicine for pre-surgical planning is already commonplace in fields such as paediatric cardiology (Noecker et al. 2006), orthopaedic oncology (Punyaratabandhu et al. 2018) and paediatric neurosurgery (Karuppiah et al. 2021).

A systematic literature review on the use of 3D models (Tack et al. 2016) analysed 227 surgical papers describing the use of 3D-printed models for surgical planning, anatomical models and custom implants, concluding that several advantages exist to 3D-printed applications; however, a formal cost-effective analysis was required.

Specific to the area of paediatric oncology and neuroblastoma, some recent studies have been conducted to evaluate the use of 3D-printed models for pre-surgical planning. A comprehensive literature review of 3D surgical planning for paediatric tumours by Pereira et al. (2022) analysed studies from 2010 to 2021, with inclusion criteria of 3D-printed models only for paediatric tumours in children from birth to 18 years. Of the 18 studies and 28 cases included, five studies (and nine cases) were specific to neuroblastoma (Table 6.3).

Souzaki et al. (2015) documented the first reported case of a 3D-printed model used in the laparoscopic adrenalectomy surgical simulation for three NB adrenalectomy cases. The patient-specific 3D-printed models enabled the insertion of trocars and optimization of the trocar layout while also providing a better understanding of patient anatomy, laparoscopic perspective and range of forceps movement preoperatively.

Krauel et al. (2016) presented three cases of tumours encasing major vessels, two of which were high-risk NB cases. Case 1 required the production of two separate files for PolyJet 3D printing by Stratasys. File 1 included bones, vessels and 'other parts' printed using a rigid white material. In contrast, the tumour was printed using a soft translucent material that (1) enabled visualisation of encased structures and (2) served as an 'operable' structure before surgery. Noted in this study is a segmentation time of 10 h under expert radiology and surgical guidance, with an approximate printing time of 24 h.

Case 2 presented greater complexity of vessel encasement, increasing the difficulty of visualising the vessels potentially compromised during resection surgery. Thus, a PolyJet 3D-printed model was complemented with a selective laser sintering (SLS) model comprising two separate parts (1) the encased vessels and (2) a semitransparent 'operable'/removable tumour.

They concluded that the 3D-printed models demonstrated precision that was comparable with surgical findings. These prototype models were to scale with a soft consistency enabling the use of true surgical instruments for surgical planning. The cost of production, however, is not declared in this study.

A further study by Sánchez-Sánchez et al. (2018) demonstrated the successful use of both a 3D-printed model and a virtual model for pre-surgical planning in neuroblastoma surgery, concluding that patient-specific 3D reconstructions help with assessing spatial relationships and anticipation of surgical complications.

Tejo-Otero et al. (2021) created a 3D-printed neuroblastoma prototype via a semi-automatic

Table 6.3 3D-printed models for surgical planning of neuroblastoma cases

Author	Tumour model	Imaging technique	Tools (segmentation and model preparation)	Techniques, materials and printers	Performers, printing time and cost
Souzaki et al. (2015)	3 cases of neuroblastoma (1 to 20 m.o)	CT	ZedView, 3D Doctor, FreeForm, and CATIA	Technique: PolyJet; materials: acrylic ultraviolet curable resin (different colour resins for tumour, veins, arteries, kidney and outer body); printer: Objet 500 Connex 3	NR
Krauel et al. (2016)	High-risk stage 4 neuroblastoma (3 y.o)	MRI or CT	VRMed DICOM Platform	Technique: PolyJet; materials: epoxy photopolymer (bones, vessels and other parts) and translucent material; Printer: Connex 500	Segmentation time: 10 h; performers: paediatric radiology and leading surgeon; printing time: 24 h
	High-risk stage 4 neuroblastoma (5 y.o)			Technique: PolyJet and SLS; materials: epoxy photopolymer (bones, vessels and other parts) and translucent material—PolyJet. Printer: Connex 500 and Vanguard	
Sánchez-Sánchez et al. (2018)	Right abdominal neuroblastoma (13 m.o)	MRI	ROVA3D, BCN3D, ORD Solutions, BCN technologies©	Technique: FFF and SLA; materials: polylactic acid, acrylonitrile butadiene styrene (ABS), polyvinyl, polyurethane and polystyrene; printer: FFF: ROVA3D, BCN3D, ORD Solutions, BCN technologies©, SLS: FORM 3D©	Performers: team of engineers
	Left paravertebral neuroblastoma (7 m.o)				
Tejo et al. (2021)	Neuroblastoma (age NR)	CT	IntelliSpace Portal (Philips), Rhinoceros or Meshmixer	Technique: FFF-DIW; materials: polyvinyl acetate (support), polylactic acid (blood vessels, spinal cord and kidney) and thermoplastic polyurethane (tumour); printer: hybrid multi-material 3D printer	Printing time: 48 h; cost: $15.84
Tejo-Otero et al. (2021)	Neuroblastoma (age NR)	CT	IntelliSpace Portal (Philips), Rhinoceros or Meshmixer	Technique: SLS and FFF; materials: polyamide (tumour, blood vessels and the kidney)—SLS; green and sand-coloured thermoplastic polyurethane and polyvinyl acetate (liver and portal system) FFF; printer: SLS: Ricoh AM S5500P, FFF: multi-material 3D printer	Performers: NR, printing time: 48 h; cost: $390.77

CT, computed tomography; MRI, magnetic resonance imaging; NR, non-reported; y.o, years old; m.o, month old; SLS, selective laser sintering; FFF, fused filament fabrication; SLA, stereolithography; DIW, direct-ink-writing; CMR, cardiac magnetic resonance; CT, computed tomography; MRI, magnetic resonance imaging; NR, non-reported
Adapted from Pereira et al. (2022)

segmentation using IntelliSpace Portal from Phillips® and a two-part-printed manufacturing process. Using selective laser sintering (SLS) and fused filament fabrication (FFF), a 3D-printed model was produced with a manufacturing time of 48 hours and a total cost for materials and labour of £299 ($390.77). This prototype was used for surgical planning and communication with family and sterilised for surgical reference in theatre, concluding that this novel printing approach enables more cost-effective printing of realistic 3D models. This paper discusses the comparative cost of material jet-printed prototypes estimated at €2000 as used by Krauel et al. (2016).

A recent study by McKay et al. (2023) presenting a case report of thoracoabdominal neuroblastoma discussed the benefits of the 3D model for pre-surgical planning stating that it was unlikely a laparoscopic procedure would have been offered without prior knowledge that the tumour was separate from the aorta and renal vasculature.

6.1.2.1 Advantages and Limitations of 3D-Printed Models

A systematic review of 158 studies assessing the advantages and disadvantages of 3D printing in surgery by Martelli et al. (2016) reported that 48.7% of studies describe the main advantages as possibilities for surgical planning, accuracy (33.5%), along with time saved in the operating room (32.9%). In contrast, 34 studies described anatomical accuracy as unsatisfactory, with production time (19.6%) and cost (19%) being the other drawbacks.

6.1.3 3D Models in Virtual Reality

In contrast to a virtual model displayed on a computer screen, virtual reality (VR) encompasses a computer-generated simulation of a 3D model that can be interacted with in an immersive, seemingly real environment using a head-mounted display (HMD), hand-held controllers and/or hand tracking (Li et al. 2017). 3D models for VR are generated similarly to 3D printing, requiring segmentation of Digital Imaging and Communications in Medicine (DICOM) files of computed tomography (CT) or MRI, with additional decimation of the 3D model and programming of specific functionalities in the real-time game engine.

Although not widely adopted in clinical practice, VR technologies have significantly advanced in recent years, with applications in surgical planning: abdominal surgery (Sampogna et al. 2017), colorectal surgery (Guerriero et al. 2018), surgical simulation (Chheang et al. 2019), patient/parent comprehension, pain management (Eijlers et al. 2019), liver surgery (Boedecker et al. 2021) and education and training (Pears and Konstantinidis 2022). However, the literature surrounding the use of 3D immersive VR models for paediatric neuroblastoma surgical planning is sparse. This potentially is due to the relatively low volume of paediatric surgical oncology patients compared to the adult population, patient variability and the greater complexity of segmentation of DICOM files in soft tissue–based pathologies requiring manual or semi-automatic segmentation.

Principal factors to consider in the use of 3D models (either printed or in an immersive virtual environment) include anatomical accuracy, cost and time of production and shipping, accessibility to the medical team including cost and technical ability and potential reusability of the model.

6.1.4 Junior Doctor Education and Immersive Technology

With medical imaging and its interpretation having such a crucial role in decision-making across many disciplines, Ayesa et al. (2021) found that the greatest proportion of post-graduate medical imaging education was provided by senior colleagues.

Eid et al. (2017) conducted a study on 74 general surgery residents in the U.S.A. using a 30-item web-based radiology imaging test. This study concluded that general surgery residents were able to accurately identify 75% of basic radiology images, with a recommendation for integrating radiological education during surgery training. A further cross-sectional study by Butler et al. (2016) across 13 teaching hospitals in the U.S.A., with a response rate of 26% and 30%, respectively, from 465 faculty and 520 residents, showed a major need for a specified radiology curriculum. A cross-sectional analysis study of 121 participants in a large teaching hospital in Australia was conducted by Glenn-Cox et al. (2019). This study reports that radiology teaching at medical school was mostly informal and infrequent, with 52% of participants feeling it was inadequate. With medical imaging and immersive technology being two dynamically evolving fields, it raises the question of where innovative approaches to radiology education may be beneficial. Concerning immersive technology in education, a systematic review of augmented and virtual reality in anatomical education by Uruthiralingam and Rea (2020) demonstrated that of 56 articles relating to VR, 45 were in favour, eight were neutral and three opposed the use of this technology.

6.1.5 Conclusion

From this review, it is clear the surgical complexity that NB diagnoses present, particularly in high-risk category cases. The literature demonstrates both the advantages and limitations of patient-specific 3D models, with most research on paediatric neuroblastoma demonstrating the use of physical 3D-printed models for pre-surgical and intra-operative use. Given the rarity of neuroblastoma and the need for integrated radiology teaching for surgery residents, this research project aims to produce a bespoke immersive VR application of a 3D NB model. This application will serve as a surgical planning tool and give the user the ability to overlay the original CT dataset, along with scientific information regarding NB for junior doctor education.

6.2 Materials and Methods

6.2.1 Materials

A range of software, hardware, data and third-party assets used in the development of this application, along with their purpose and developer/source, are listed in Table 6.4.

6.2.2 Concept and Workflow

The concept of this project was to create an anatomically accurate 3D virtual reality model of a large abdominal neuroblastoma demonstrating spatial relationships to major vessels and surrounding organs. An expected timeframe requirement for VR 3D model production, as advised by surgical supervisors at the Royal Hospital for Children, Glasgow (RHCG), compared to a 3D-printed model received pre-surgery is illustrated in Fig. 6.1.

This prototype development would be tested at the Royal Hospital for Children, Glasgow to determine its efficacy for surgical planning and junior doctor education. A basic overview of the developmental workflow is shown in Fig. 6.2. On completion of the 3D models, the application was built in Unity and displayed on a Meta Quest 2 headset.

6.2.3 Dataset Acquisition

This research is delivered retrospectively of surgery, with anonymised CT and MRI DICOM datasets of a large abdominal paediatric neuroblastoma provided by project supervisor Dr. Michael Jacovides (FRCS Consultant Paediatric Surgeon), Royal Hospital for Children, Glasgow. CT imaging provided for this project was performed using a GE Revolution™ CT, with MRI imaging performed using a Siemens MAGNETOM Aera 1.5T MRI | Siemens MAGNETOM Avanto 1.5T MRI.

Table 6.4 Software, hardware, data and third-party assets used in this VR development

Software	Purpose	Developer
3D Slicer	Direct volume rendering | segmentation	3D Slicer
Adobe Acrobat	Form creation—user testing	Adobe, Inc.
Adobe Illustrator	2D asset creation	Adobe, Inc.
Adobe Substance Painter	Texturing 3D models	Adobe Inc.
Autodesk 3DS Max	3D modelling | retopology | texturing	Autodesk, Inc.
Microsoft Office Excel	Data collation	Microsoft
MITK	Dataset registration	MITK
PSPP Statistical Software	Statistical analysis	PSPP
SCRCPY (Screen Copy)	Screen mirroring VR to laptop screen	SCRCPY
Unity	Application development engine	Unity Technologies
Visual Studio Code	Source-code editor	Microsoft

Hardware	Purpose	Developer
Surface Studio Laptop i7	Segmentation | 3D modelling | App Dev.	Microsoft
Oculus Quest 2	Virtual reality	Meta

Data | resources	Purpose	Source
Anonymised DICOM CT	Segmentation | 3D models	Royal Hospital for Children, Glasgow
Anonymised DICOM MRI	Segmentation | 3D models	Royal Hospital for Children, Glasgow
Annotated Radiological Imaging	Anatomical referencing for segmentation	Radiopedia.org

Third-party assets	Purpose	Source
Neuroblastoma reference image	Texturing neuroblastoma model	Pediatric Imaging
Office with conference room	Virtual reality environment	Unity Asset Store
Digestive System Prefab	Materials—abdominal organs	Unity Asset Store

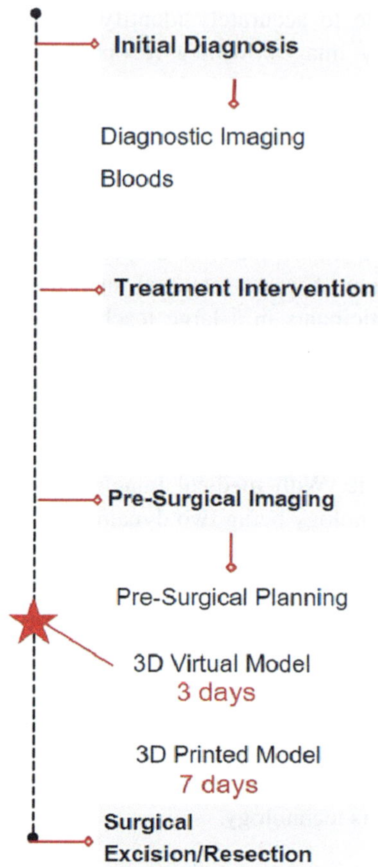

Fig. 6.1 Timeframe requirement 3D VR vs. 3D-printed model

6.2.4 DICOM Dataset Analysis

A comprehensive evaluation of the radiology report and key images was undertaken to prioritise the segmentation workflow sequence in 3D Slicer and MITK (Fig. 6.3).

6.2.4.1 Direct Volume Render (Spatial Relationship)

Direct volume rendering (DVR) was utilised to get a 3D representation of the volume data directly and a greater understanding of the spatial relationship between the MRI and CT dataset volumes. The MRI dataset contained four individual volumes as presented in Fig. 6.4, along with their equivalent volume dimensions. Comparing the spatial relationship between the MRI and CT demonstrates that vol. 2 and vol. 3

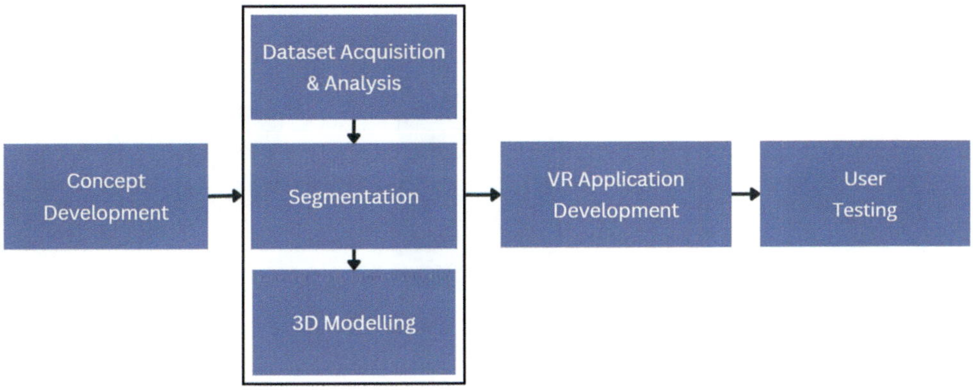

Fig. 6.2 Developmental workflow

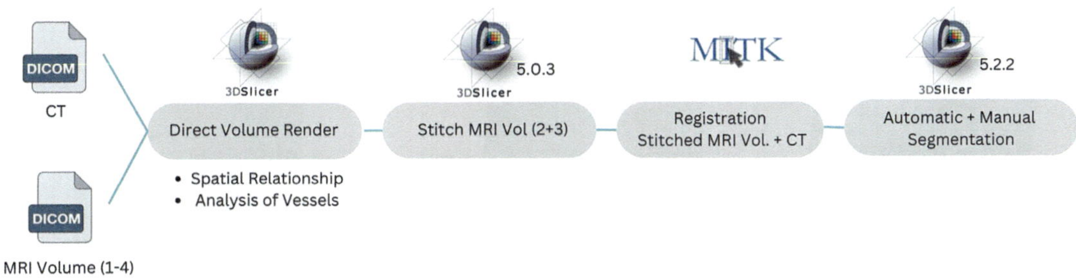

Fig. 6.3 Segmentation workflow

of the MRI dataset would be most suitable for registration to the CT dataset, although prior stitching of volumes would be required.

6.2.4.2 Direct Volume Render (Vessel Analysis)

DVR of both the CT and MRI datasets assisted with the analysis of specific structures and enabled focused decision-making on which dataset was best suited to produce the required segmentations. The IVC is most prominent in MRI volumes 2 and 3 (Fig. 6.5), demonstrating that these two MRI volumes would be most suitable for IVC segmentation, along with volume stitching and registration to the CT dataset.

Within the CT dataset; the abdominal aorta includes prominent paired and unpaired branches, iliac arteries, skeletal structure, calcification within the NB and right renal stent in situ, while a CT dataset overlay was utilised to assess the artery surrounding the NB anteriorly for segmentation planning (Fig. 6.6). An MRI dataset overlay (vols. 2 and 3) on the DVR was used to assess the IVC for segmentation planning (Fig. 6.7).

Auto-segmentation of the skin and abdominal organs from CT would be performed using the 3D Slicer (v5.2.2) TotalSegmentator module, with subsequent manual refinement.

6.2.4.3 Stitching of MRI Volumes

The Stitch Volume module (3D Slicer 5.0.3) allows the stitching of two or more image volumes, which produces an output volume in which the input volumes have been cropped, resampled and stitched together. Given that the two volumes being stitched are of the same resolution and orientation in this case, nearest neighbour interpolation is used to avoid resampling. Initially, a region of interest (ROI) is created in the 'Crop Volume' module, with this ROI used in Stitch Volumes

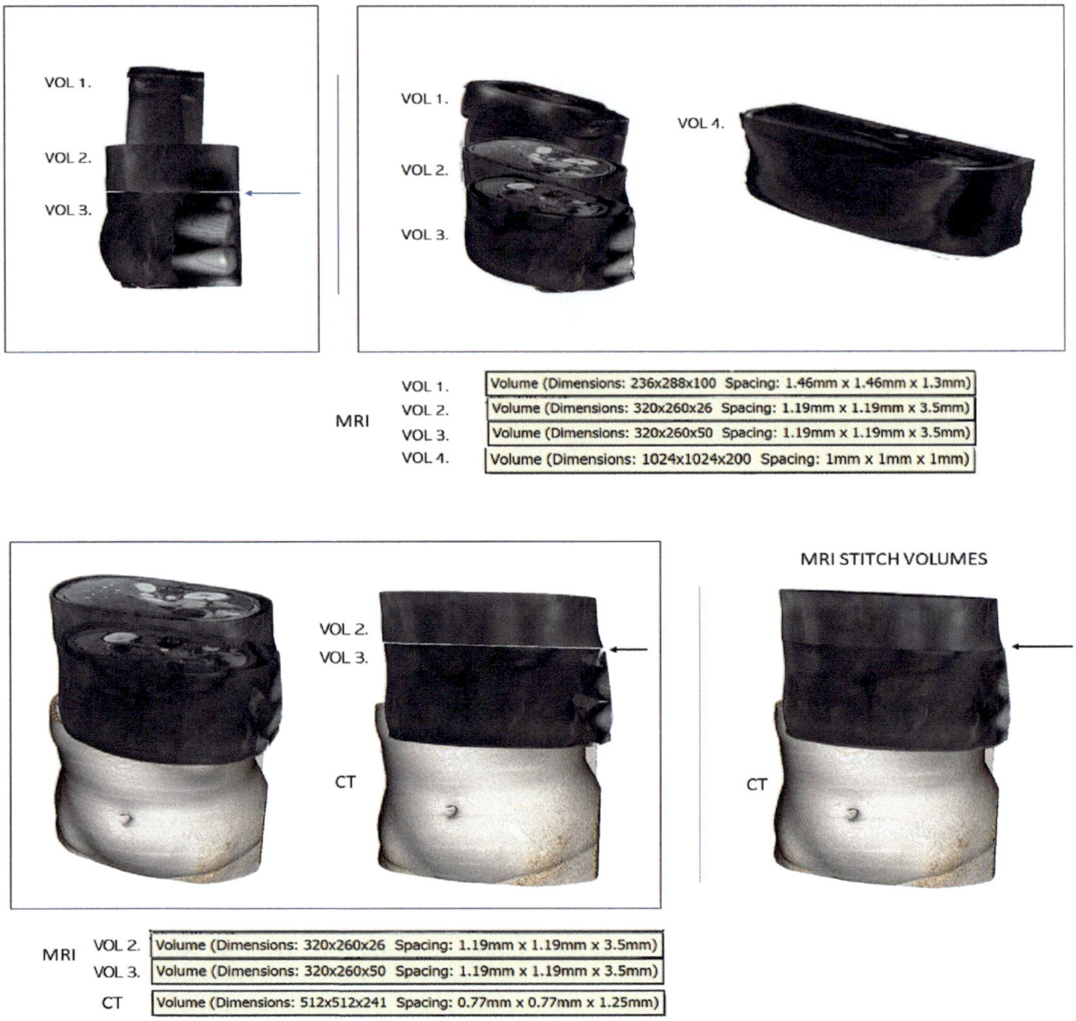

Fig. 6.4 (Top) DVR of MRI volumes 1–4 showing their spatial relationship and volume dimensions. (Above left) A sequence of MRI slices that are absent between volumes 2 and 3 (blue arrow). (Bottom) DVR comparison of MRI volumes 2 and 3 and CT volume, with volume dimensions. (Below right) Stitched MRI volumes 2 and 3 spatial relationships to CT volume

modules to generate the new stitched output volume.

6.2.4.4 Dataset Registration

With a new stitched volume created from the MRI dataset, the goal of dataset registration is to align the MRI volume to the position and orientation of the CT dataset. This was achieved in MITK software by importing a .nrrd file of the MRI stitched volume and the CT. Automatic registration was performed using Affine Registration, with the MRI volume set as the moving dataset, while the CT was fixed. Analysis of this registration was performed using a checkerboard overlay and presented a marginal offset in the dimensions of the aorta, likely resulting from the stitching of MRI volumes with an absence of a sequence of slices (Fig 6.8). The registered dataset was then

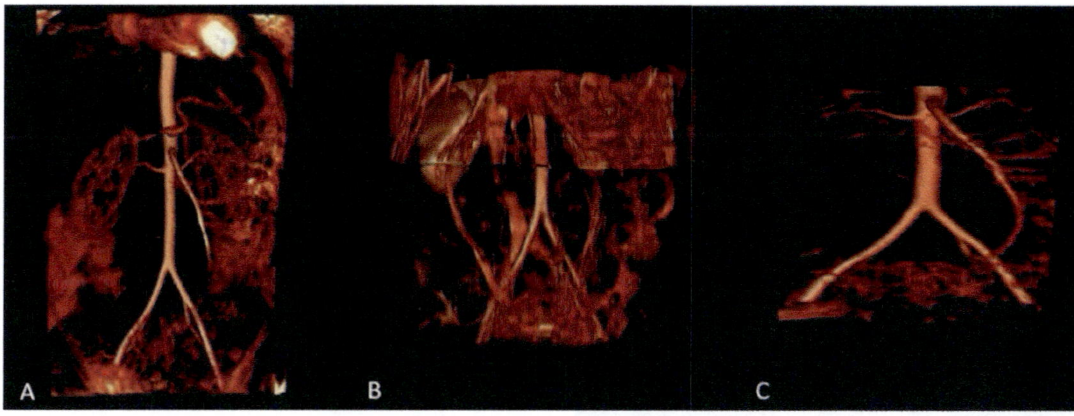

Fig. 6.5 DVR of MRI (**a**) vol. 1—coronal, (**b**) vols. 2 and 3—axial, (**c**) vol. 4. Scaled

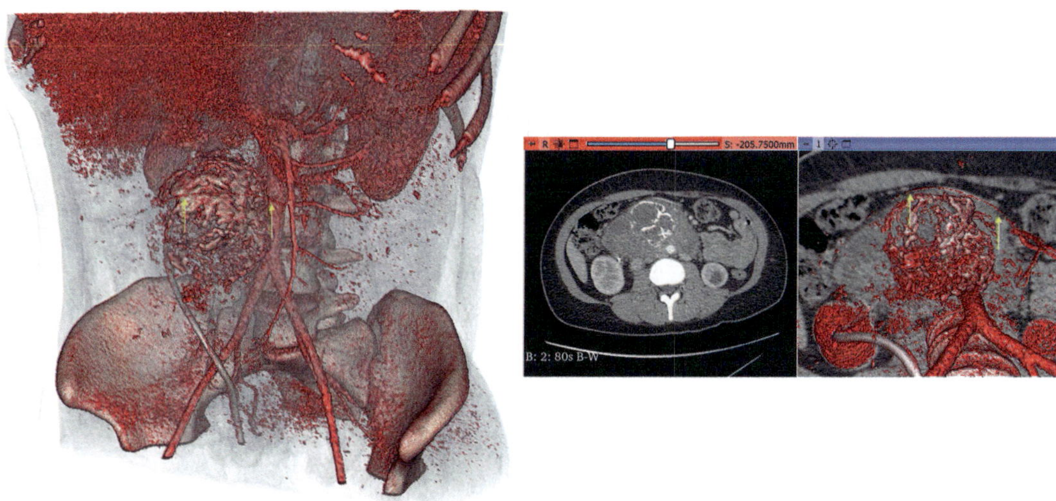

Fig. 6.6 (Left) DVR of CT—showing right ureter stent in situ, calcification within the neuroblastoma, skeletal structure, abdominal aorta with clear paired and unpaired arterial branches and iliac arteries. (Right) CT dataset overlay for segmentation planning of the artery surrounding the neuroblastoma anteriorly (yellow arrows)

exported as a .nrrd file and imported back into 3D Slicer for segmentation.

6.2.5 Segmentation of DICOM Datasets

6.2.5.1 Automatic Segmentation with Manual Refinement

Segmentation of the skin and abdominal organs was achieved using the CT dataset and 3D Slicer (5.2.2) TotalSegmentator module. This module generates an automatic whole-body '*total*' segmentation of 52 segments, of which eight were retained for this project: liver, stomach, spleen, duodenum, pancreas, kidneys and portal vein (Fig. 6.9). While enabling speed of segmentation, inaccuracies are present in these segmentations, as stated in the 3D Slicer documentation and evident in some of the segmentations produced. A further '*body*' segmentation was produced, with the trunk segment retained and the colour

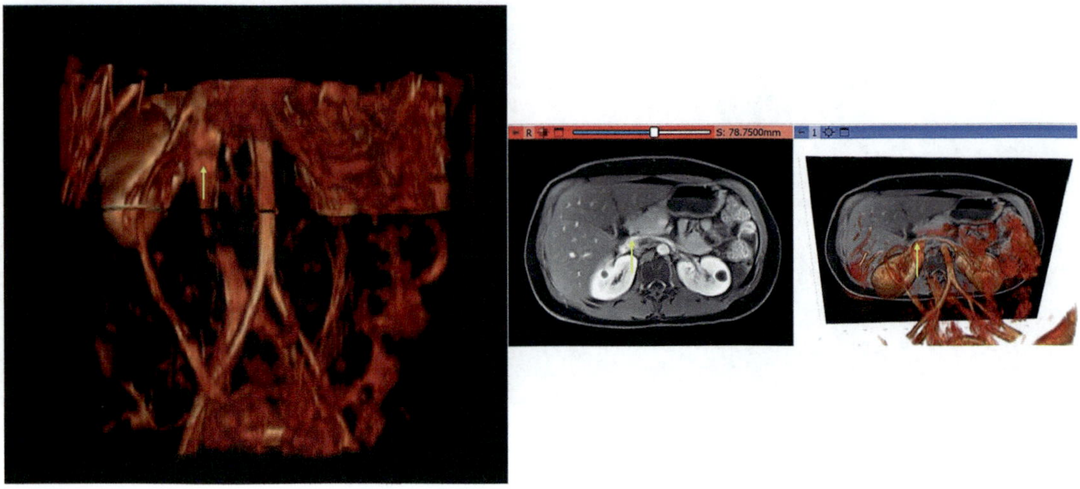

Fig. 6.7 Overlay of the MRI dataset on the respective DVR for segmentation planning of the IVC

#f5d9b8 assigned, which was then manually refined to produce the skin model.

Manual refinement of the segmentations produced in the TotalSegmentator module included the following:

- Refinement of organ segmentations
- Surface smoothing of organs—median smoothing of 3.0 mm
- Skin segmentation

6.2.5.2 Manual Segmentation

Image segmentation of the DICOM datasets was performed in 3D Slicer, utilising the 'threshold effect', with source data, threshold values, initial 3D reconstructions and a list of 3D models from each segmentation shown in Fig. 6.10.

6.2.5.2.1 Skeletal | Right Ureter Stent | Tumour Calcification

The backboard of the CT and bony protrusions on the ribs were removed using the scissors tool, followed by the islands tool 'remove small islands—1000 voxels' to remove artefacts. The distal surface of the ilia was filled using the level tracing tool. The ilia were then separated as individual segments to optimise the retopology of the models.

A right urethral mesh stent is in situ to maintain the patency of the ureter. Mesh stents are composed of very delicate metal mesh structures that support the integrity of the tubular ureter, which allows for safe stent placement and post-placement urethral movement. Given its metal composition, it segments at a similar isodensity to the bone. To isolate the right ureter as a separate structure, a new segment was created, a new colour was selected and the threshold effect 'use for masking' was applied; increasing the editable intensity range to 180–2940. The paint tool was utilised to mark the right ureter. Once segmented, the smoothing tool (remove extrusions 2 mm) was used to remove surface extrusions.

The calcification present in the centre of the neuroblastoma shares a similar isodensity to that of the bony structures. This calcification can result from tumour necrosis or as a response to chemotherapy (Papaioannou and McHugh 2005). To isolate the neuroblastoma calcification, a new segment was added and isolated as above.

6.2.5.2.2 Abdominal Aorta and Branching Arteries

The rationale for utilising a large threshold range for arterial segmentation was to produce an extensive vessel segmentation including the mesenteric vein, which would later be isolated as a separate segment and merged with the portal vein from the automatic segmentation produced in the TotalSegmentator module. A new 'spine' seg-

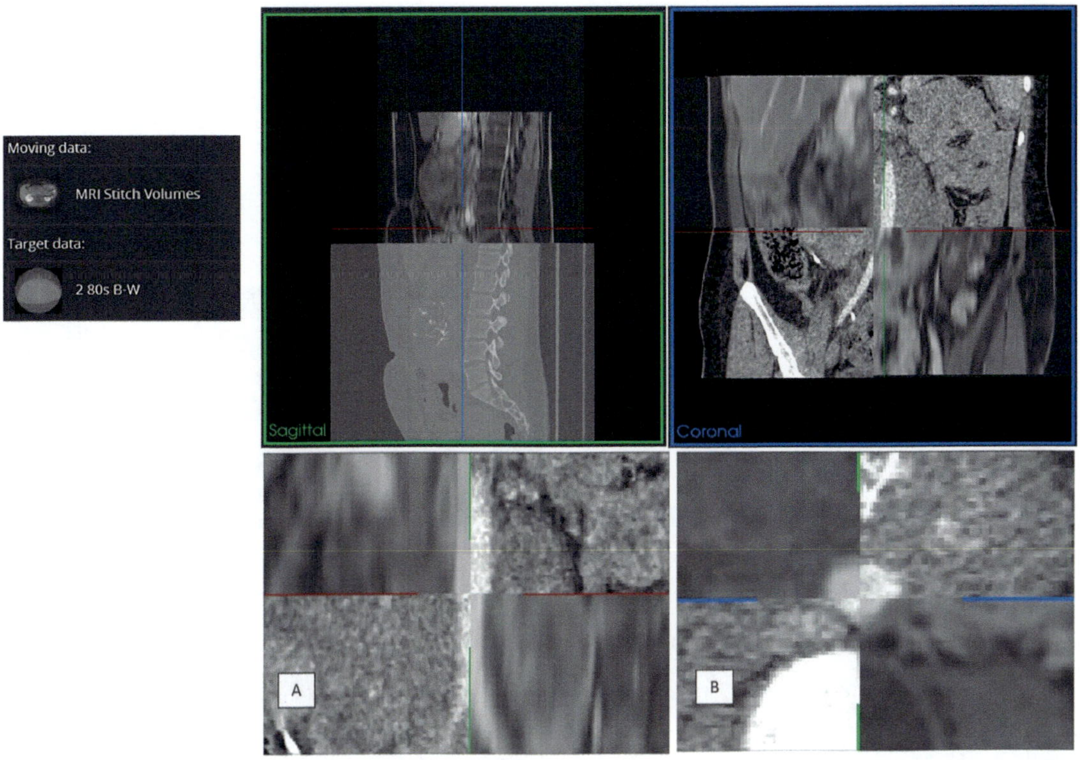

Fig. 6.8 Dataset registration in MITK, with the stitched volumes MRI set as the moving data and the CT as the target data. (Sagittal) Pre-Registration (Coronal) Post-Registration. Marginal offset in the aorta (**A**) Coronal View (**B**) Axial View

ment was created at threshold value [220–2940] to preserve the abdominal aorta. The logical operator tool was used to subtract this 'spine' segmentation from the vessels, with the scissors tool utilised to remove the backboard of the CT, separate the iliac arteries from artefacts of the ilia and separate the lumbar artery from artefacts of the spinal vertebra. Islands tool 'keep selected island' was used to isolate the abdominal aorta and branching vessels, while the liver and spleen were separated using the eraser and scissors tool both in the slice view and 3D viewer, with the islands tool chosen to 'remove selected islands'. Refinement of the iliac arteries was achieved by carefully tracking the course of the arteries along the ilia and using paint and eraser tools for definition. Refinement of the major aortic branches, celiac trunk and superior mesenteric artery was achieved using the eraser tool in slice and 3D view.

6.2.5.2.3 IVC (Comparative Analysis and Transform Function)

Comparative analysis was conducted on a gross segmentation of the IVC from both the registered dataset (MRI–CT) and the standalone MRI stitched volume dataset to determine the quality of segmentation and establish if one proved more beneficial as part of a methodological framework. A segmentation of the registered dataset utilising a threshold range [155–402.57] demonstrates a rotation of the dataset in both axial (red) and sagittal (yellow) slice views, with a subtle misalign-

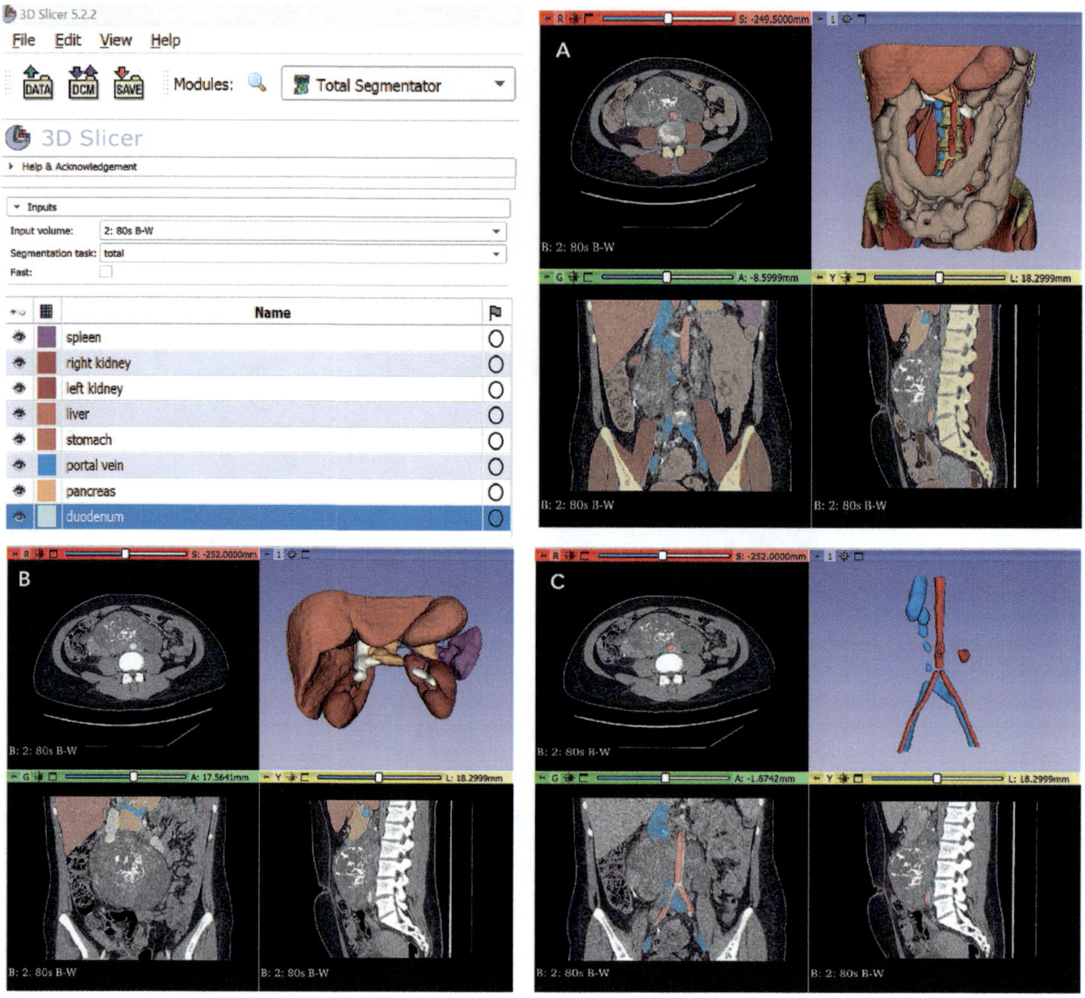

Fig. 6.9 3D Slicer (5.2.2) TotalSegmentator module (**a**) 'total' segmentation from CT dataset, (**b**) with eight structures retained for further refinement, (**c**) automated abdominal aorta and IVC segmentation deemed inadequate for this development

ment present (yellow arrow) where the MRI datasets have been stitched (Fig. 6.11).

The purpose of registering the MRI stitched volume to the CT dataset was to enable an accurate segmentation of the IVC in the same space as the previously segmented structures, most importantly the abdominal aorta. However, as is apparent in Fig. 6.12, there is an offset present in the alignment of the aorta, which would require a transform applied to the registered segmentation, while a similar, yet larger, transform would be required to orient the IVC relative to the aorta (B) from the MRI stitched segmentation.

On critical evaluation, a decision was reached to proceed with the MRI stitched volumes for IVC segmentation and transform it to the CT segmentations for the following reasons:

1. As a prospective workflow, the step of automatically registering two datasets in another software application (MITK) may be omitted; although the software is free and open source, it may prove time-saving.

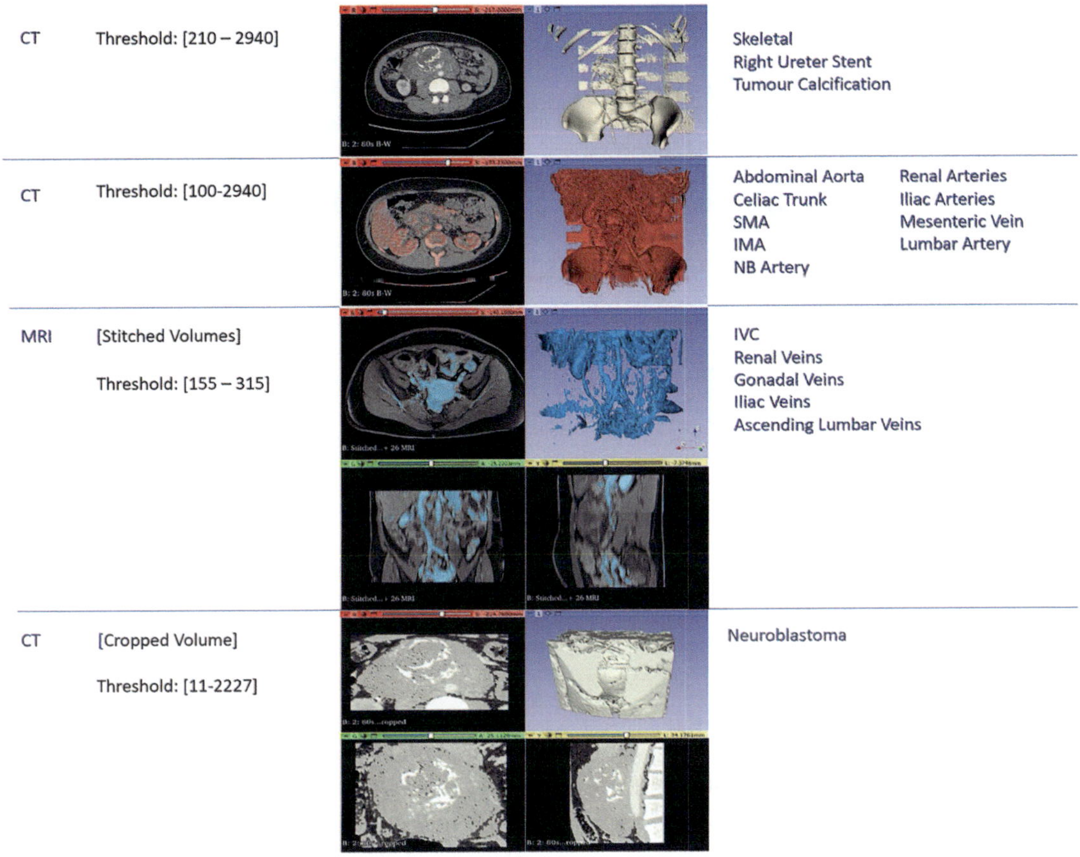

Fig. 6.10 Demonstrates the data source, 'threshold effect' values and initial segmentations in 3D view along with the structures segmented from each

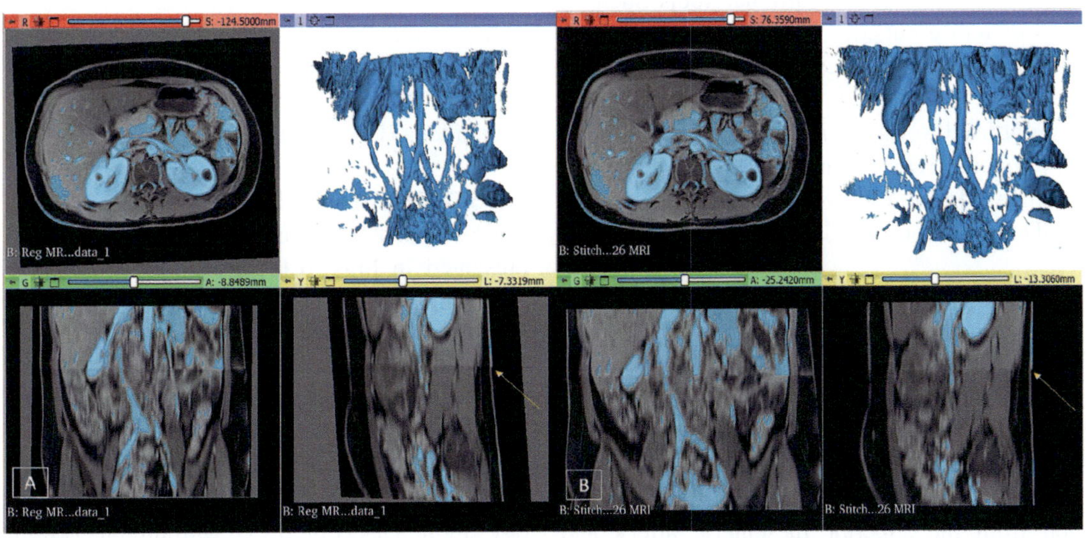

Fig. 6.11 Comparative analysis of a gross IVC segmentation: (left) registered MRI stitched volumes with CT [115–402.57], (right) MRI stitched volumes [150–315] with the line of stitching (yellow arrow)

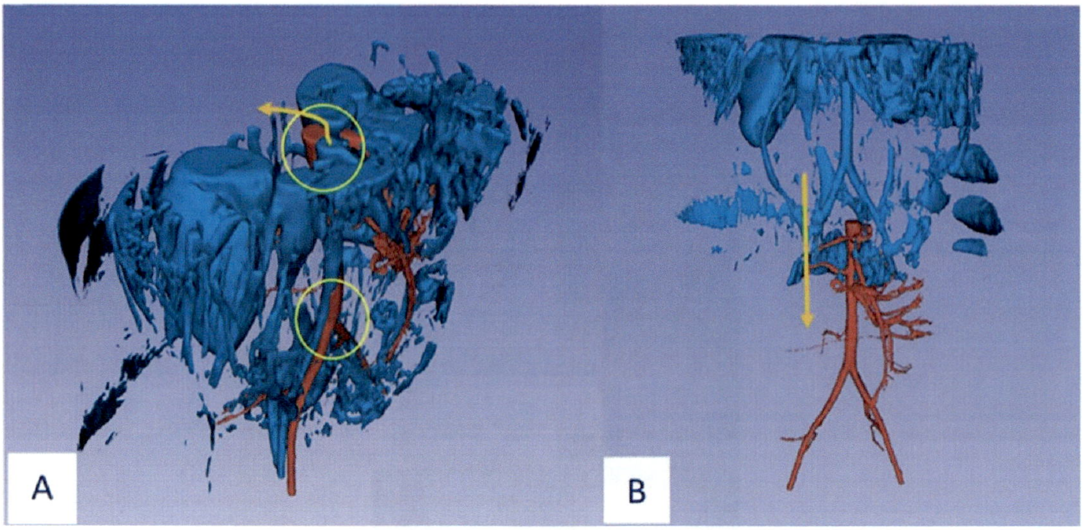

Fig. 6.12 Analysis of transforms required for the IVC segmentations (blue) to align with the aorta segmentation: (**a**) registered datasets—subtle posterior rotation, (**b**) MRI stitched volumes—requiring linear transform

2. The resolution and orientation of the MRI stitched volume dataset prove easier for refined segmentation.
3. Alternatively, manual registration of the MRI and CT could be trialled in 3D Slicer.

6.2.5.2.4 Neuroblastoma

Initially, the Crop Volume module was utilised to isolate the neuroblastoma for segmentation at the threshold [11–2227]. Additional tools such as scissors (erase outside), manual erase and point lists were used to create perimeter boundary markings, while paint and level tracing tools were utilised to fill the inside of the solid mass. To refine the 3D segmentation, a smoothing tool (median 1.5 mm) followed by manual smoothing in 3D view was used.

6.2.5.2.5 Portal–Mesenteric Vein

Separation of the mesenteric vein from the superior mesenteric artery required extensive cross-referencing between a DVR of the CT dataset and the aorta segmentation. To separate the two structures, the eraser and scissors tool was carefully utilised in both slice and 3D view. Upon separation from the superior mesenteric artery and intestinal arteries, the mesenteric vein was created as a new segment using the islands tool 'add selected island' and given a blue colour. The portal vein which had been retained as one of the eight initial segmentations achieved in the TotalSegmentator module was then used to merge it to the mesenteric vein. In the Segment Editor module, paint and level tracing tools were used to form the absent venous section between the mesenteric and portal veins. The portal vein was then moved under the segmentation containing the mesenteric vein, and the two segments were merged. The original portal vein segment was then hidden (Fig. 6.13).

6.2.5.3 Segmentation Outcomes

Final segmentation outcomes in 3D Slicer are presented in Figs. 6.14, 6.15, and 6.16 before exporting .obj models to 3DS Max for retopology.

6.2.5.4 Cross-reference Radiology Imaging | Anatomical Accuracy

Anatomical accuracy was gauged by using fiducial line measurements compared against radiology key images (Fig. 6.17), with tumour volume

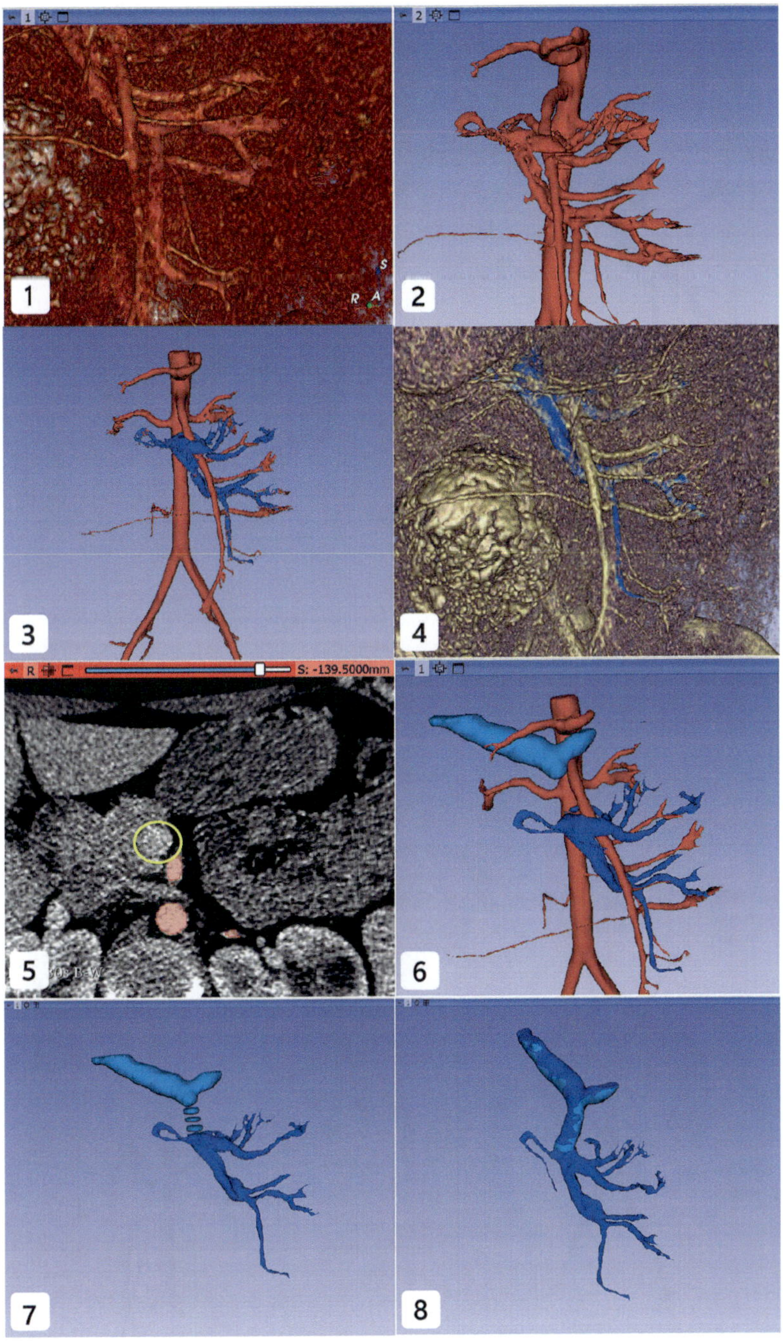

Fig. 6.13 (1) CT DVR to assist with separation of jejunal-ileal arteries from the mesenteric veins (2) abdominal aorta segmentation before venous differentiation (3) mesenteric vein separated as a new segment with the colour blue assigned (4) Cross reference to CT DVR for anatomical accuracy (5) manual segmentation of the inferior portion of the portal vein (6) portal vein (light blue) retained from Total Segmentator (7) bridging the segmentation between the portal and mesenteric veins (8) merging of the portal and mesenteric veins

measured in the Segment Statistics module at 978 cm^3 compared to radiology measurement of ~1000 ml. Geometric accuracy was assessed by overlaying cross-sectional slices in axial, coronal and sagittal planes on the 3D segmentation in 3D view (Fig. 6.18).

6.2.6 Retopology

The individual 3D models generated from segmentation required retopology to decimate the individual mesh to be suitable for real-time game engine rendering. Individual models were

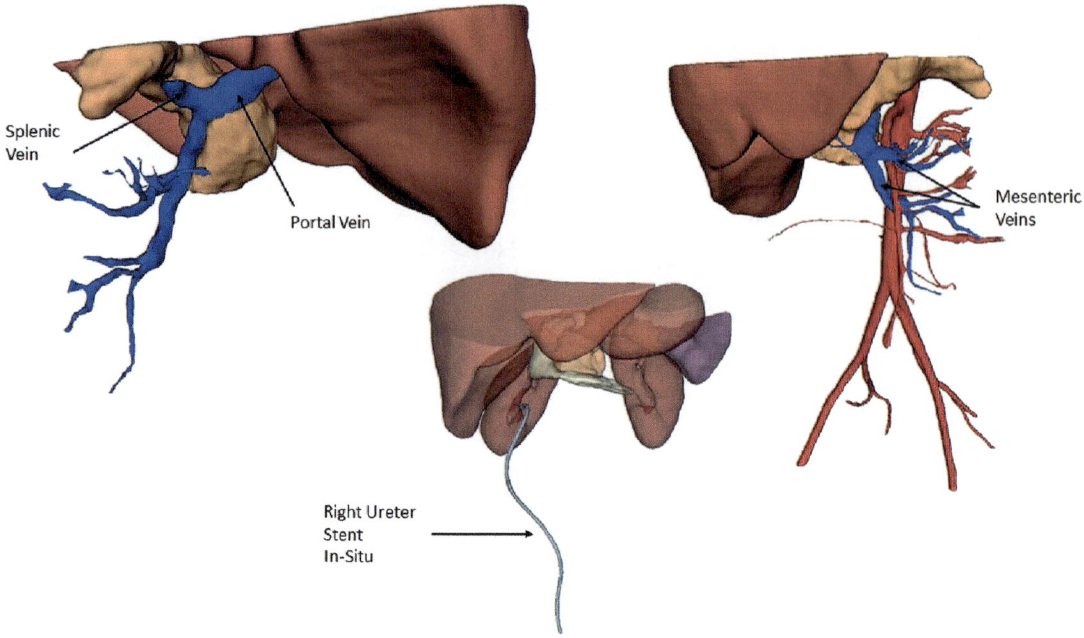

Fig. 6.14 Segmentation outcome of abdominal organs

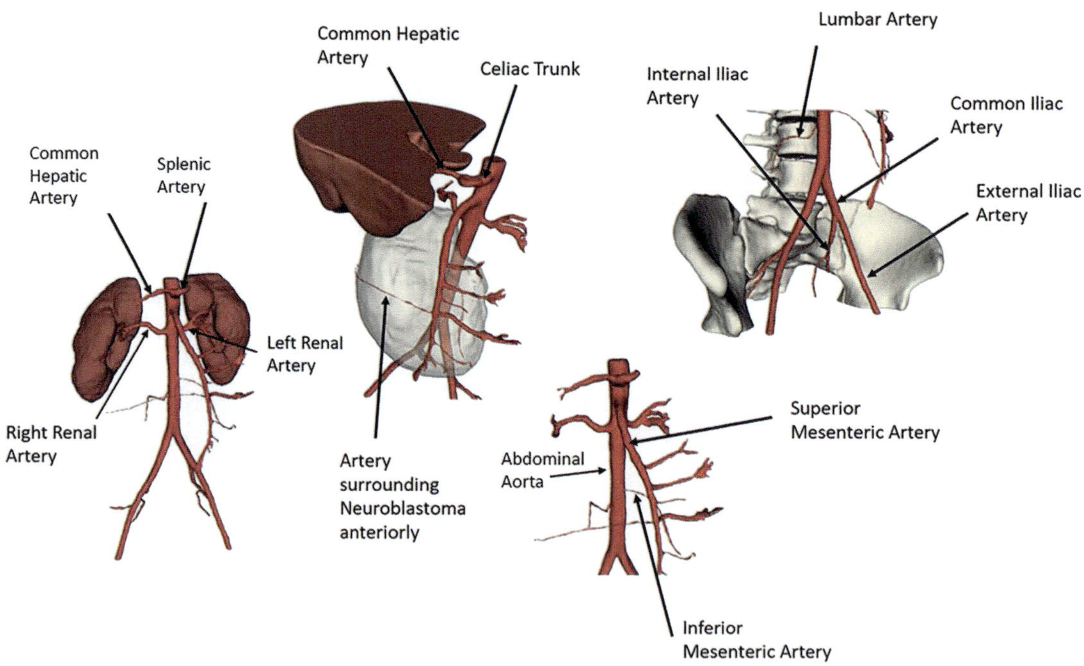

Fig. 6.15 Arterial segmentation outcomes

imported into 3DS Max as exported wavefront object (.obj) meshes, converted to editable poly, with pivots centred to enable unified rotation of the model in Unity. A retopology modifier was utilised to automatically decimate the mesh, with specific face counts chosen for individual meshes,

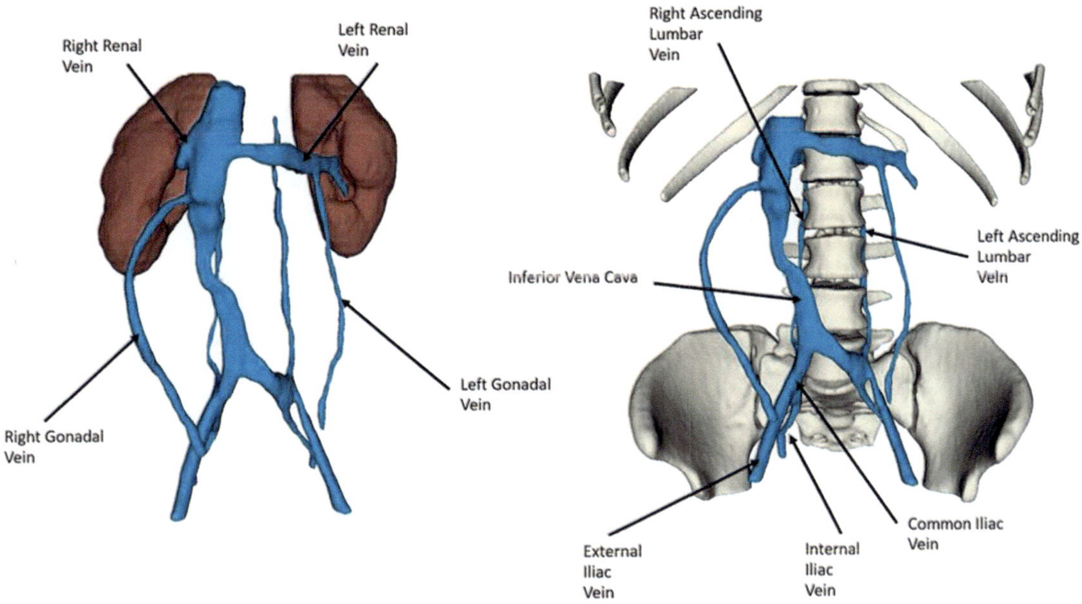

Fig. 6.16 Venous segmentation outcomes

ranging from 1000 polygons (right ureter stent) to 70,000 polygons (skin). Retopology of the IVC and abdominal aorta mesh is shown in Fig. 6.19, with a higher face count chosen for the decimation of the abdominal aorta to retain the artery surrounding the neuroblastoma anteriorly. Retopology of the abdominal organs is demonstrated in Fig. 6.20. An overview of the original polygon counts for each anatomical structure and the lower poly count achieved with retopology is displayed in Table 6.5.

6.2.7 Texturing

Texturing of 3D models was completed in both 3DS Max and ZBrush. The low poly skin mesh was UV unwrapped in 3DS Max to prepare for texturing in substance painter. This was achieved by marking seams along the sides and top of the mesh and reoriented within the UV map editor. This UV map would be exported along with the model as an .fbx file for texturing in substance painter.

To generate photorealistic texturing for the neuroblastoma model, the model was centred within the UV map, with a bitmap base colour material applied, and the baked texture was later exported with the model (Fig. 6.21). The bitmap used is a small, cropped section of a neuroblastoma reference image.

A photorealistic texture for the aorta was trialled in Substance Painter. Auto-unwrap was utilised given the complexity of the structure and two paint layers applied 'organic flesh' with a paler pink undertone (Fig. 6.21). However, it was felt that given the likeness in colour to that of neuroblastoma, this may detract from the overall user experience. Furthermore, for pre-surgical planning, it is commonplace for the surgeon to request stark contrast in colours for identification, so this texture was omitted from the final production. Materials obtained from the Unity Asset Store were applied to the abdominal organs within the Unity application.

The final output model generated in 3DS Max is demonstrated, with well-retained anatomical structures (Fig. 6.22).

6.2.8 3D Modelling

A whiteboard marker, a 3D cube displaying the orientation of the 3D model and a display tablet

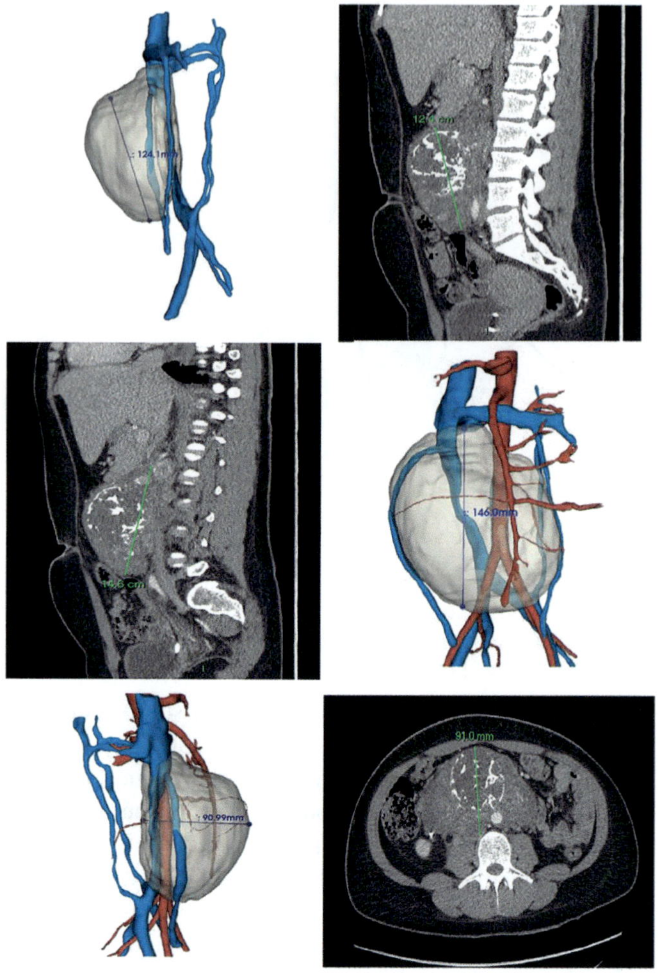

Fig. 6.17 Fiducial line measurements compared to key radiology measurements

were created in 3DS Max modelling software for use in the VR development (Fig. 6.23).

6.2.8.1 Whiteboard Marker (Handle)

A whiteboard marker was modelled in 3DS Max from a cylinder with genuine marker dimensions: height 90 mm, radius 15 mm, sides 30. Processes of inset and extrude, edge chamfering, scaling and bevelling were utilised. The tip of the marker was created by inserting a cone and scaling it accordingly to fit inside the handle. A more rounded appearance was created by outward scaling of the individual edge loops and inserting additional edge loops towards the point of the tip. The base of the marker was completed through processes of inset, extrude, edge chamfering and the placement of additional edge loops to round the base of the marker.

6.2.8.2 3D Cube

The concept of producing a 3D cube was derived from the 3D Slicer software which rotates in sync with the 3D segmentation produced in the slice view. To recreate this model, individual letters were generated using snipping tool software and combined in a .png with a dark grey background.

In 3DS Max, a standard cube was created, to which a bitmap material was added in the material editor. The result of this process is the .png added to each cube face as shown, which was then adjusted to each cube face using box mapping in the UV editor.

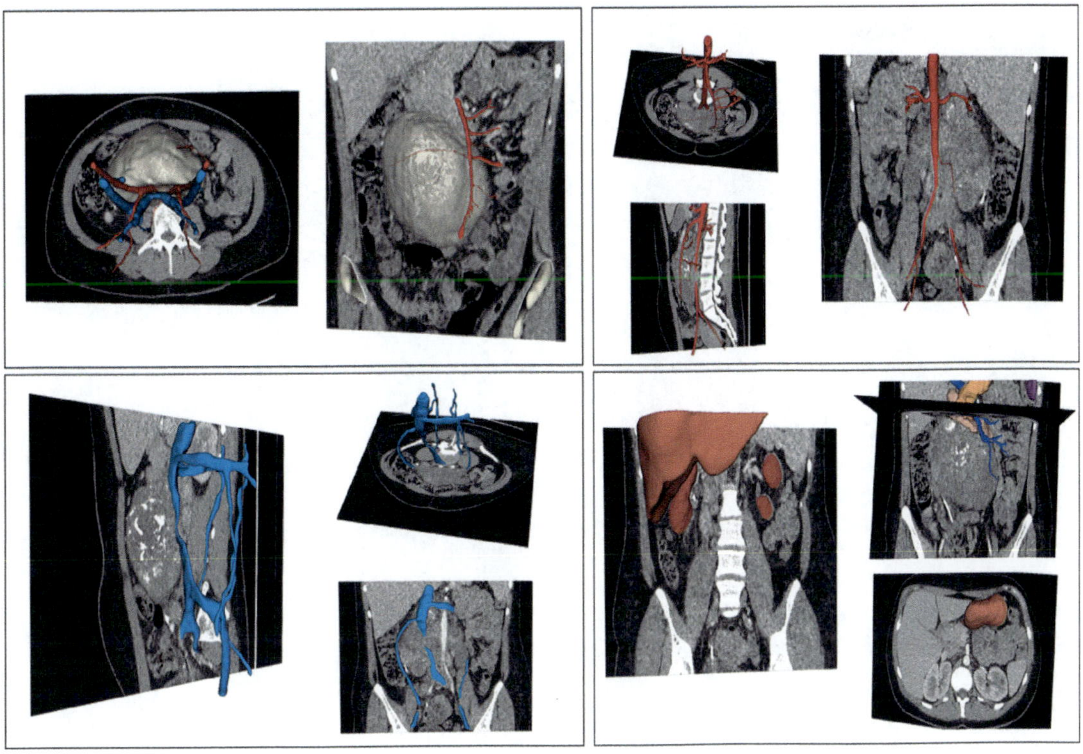

Fig. 6.18 Geometric accuracy using cross-sectional slice overlay in axial, coronal and sagittal plane on the 3D segmentation in 3D view

6.2.8.3 3D Tablet

A realistic display tablet was created in 3DS Max by inserting a box of dimensions: L 244.5 mm, W 177.3 mm and H 5.7 mm, like a Samsung S8 Tablet, with the corner edges chamfered 1.803 mm with five edge segments. The screen was created by inserting a simple plane aligned with the top surface of the cube, along with a cylinder embedded in the box representing a 'home button'. The purpose of the tablet is to serve as a placeholder for a multiple-layered user interface (UI) canvas with toggle buttons in Unity.

6.2.9 2D UI Graphics

Sample 2D graphics were created in Adobe Illustrator, which was trialled early in Unity development as a background image for the UI toggle buttons. However, due to notable pixelation, the use of graphics was refined to the DICOM button to create a feature button.

6.2.10 Interactive Application Development

Unity version 2021.3.4f1 was used in the development of this project application with the implementation of the OVR Interaction Rig—Full Synthetic prefab for base VR interactions including UI interaction and hand grabbing.

6.2.10.1 3D Model Position

During initial development, an .fbx file of the 3D model was imported into Unity; for which a cubic stand was created, centred on (0,0,0) coordinates and set at a height of 1.5 m to account for the eye-level placement of the 3D model.

6.2.10.2 Overlay CT Dataset on 3D Model

A unique feature of this application is the ability to overlay the CT dataset on the 3D model, which was next considered in the development process. This was achieved by utilising a canvas with a

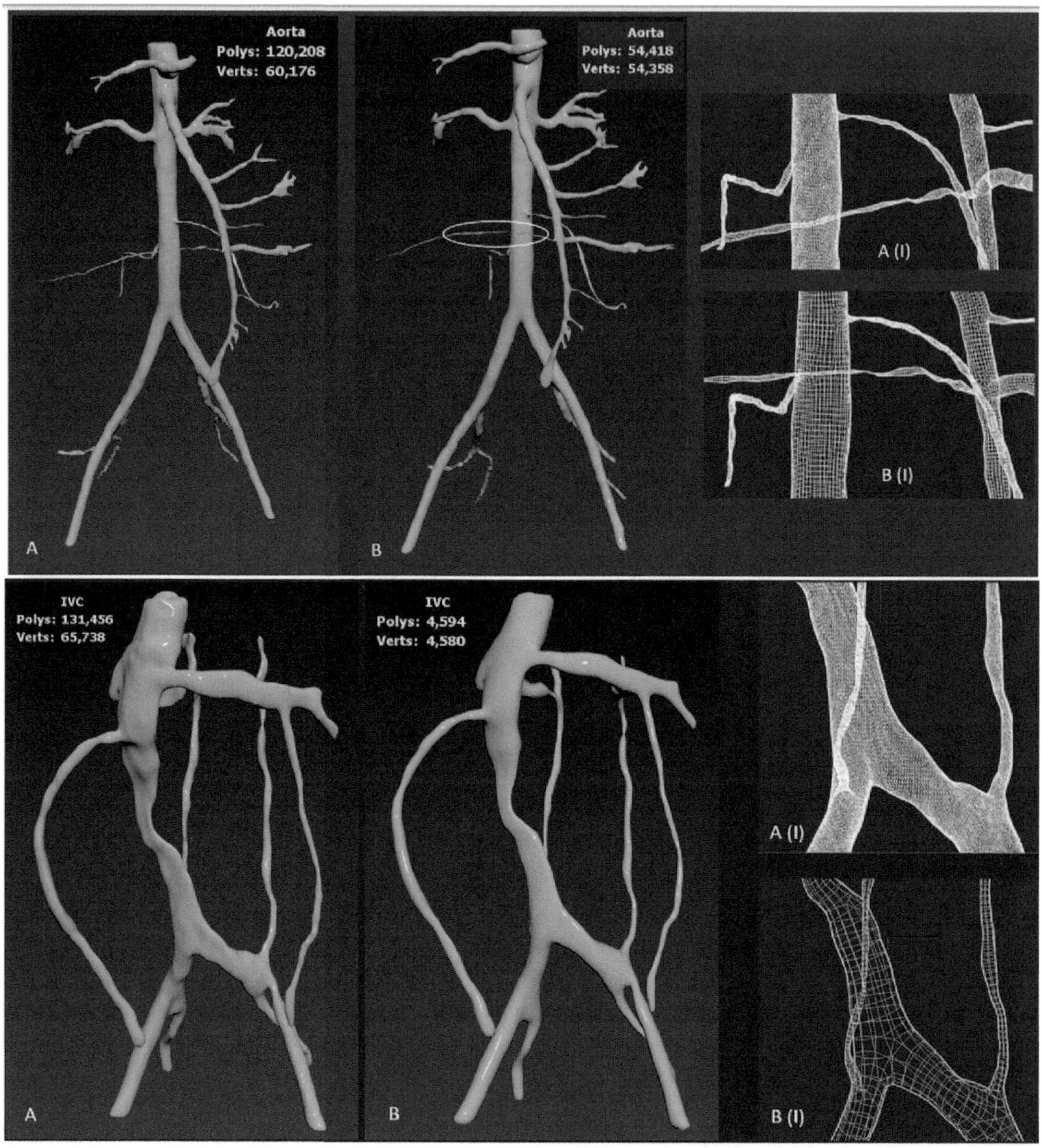

Fig. 6.19 Retopology outcome of the IVC and abdominal aorta (**a**) high poly, (**b**) low poly, **a (i)** high poly triangular mesh, **b (i)** low poly quad mesh

raw image as a placeholder. Three specific C# scripts were created to populate and contain the complete series of CT dataset .jpeg images, which are controlled by a slider on the world space canvas. Once the 241 CT dataset .jpeg images were loaded, the canvas on which these images would be displayed was scaled and positioned to align with the 3D model (Fig. 6.24).

6.2.10.3 Interactive Tablet Display

To create the interactive tablet display used in this application, a flat unity canvas prefab was added to the scene, which comes populated with toggle buttons as a horizontal layout group. This was adapted and arranged according to the required functionality of this application, with multiple canvases overlaid on the 3D tablet in the

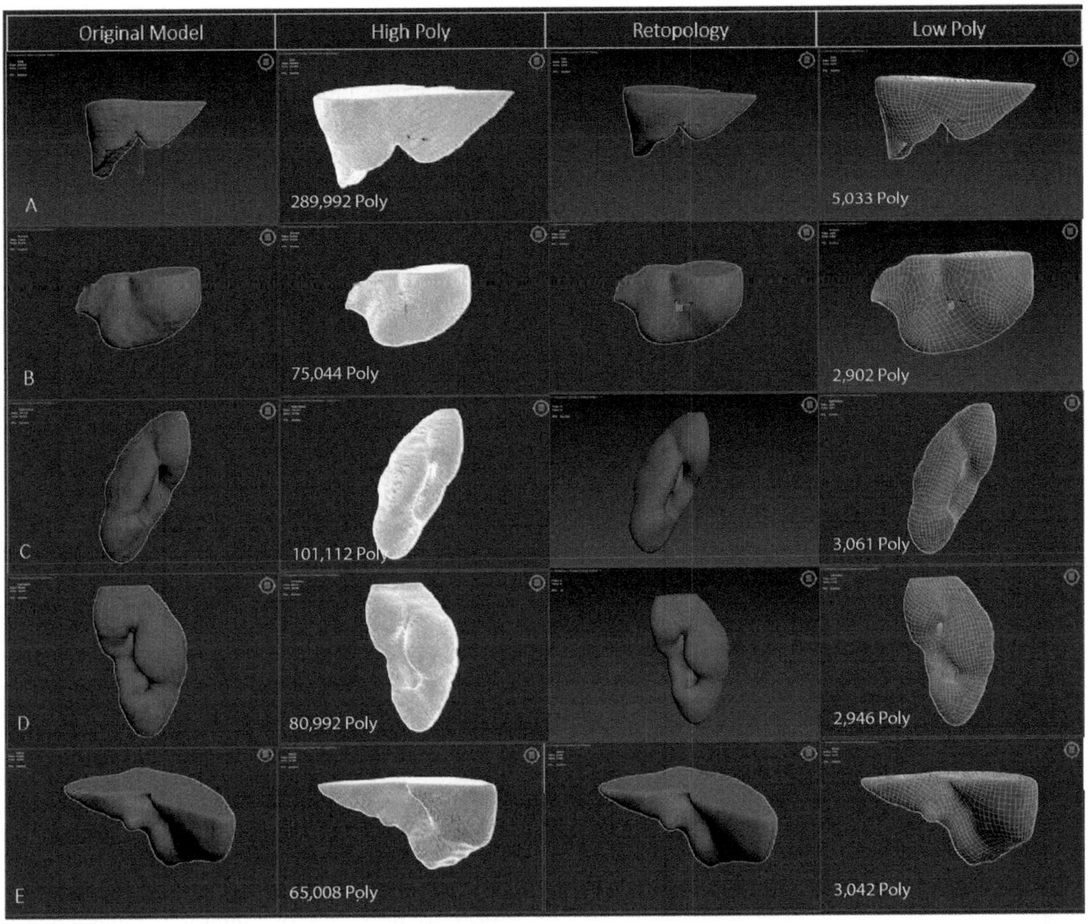

Fig. 6.20 Retopology outcomes of abdominal organs, displaying high and low poly mesh

final display. All toggle buttons were assigned a specific anatomical structure or alternative canvas to 'setActive' on value change.

Subsequently, additional C# scripts were created to control other key functionalities within the application. These scripts included tumour transparency control using a slider, rotation of the 3D model and cube and notation using the whiteboard marker and whiteboard (Table 6.6).

6.2.10.4 Virtual Environment

The virtual environment for this application was created with a prefab of a conference room purchased from the Unity Asset Store (Table 6.4). Key furniture and furnishings utilised from this office-conference room package include a conference table and chairs, computer, mouse, office folder, pen, notepad, water cooler, whiteboard and whiteboard eraser, blinds and ceiling lights.

6.3 Developmental Results

6.3.1 3D Model

The completed 3D model presented in Fig. 6.21 demonstrates the user perspective from within the Oculus Quest 2 headset. The 3D model is positioned on a cubic stand (height 1.27 m) to place the centre of the model at eye level (average user height 5 ft 7 in.), accounting for male and female participant height.

Table 6.5 Displays the original polygon count and the lower poly count achieved with retopology for each 3D anatomical model

Anatomical structure	High poly	Low poly
Neuroblastoma	198,480	20,757
Tumour calcification	115,212	57,479
Abdominal aorta + arteries	120,208	54,419
IVC + veins	131,456	4594
Portal—mesenteric vein	49,916	20,071
Skin	1,802,311	70,000
Spine	594,784	60,250
Ilia	263,192	50,755
Right ureter stent	13,552	1045
Liver	289,992	5033
Stomach	74,044	2902
Spleen	65,008	3042
Pancreas	56,044	2854
Duodenum	42,072	4146
Right kidney	101,112	3061
Left kidney	80,992	2946
Total	**3,898,263**	**363,354**[a]

[a]9.08% of the original polygon count

An isolated view of the more pertinent structures of the 3D model, namely, the abdominal aorta, inferior vena cava and neuroblastoma including calcification, is also shown (Fig. 6.25).

6.3.2 Virtual Environment

The virtual environment chosen for this application was representative of that in which user testing was to be conducted—a seminar room within the Royal Hospital for Children, Glasgow. The purpose is to maintain a sense of presence for the participant transitioning from a real to a simulated environment.

Typical features such as a pen, notepad and folder, alongside a computer and mouse, were included to create a sense of realism. Additionally, a water cooler, exit sign and chair positioning were considered to enable a more immersive environment. A wall poster of the Glasgow Children's Hospital Charity was added, for further realism.

6.3.3 Interactive Display Panel

An interactive tablet display (Fig. 6.26), with toggle feature buttons, is available to users to transition between two specific sections within the main scene:

1. Anatomical identification to identify five specified structures
2. Neuroblastoma to explore additional functionalities of the application (Fig. 6.27)

Key features of the application include the following:

- Tumour transparency (Fig. 6.27)
- Interactive toggle buttons to show/hide individual structures (Fig. 6.28)
- Ability to overlay the CT dataset on the 3D model (Fig. 6.29)
- Medical information related to neuroblastoma including IDRFs (Fig. 6.29)
- Tumour volume (radiology measurement compared with 3D model)
- 360° (left to right) and 180° (supine/prone) rotation of 3D model (Fig. 6.30)
- Notation: the whiteboard marker enables the user to write on the interactive whiteboard (Fig. 6.31)

The 3D cube labelled (A|P, R|L, S|I) rotates in sync with the 3D model to provide a visual cue to the user regarding the anatomical view of the model (anterior | posterior, right | left, superior | inferior).

6.4 Evaluation

6.4.1 User Testing

Participants

Twenty participants were recruited for this study (♂ 7, ♀ 13, aged between 24 and 57 $M = 35.2$, $\sigma = 10.3$), all qualified doctors/medical profes-

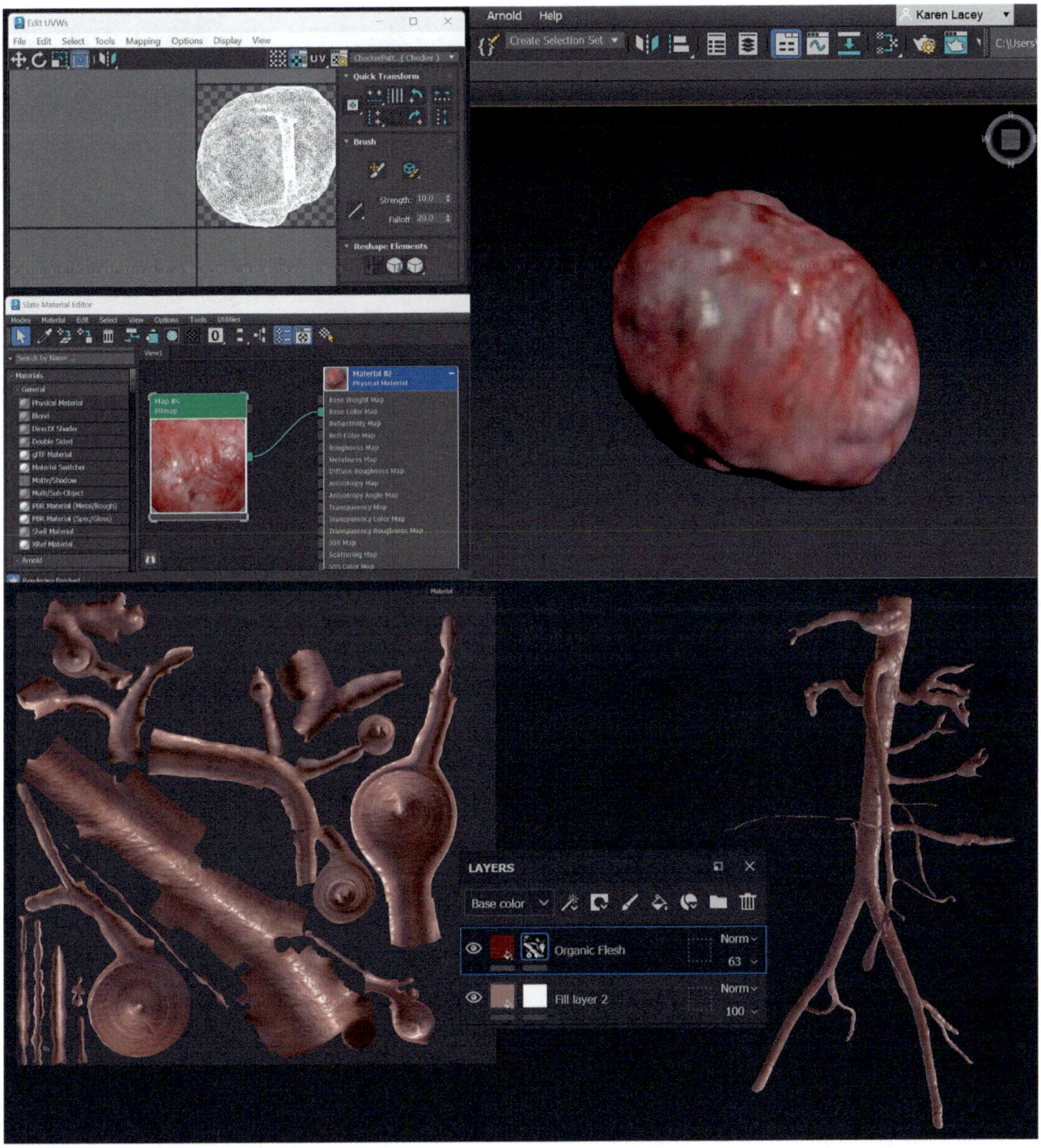

Fig. 6.21 (Top) UV unwrap and texturing of neuroblastoma (3DS Max); (bottom) texturing (trial) of abdominal aorta (substance painter)

sionals at the Royal Hospital for Children, Glasgow. Seven identified as male and 13 as female. All participants were recruited via email distribution from one of the project supervisors, Dr. Giuliana Torpiano, which contained a participant information sheet and consent form, provided by the researcher. Participation was anonymized using a unique identifier code, and participants were assigned to two experimental groups: group 1—2D dataset anatomical identification test followed by 3D VR anatomical identification and group 2—3D VR anatomical identification test followed by 2D dataset anatomical identification, based on educational level to ensure similar initial knowledge in each test group.

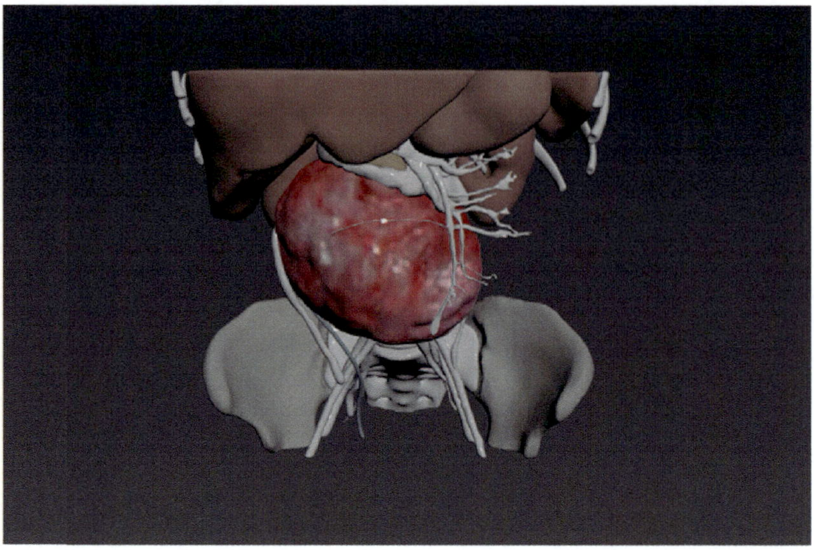

Fig. 6.22 Post-process models (3DS Max)

The educational standard of the participants ranged from foundation year 1 (FY1) to consultant paediatric surgeons. Overall, 85% ($n = 17$) of participants showed little to no knowledge of VR/3D image production; 90% ($n = 18$) of participants had viewed stereoscopic 3D images, while 30% ($n = 6$) had used experimental VR prior.

Procedure

The experimental test was conducted in a safe controlled environment within a seminar room of the Royal Hospital for Children in Glasgow, Scotland. Participants were provided with a printed participant information sheet and instructed on health and safety guidelines while using VR, ensuring no contraindications to use. Additionally, participants were informed of the guardian boundary concept within VR, basic interactions such as finger poke UI and whiteboard use and instructed to begin with the 'anatomical identification' modality. The VR headset was sanitised between participants, and participant safety was monitored, while the headset was connected to the laptop via a lead.

A counterbalanced experimental design (Fig. 6.32) was adopted; group 1 commences with a 2D anatomical identification test of five anatomical structures: abdominal aorta, inferior vena cava, neuroblastoma, right ureter and left kidney.

Participants were provided with axial, coronal and sagittal slice views, instructed on sliders to scroll through the dataset and zoom function and asked to place the mouse cursor on the selected structure for verification. The axial view presents the registered volume of both MRI and CT, with coronal and sagittal views (CT only). Responses were recorded as yes (accurate) or no (inaccurate).

On completion, group 1 participants were handed a VR headset with the application running and instructed to commence with the 'anatomical identification' modality. Participants were asked to identify the same five anatomical structures by pointing to the 3D structure within the virtual environment. Response verification was possible in real time by mirroring the VR headset display to a laptop using the SCRCPY software projection. Participants were then encouraged to explore the 'neuroblastoma' interactive functionalities further. If required, guidance could be given by voice only.

Group 2 participants performed the test procedure, commencing with 3D virtual reality and proceeding to 2D anatomical identification.

6.4.2 Data Analysis

All test data was collated in Microsoft Excel, with statistical analysis conducted using PSPP.

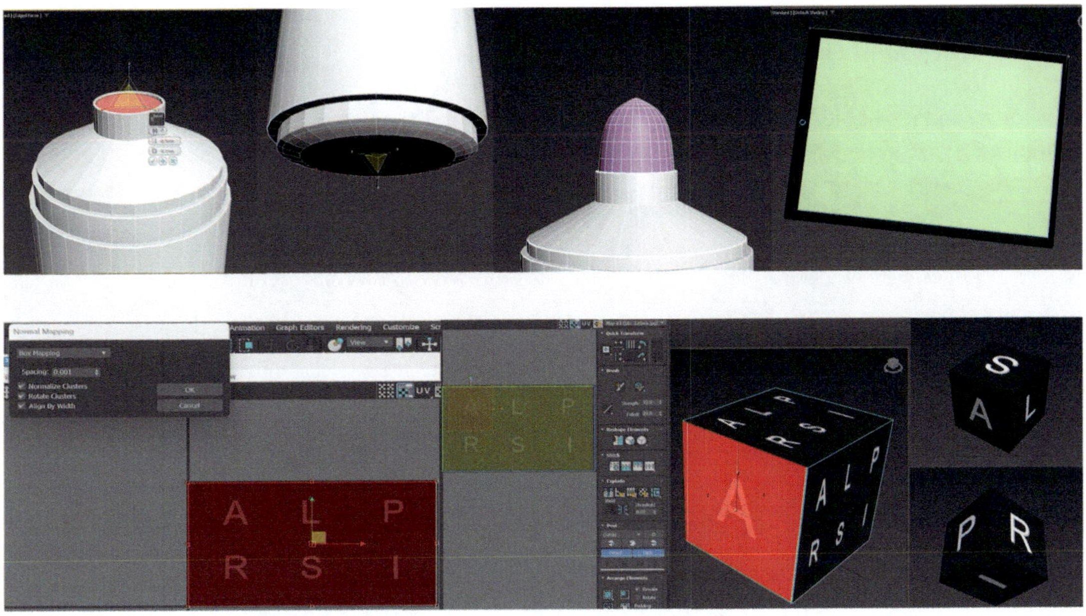

Fig. 6.23 Development of the whiteboard marker, display tablet and 3D cube with box mapping in 3DS Max

Anatomical Identification (2D vs. 3D VR)
Individual participant responses—accurate (yes) and inaccurate (no)—were collated in Excel for both groups. Responses were then assigned a 0/1 value, yes (0) and no (1), to calculate the total error for each participant and delta (Δ) value. As data is not normally distributed, non-parametric analysis was performed to test for significant differences and potential order effects.

System Usability Scale
The System Usability Scale (SUS) standardised questionnaire comprises a simple, 10-question Likert scale format used to measure the usability of an interactive system, with the SUS guidelines used to analyse results (Brooke 1996). SUS scores can be converted to percentile ranks, with a standard SUS score of 68 ranking in the 50th percentile.

A grading system can also be used which closely relates to percentile rank, with an A grade indicating a superior performance and a C grade representing the standard SUS score. Further grading can be used in terms of acceptability (Bangor et al. 2008): acceptable (≥ 70), marginal (50–70) and unacceptable (<50). Based on SUS scores, an application may also be termed a promoter or detractor. Promoters mean the user is likely to recommend the application to a friend/colleague, achieving an average SUS score reasonably close to 81, while detractors show an average SUS score ≤ 53.

Cross-media Presence Questionnaire: The ITC-Sense of Presence Inventory Questionnaire (ITC-SOPI)
The ITC-SOPI questionnaire presents a two-part series of 44 questions: part A (Q1–6) assesses the participants' thoughts/feelings once the displayed environment is over and part B (Q1–38) assesses the participants' thoughts/feelings while they were experiencing the displayed environment (Lessiter et al. 2001). Utilising a 5-point Likert scale, 1 (strongly disagree) to 5 (strongly agree), participant scores are analysed according to the scoring instructions. Spatial presence implies the sense of 'being there' or 'in the physical space'. Engagement refers to the participants'

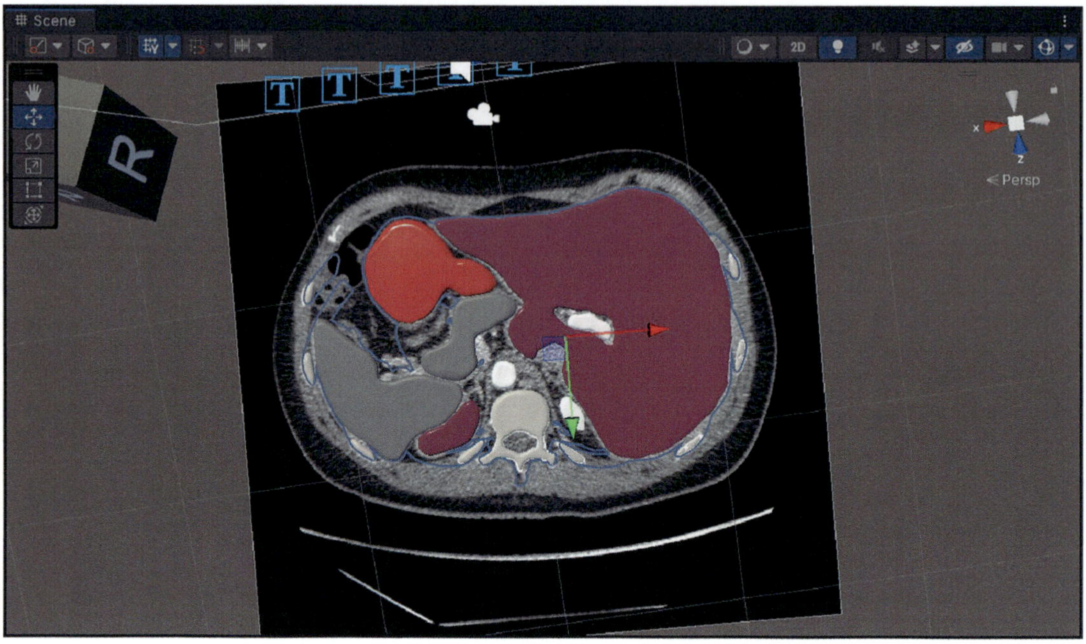

Fig. 6.24 Alignment and scaling of the CT dataset on the 3D model in unity

Table 6.6 The purpose and sources of all scripts used in the development of the interactive application

Script	Purpose	Source
Overlay CT dataset	Create scriptable test object, load .jpeg images of CT dataset, control dataset Slice with Slider	Custom Script—Dr. Matthieu Poyade
Object transparency	Tumour transparency control with Slider	Khan (2020), https://www.youtube.com/watch?v=ALE9Z_wxavg&t=58s
Rotate 3D model with 3D cube	Synchronise rotation of 3D model and cube using Slider	Liam Pearce
Whiteboard marker | whiteboard	Notation using a whiteboard marker	J.P Barnett (2021), https://www.youtube.com/watch?v=sHE5ubsP-E8&t=1246s

psychological experience of the environment. Ecological validity encompasses the naturalism of the virtual environment and its elements, while negative effect accounts for displeasing elements of the VR experience.

Participants Comments

Participants could also voluntarily provide feedback on the application.

Surgical Planning—Paediatric Consultant Feedback

Feedback was sought from paediatric consultants regarding the anatomical accuracy and efficacy of the 3D virtual model as a prototype development for surgical planning.

6.5 Results

6.5.1 Anatomical Identification (2D vs. 3D VR)

Results of anatomical identification tests for group 1 and group 2 were collated in Excel with successful identification rates per anatomical structure displayed in Fig. 6.33.

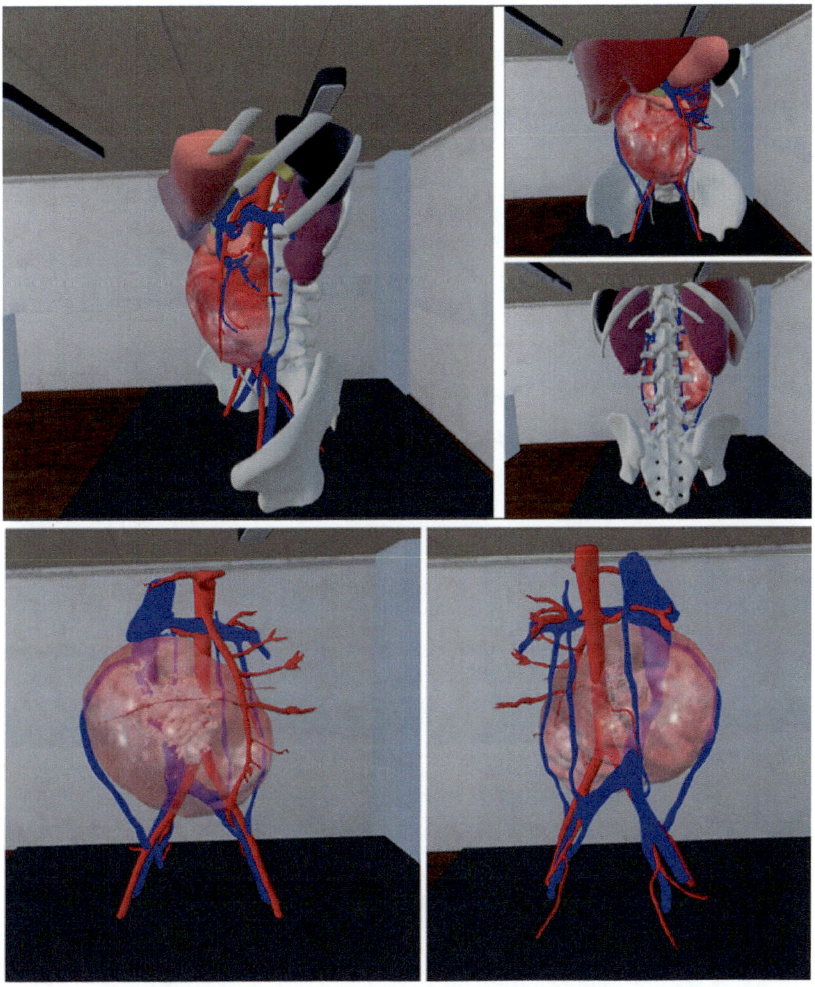

Fig. 6.25 (Top) 3D virtual reality model, (bottom) isolated view of the abdominal aorta, IVC and neuroblastoma model

Due to data being non-normally distributed, a Mann-Whitney U test was conducted in the first instance to explore potential order effects between groups. No significant difference in the total errors between groups was found U ($N\text{control}_{2D(1)} = 10$, $N\text{control}_{2D(2)} = 10$) = 30, $Z = -1.62$, $p = 0.106$ and U ($\text{Nvr}_1 = 10$, $\text{Nvr}_2 = 10$) = 48.5, $Z = -0.14$, $p = 0.888$ (Table 6.7).

These results show that, overall, more errors were committed when analysing 2D imaging, however, to a lesser extent when preceded by VR (group 2). Although a significant difference was not noted in the order of experimental conditions, this suggests that VR could potentially support greater anatomical identification.

Further descriptive analysis between groups for 2D (control) and 3D (VR) demonstrates that group 1 who performed the 2D (control) condition as the first experimental treatment has a higher mean error value ($M = 1.2$) compared to group 2 ($M = 0.5$) (Table 6.8).

Considering the absence of order effect, a Wilcoxon-signed rank test was conducted to contrast the two experimental conditions: control and VR. Results demonstrated that there was a significant difference in errors committed between 2D (control) and 3D VR conditions ($Z = -2.16$, $p < 0.05$). Descriptive statistics demonstrated that participants performed better in VR (MVR = 0.35, $\sigma = 0.59$) compared to 2D (Mcontrol = 0.85, $\sigma = 0.93$) (Table 6.9).

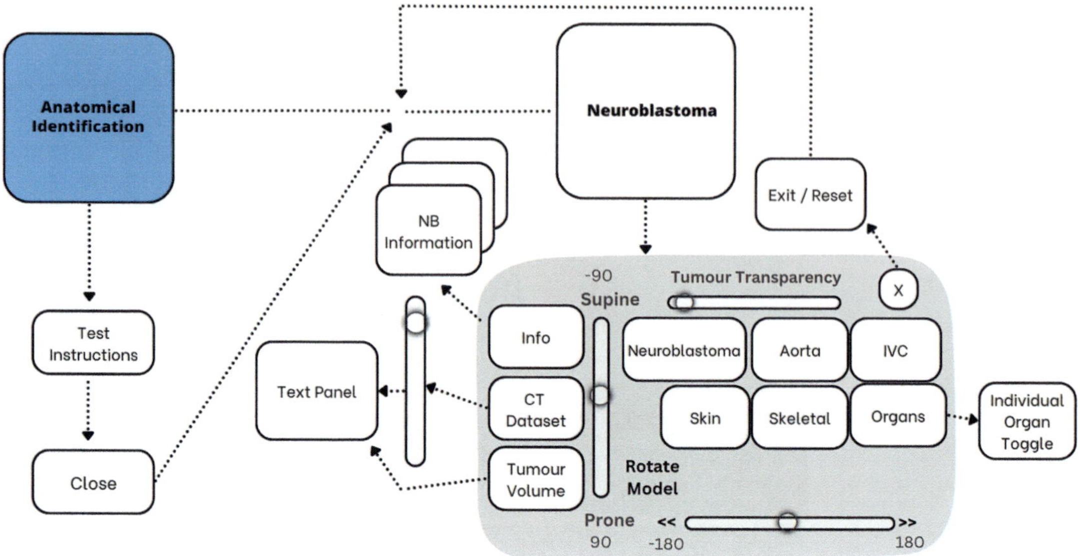

Fig. 6.26 Interactive panel display functionality

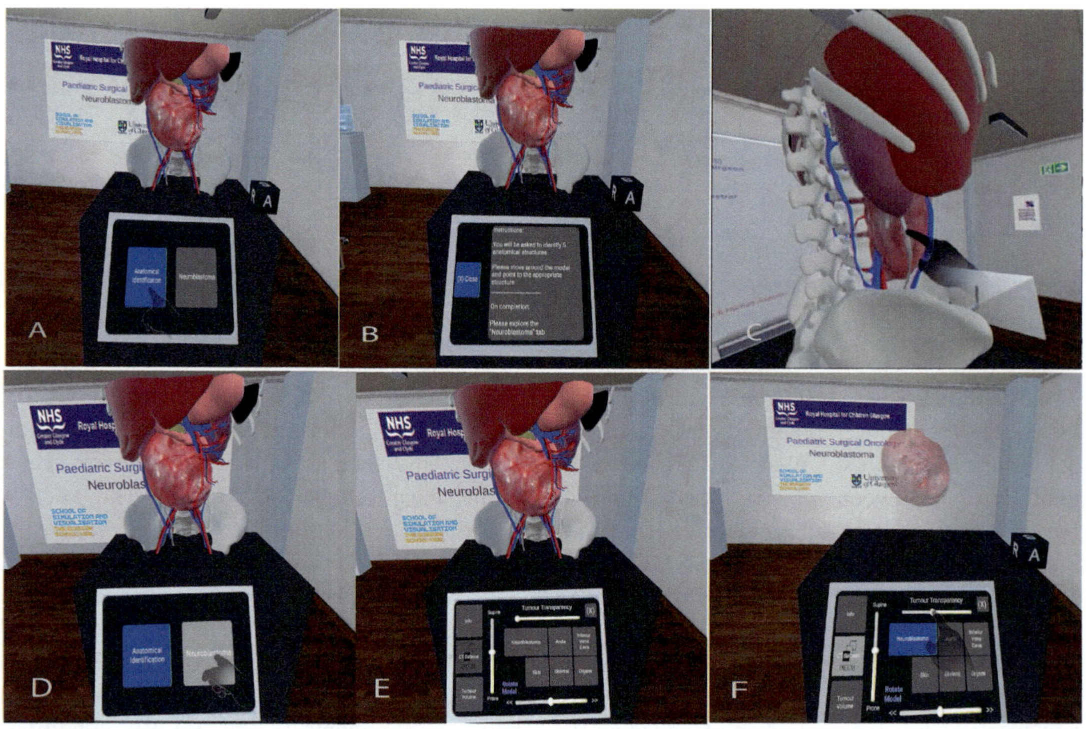

Fig. 6.27 (Top) 'Anatomical identification' modality with instructions and close button. (Right) User perspective inside the VR headset during 3D anatomical identification test. (Bottom) 'Neuroblastoma' tab with pop-up interactive panel. (Right) Tumour transparency function

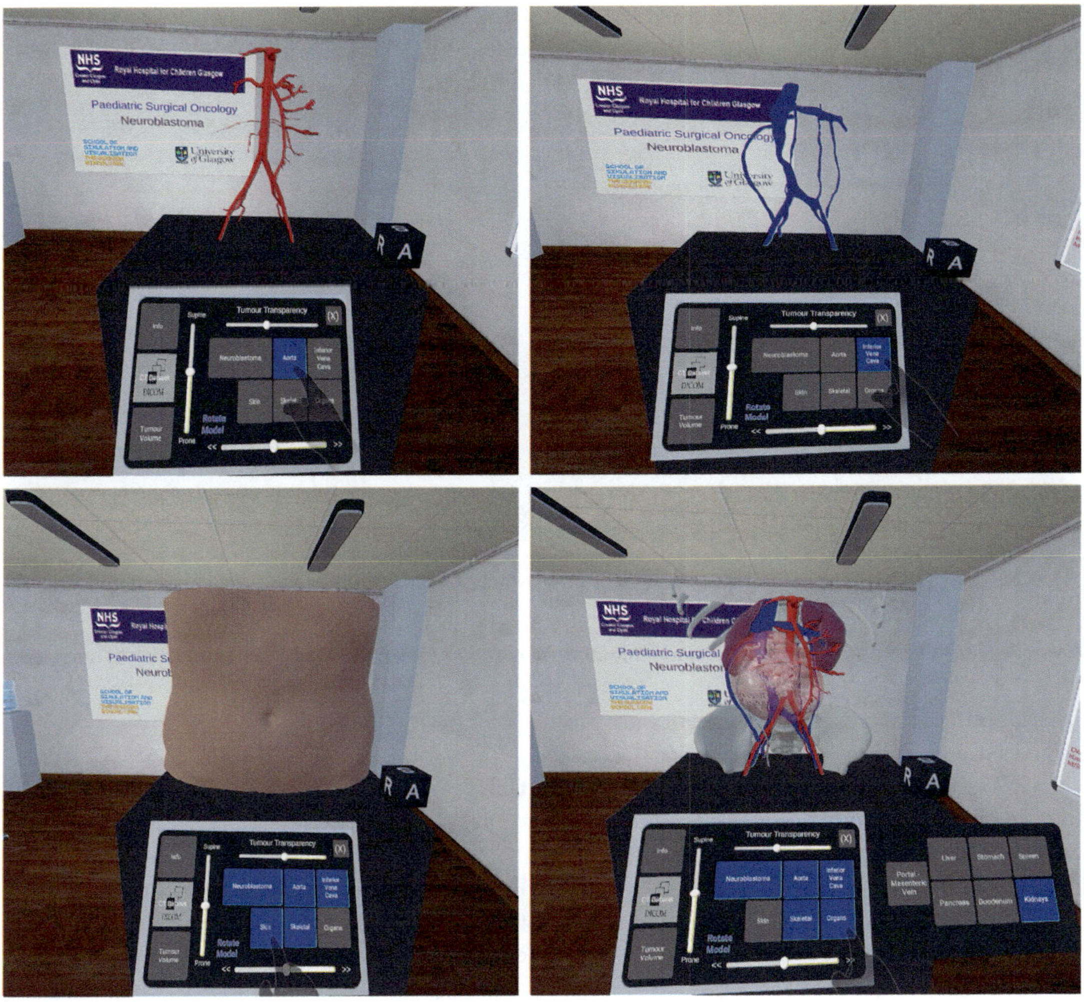

Fig. 6.28 Interactive toggle display to show/hide structures. (Top) Isolated view of abdominal aorta and IVC, (bottom) multi-structure selection

A Mann-Whitney *U* test was carried out to contrast the evolution of errors committed by participants throughout the experimental procedure. Results reported that there was a significant difference ($Z = -2.23$, $p = < 0.05$) between groups (Table 6.10). Descriptive analysis showed a decrease in error for group 1 which undertook the 2D condition first and then the 3D VR condition ($M = -0.8$) (Table 6.8).

Further analysis of the mean delta values between groups shows that group 1 showed a decrease in error from 2D to 3D VR ($M = -0.8$, $\sigma = 1.03$), while group 2 showed a slight increase in error ($M = 0.2$, $\sigma = 0.79$) (Table 6.8).

6.5.2 Application Usability

Individual participant SUS score, SUS standard score and application SUS score are illustrated in (Fig. 6.34), along with SUS score 'grading'. The VR application SUS score measured 79.75.

6.5.3 Presence

Results of the ITC-SOPI questionnaire were collated in Excel and categorised into the four recommended categories: 'spatial presence',

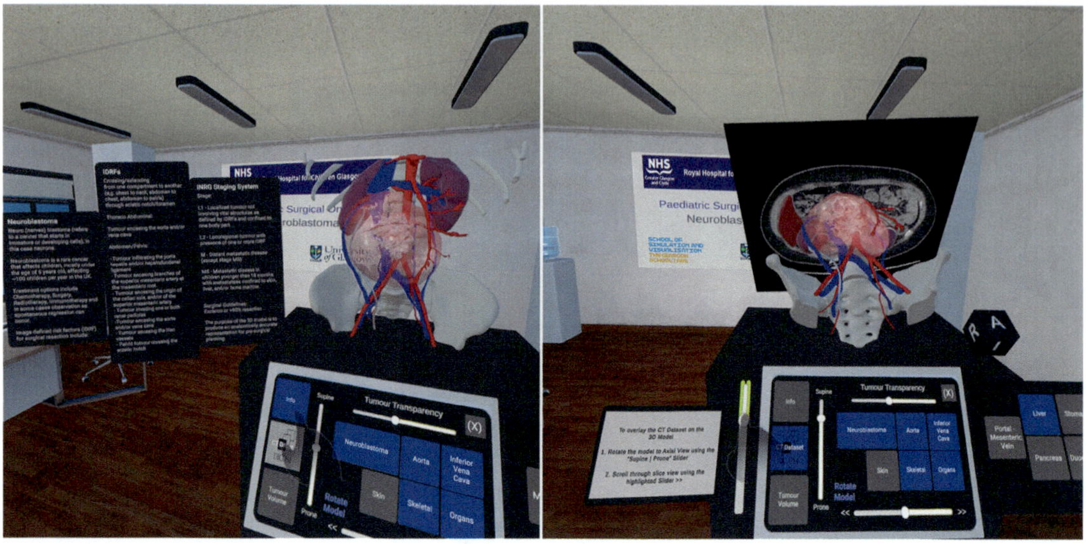

Fig. 6.29 Info panel with scientific information on neuroblastoma. Overlay CT dataset instructions and function

'engagement', 'ecological validity' and 'negative effect'.

The resulting scores in each category are presented in Fig. 6.35: sense of physical space ($M = 3.75 \pm 0.55$ SD), engagement ($M = 4.08 \pm 0.4$ SD), ecological validity ($M = 3.72 \pm 0.83$ SD) and negative effect ($M = 1.77 \pm 0.78$ SD).

6.5.4 Participant Comments

Provision of additional comments was optional at the end of the ITC-SOPI questionnaire received by both participant groups. Of the 20 total participants, 10 participants provided qualitative feedback.

Of the 10 comments received, eight had positive feedback, describing the application as '*excellent*', '*surprisingly intuitive*' and '*really helpful*'. Others remarked that they '*liked the interactive display panels*' and '*enjoyed superimposing the CT dataset over the 3D Model*', while more were '*thankful to see what the future of learning could be*' and noted that they '*could see real teaching and clinical applications for this*'.

Two constructive feedback comments were received, providing useful usability insights. These described the '*glitching*' of images if moving suddenly around the 3D model and the '*blurring of written text*' irrespective of wearing glasses.

6.5.5 Paediatric Consultant Feedback

Paediatric consultant feedback demonstrates that the virtual model provides greater versatility compared to a pre-operative 3D-printed model given specific functionalities such as adding/removing structures or isolation/emphasis of specific structures as well as the opacity of the tumour for clear identification of encased vessels.

6.6 Discussion and Conclusion

6.6.1 Critical Review of 3D Model Development

The process of reconstructing the 3D neuroblastoma model with surrounding structures was relatively straightforward given the quality of the DICOM images acquired. However, given that both patient CT and MRI were used for segmentation, a comprehensive segmentation workflow was needed to be established at the outset for the

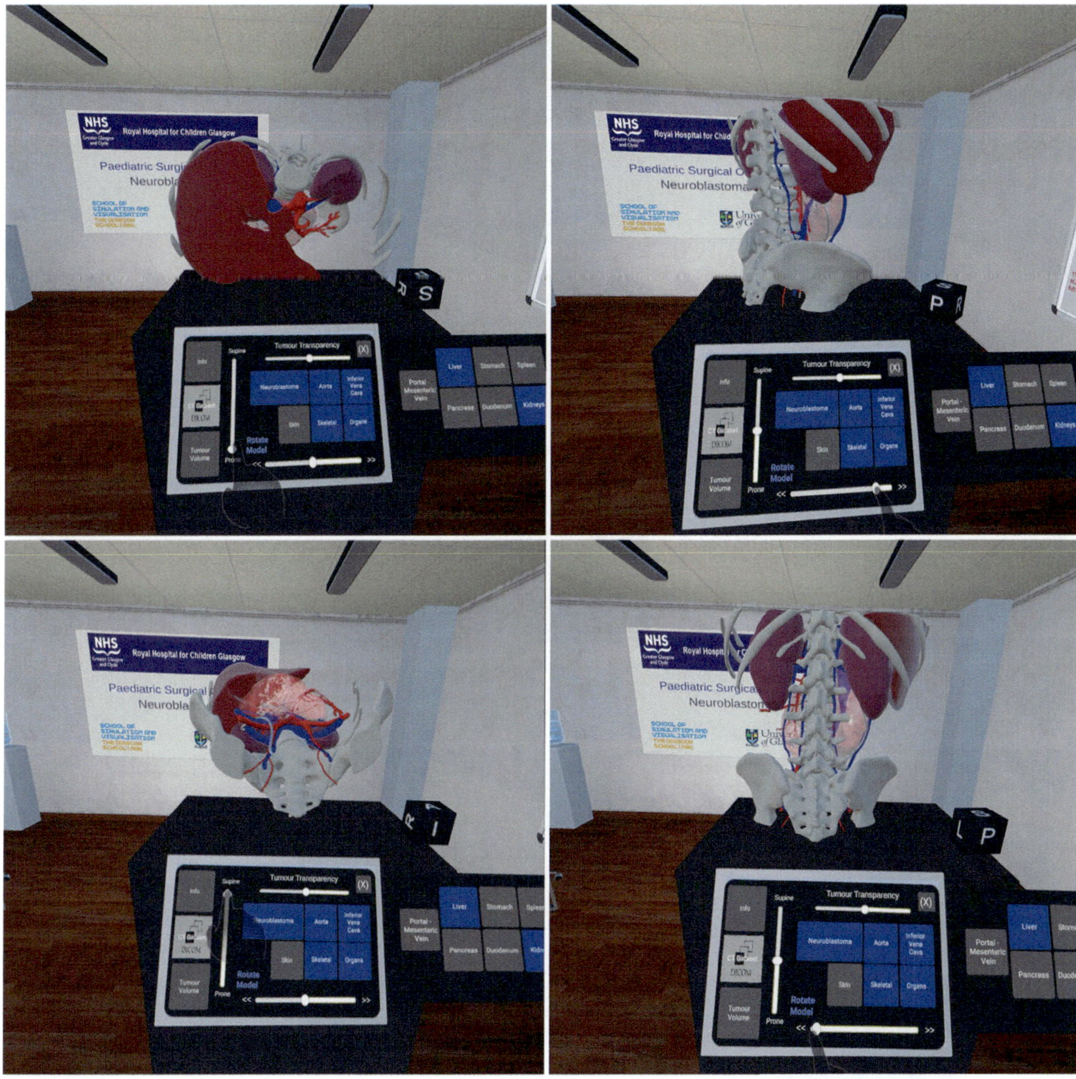

Fig. 6.30 Slider function to rotate the 3D model 360° right to left and 180° supine/prone. Rotation of 3D cube in sync with the 3D model indicating superior, inferior, left and right view

accurate spatial relationship of the 3D models produced. Additionally, as the major vessels and tributary vessels segment at a similar threshold to that of other abdominal structures, a more inclusive segmentation was initially required to achieve a detailed arterial and venous 3D model. This resulted in greater time spent manually removing structures not required, with cross-reference to DVR for smaller vessels and separation of the jejunal arteries from the mesenteric veins.

As this research was delivered retrospectively of surgery, there was no specific time restriction on the production of the 3D models for this prototype development, yet the goal of this research was to produce a framework in which a 3D VR model with interactive functionalities could be executed for future cases within a 3-day working

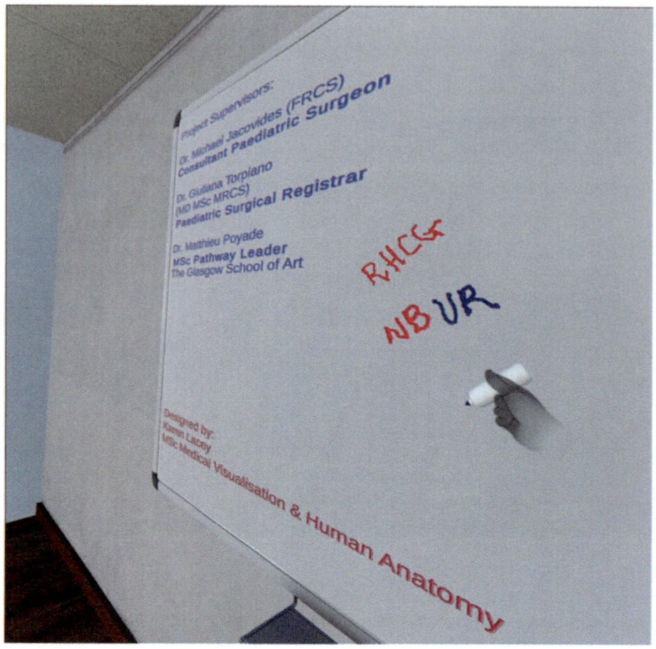

Fig. 6.31 Interactive whiteboard and marker for notation

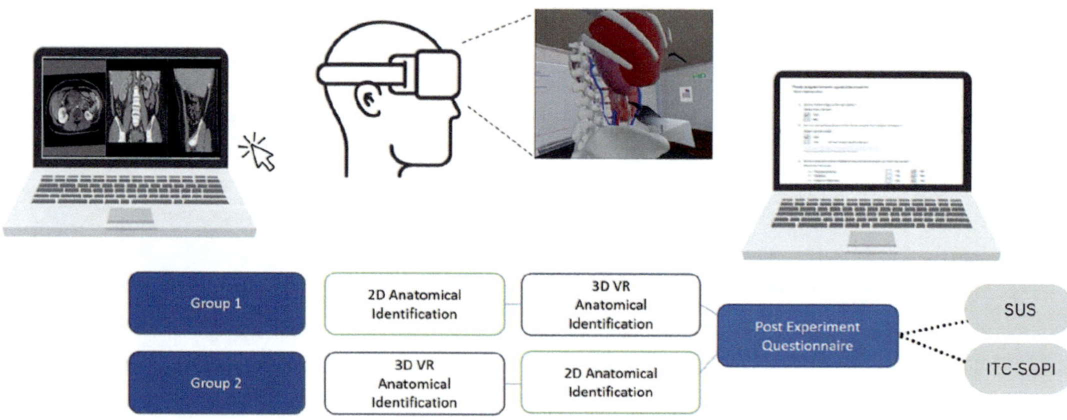

Fig. 6.32 Counterbalanced experimental design

timeframe. The efficacy of this would require testing on further and varied paediatric oncology cases. Although the 3D Slicer module TotalSegmentator was utilised for automatic segmentation of abdominal organs, improvements to AI-based medical image segmentation would significantly reduce 3D model production time, yet the variability in NB size and location may prove more difficult to achieve.

As discussed in the literature, anatomical accuracy, cost and time of production/printing, shipping and accessibility to the surgical team are important when using 3D models for surgical planning. Both VR and 3D-printed models offer valuable tools for surgical planning, education and communication in the medical field. Each approach has its advantages, and the choice between them often depends on the specific goals and requirements of the medical application.

VR provides a dynamic, interactive and real-time manipulation of 3D models. This allows for the integration of real-time medical imaging data,

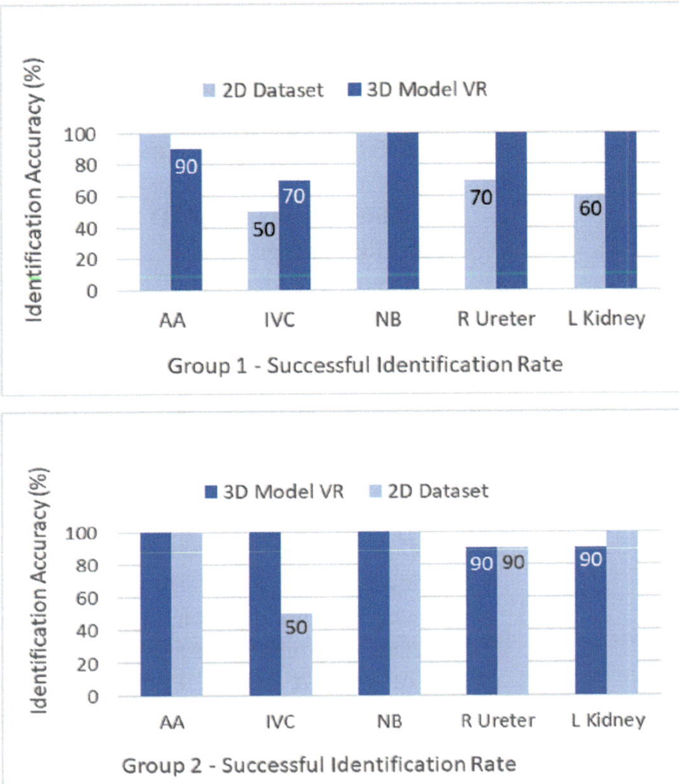

AA = Abdominal Aorta

IVC = Inferior Vena Cava

NB = Neuroblastoma

Right Ureter

Left Kidney

Fig. 6.33 Successful anatomical identification rate—(top) group 1 mean; (bottom) group 2 mean

Table 6.7 Mann-Whitney *U* test between groups

Ranks				
		N	Mean rank	Sum of ranks
Control	1	10	12.5	125
	2	10	8.5	85
	Total	20		
VR	1	10	10.65	106.5
	2	10	10.35	103.5
	Total	20		

Test statistics				
	Mann-Whitney *U*	Wilcoxon *W*	*Z*	Asymp. Sig. (2-tailed)
Control	30	85	– 1.62	0.106
VR	48.5	103.5	– 0.14	0.888

Table 6.8 Between-group descriptive analysis represented as mean error value ± standard deviation

	Mdelta	σ	Mcontrol	MVR
Group 1	–0.8	1.03	1.2	0.4
Group 2	0.2	0.79	0.5	0.3

providing surgeons with the most up-to-date information for surgical planning, and may prove more cost-effective in the long run as it eliminates the need for physical model production. The current cost of an Oculus Quest 2 headset or the newer Quest 3 ranges from £249.99 to £479.99. VR offers accessibility from various locations with the transfer of a .apk file of the application development, as users can access VR models with VR headsets and compatible devices. Supporting real-time collaboration among multiple users in different locations may foster communication and consultation among healthcare professionals. Additionally, VR allows for rapid modifications and adaptations to the 3D models based on feedback or new information, providing a flexible and iterative planning process.

While 3D-printed models offer a tangible representation, they lack the dynamic interactivity of VR. Once a physical model is printed, any updates or changes in patient data would require

Table 6.9 Wilcoxon-signed rank analysis, (p) 0.031, ($p < 0.05$)

Ranks

		N	Mean rank	Sum of ranks
Control-VR	Negative ranks	1	3	3
	Positive ranks	7	4.71	33
	Ties	12		
	Total	20		

Test statistics

	Control-VR
Z	−2.16
Asymp. Sig. (2-tailed)	0.031

Frequencies

		N
Control-VR	Negative differences	1
	Positive differences	7
	Ties	12
	Total	20

Test statistics

	Control-VR
Exact sig. (2-tailed)	0.07
Exact sig. (1-tailed)	0.035
Point probability	0.031

Table 6.10 Mann-Whitney U test contrasting evolution of error between groups

Ranks

		N	Mean rank	Sum of ranks
Delta	1	10	7.9	79
	2	10	13.1	131
	Total	20		

Test statistics

	Mann-Whitney U	Wilcoxon W	Z	Asymp. sig. (2-tailed)
Delta	24	79	−2.23	0.026

the creation of a new model, which can be time-consuming and costly. Printing high-quality anatomical models can be expensive, especially for complex structures ranging from £311.37 to an estimated £2000 (Krauel et al. 2016), while collaboration may be limited to physical presence or require the transportation of models.

Concerning use as an educational tool, VR serves as a powerful educational tool, offering immersive experiences for both surgical planning and education as echoed in user feedback: '*thankful to see what the future of learning could be*' and noted that they '*could see real teaching and clinical applications for this*'. In contrast, 3D-printed models provide a tactile learning experience but may not provide the same level of interactivity or engagement as VR.

Anatomical Accuracy of 3D Model/Pre-surgical Planning

The anatomical accuracy of this 3D model was determined retrospectively, with overlays of the original dataset on the model demonstrating a high degree of accuracy (Figs. 6.17 and 6.18). Further exploration of this may be achieved through independent validation from radiology experts.

Participant feedback demonstrates that the VR model provides greater versatility compared to a 3D-printed model with features such as adding/removing organs, isolation of specific structures and control of tumour opacity for clear identification of encased vessels. Further advantages to this 3D VR model include the facilitation of patient/parent-physician communication.

6.6.2 Evaluation Results

6.6.2.1 Usability

With an SUS score of 79.95, this indicates that the VR application is intuitive and easy to use. Ranking within the 85–89th percentile, marginally below an excellent grade of 80.8, deems the application acceptable and qualifies it as a 'promoter', indicating the users' likelihood to recommend the application to a peer (Brooke 1996; Bangor et al. 2008).

6.6.2.2 ITC-SOPI

The ITC-SOPI questionnaire assessed four specific parameters: spatial presence, engagement, ecological validity and negative effect.

Presence is related to the users' evaluation of the appeal and believability of the content within the displayed environment. Results of user testing show that the participants' sense of presence scored reasonably well ($M = 3.75 \pm 0.55$ SD), with 5 being the maximum score. Factors such as being able to interact with the displayed environ-

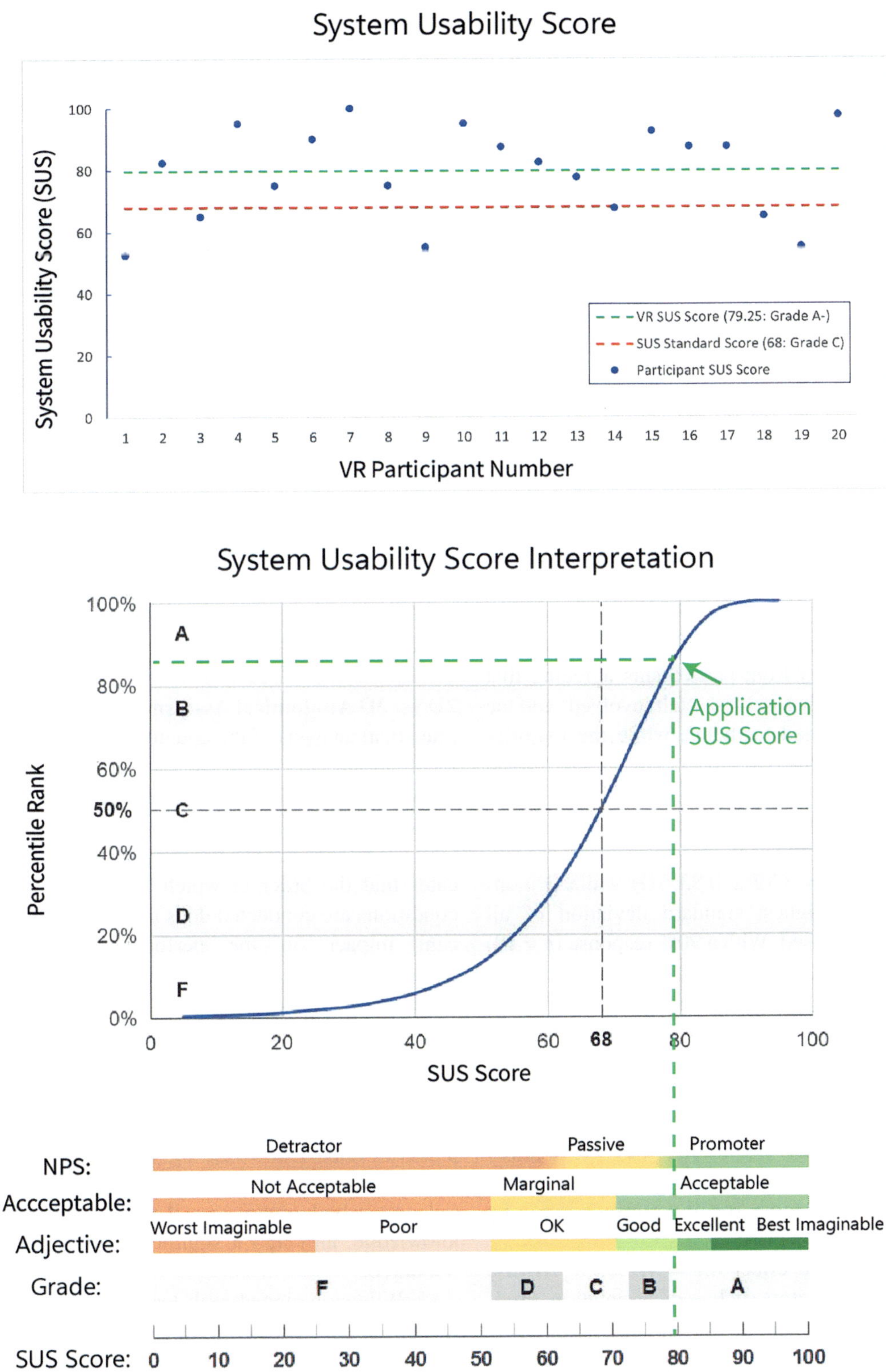

Fig. 6.34 System usability score and interpretation

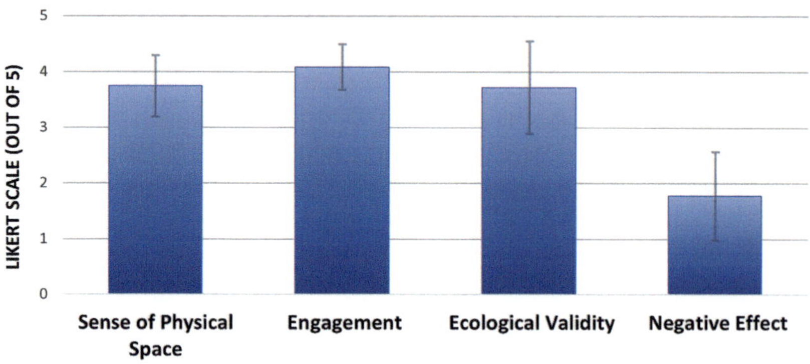

Fig. 6.35 ITC-SOPI results expressed as mean ± standard deviation

ment scored well with 95% (n = 19) of participants 'agreeing/strongly agreeing'. The ability to move objects (n = 18, 90%) and reach out and touch them (n = 19, 95%) showed a high consensus rating.

Participant results for engagement scored best of the four parameters measured, with an average score of $M = 4.08 \pm 0.4$ SD. Engagement represents the users' overall experience and interest in the content displayed, with a unanimous response (n = 20, 100%) from participants agreeing that they 'enjoyed themselves', 'felt involved' and the 'content appealed to them', while the majority (n = 18, 90%) of participants would have 'liked the experience to continue'.

Ecological validity relates to the realism and believability of the content, which scored reasonably well ($M = 3.72 \pm 0.83$ SD) while demonstrating the highest standard deviation of all measures assessed. With a 90% response (n = 18) that the content seemed believable, a greater variation in response was received to whether the displayed environment 'could occur in the real world', with n = 6 in disagreement, n = 5 neutral response and n = 9 in agreement. Although the environment represents a real patient clinical presentation, further exploration may be required regarding photorealism and case presentation. Additional and more specific questions may be necessary to gain clarity.

The negative effect ($M = 1.77 \pm 0.78$ SD) encompasses factors such as disorientation, tiredness, dizziness and eyestrain. No participants reported feeling nauseous/having a headache, while 15% (n = 3) participants reported dizziness, and 30% (n = 6) 'agreed' that they experienced eyestrain. Further exploration of UI elements including text/image resolution and lighting/texturing would be required.

Overall, the application scored well in the ITC-SOPI presence questionnaire, which suggests the plausibility of the VR environment, while demonstrating that this application may prove an effective tool for pre-surgical planning and education.

2D vs. 3D Anatomical Assessment

Statistical analysis of the counterbalanced experiment group 1, 2D–3D, and group 2, 3D–2D, demonstrates that an order effect was not present, as no statistical difference was found between total errors committed between groups. This indicates that the order in which the experimental conditions are conducted does not have a significant impact on the performance of the participants.

However, when comparing the 2D mean error value between groups, group 1 who undertook the control condition as a first experimental treatment shows a higher error value (M = 1.2), compared to group 2 (M = 0.5). This suggests a potential impact of using 3D VR before undertaking the control condition, assuming that participants in both groups have the same initial base knowledge, although a significant difference is not noted.

A Wilcoxon-signed rank test comparing two related samples demonstrates a significant difference ($p < 0.05$) in error committed between the control and VR groups, with descriptive statistics showing that participants performed better in VR (MVR = 0.35, σ = 0.59) compared to 2D (Mcontrol = 0.85, σ = 0.93).

A further Mann-Whitney test between group analysis to assess the evolution of error committed throughout the experiment shows a significant difference ($p < 0.05$). This suggests that the group 1 participants who have first undertaken the control condition and then VR have seen the number of errors decreasing indicating that the VR condition promotes greater accuracy for anatomical identification.

6.6.2.3 Critical Review of Experimental Outcomes

In future research, it would be beneficial to increase both the number of participants and experimental questions to ascertain if these parameters impact the results of this experiment. Additionally, refining the participant demographic to FY1 participants in their first year of clinical training may give greater insight into some of the present study's findings.

6.6.2.4 Improvements to Application

On reflection of participant feedback, the most notable feature of the application that warrants consideration for future development is the clarity of images and text in the user interface. Although measures were taken to mitigate this in the application development by minimising UI sprites and utilising plain text on toggle buttons, further consideration will be given to provide solutions by improving image resolution, font size and style. It would be beneficial to evaluate this across a spectrum of glass wearers and determine the potential limitations of virtual reality while wearing a headset over prescription glasses.

Further consideration would also be given to inclusivity and aspects of this application that could be redesigned to make the application accessible to all users. Redesign elements would include a function to alter the height of the model and secondly to change the stationary tablet UI to a portable version that would 'snap' to the user's hand while moving around the model. Optimising the functionality of the whiteboard marker to allow surgical markings on the skin model, along with the potential for a multi-user experience, may prove beneficial for medical training.

The next steps in this technology would include junior doctor education, using scenario-based learning that simulates various presentations of NB and tests clinical decision-making as well as technical simulation with haptic feedback. Involvement of the multidisciplinary oncology team can be useful in developing these tools to ultimately improve patient experience and outcomes.

6.6.3 Summary of Key Experimental Findings

User testing was conducted at the Royal Hospital for Children, Glasgow, with 20 participants ranging in professional experience from FY1 (foundation year 1), junior doctor to consultant surgeon. The application received a good SUS usability rating of 79.75, deeming it a promoter and likely to be recommended to a colleague.

ITC-SOPI questionnaire results were reasonably good across the four parameters tested: sense of physical space (M = 3.75 ± 0.55 SD), engagement (M = 4.08 ± 0.4 SD), ecological validity (M = 3.72 ± 0.83 SD) and negative effect (M = 1.77 ± 0.78 SD).

A counterbalanced anatomical identification experiment between the 2D dataset and 3D VR model showed no order effect. A significant difference ($p < 0.05$) in errors committed between the control and VR groups demonstrated that participants performed better in VR (MVR = 0.35, σ = 0.59) compared to 2D (Mcontrol = 0.85, σ = 0.93). A significant difference ($p < 0.05$) was also noted in the evolution of error between groups, suggesting that group 1 participants who have first undertaken the control condition and then VR have seen the number of errors decreasing indicating that the VR condition promotes greater accuracy for anatomical identification.

In summary, the 3D neuroblastoma model presented in this study, particularly when implemented through VR technology, holds promise as an effective tool for enhancing pre-surgical planning, medical education and overall patient care in the field of paediatric oncology. The positive outcomes and user feedback provide a foundation for continued research and development in this innovative area of medical technology.

This research was approved by the Teaching and Learning Ethics Committee at The Glasgow School of Art.

Anonymized datasets provided for this study by the Royal Hospital for Children, Glasgow received prior patient consent for their imaging to be used in this manner. Authorization to access willing participants and conduct testing within the surgical innovation and simulation office of the Royal Hospital for Children, Glasgow was granted, with a statement of informed consent received from all participants.

References

Ayesa S, Katelaris A, Brennan P, Grieve S (2021) Medical imaging education opportunities for junior doctors and non-radiologist clinicians: A review. J Med Imaging Radiat Oncol 65(6):710–718. https://doi.org/10.1111/1754-9485.13266

Bangor A, Kortum PT, Miller JT (2008) An empirical evaluation of the system usability scale. Int J Hum Comput Interact 24(6):574–594. https://doi.org/10.1080/10447310802205776

Barr EK, Applebaum MA (2018) Genetic predisposition to neuroblastoma. Children 5(9):119. https://doi.org/10.3390/children5090119

Boedecker C, Huettl F, Saalfeld P, Paschold M, Kneist W, Baumgart J, Preim B, Hansen C, Lang H, Huber T (2021) Using virtual 3D-models in surgical planning: workflow of an immersive virtual reality application in liver surgery. Langenbeck's Arch Surg 406(3):911–915. https://doi.org/10.1007/s00423-021-02127-7

Brooke J (1996) SUS: A 'quick and dirty' usability scale. CRC, London

Butler K, Chang Y, DeMoya M, Feinstein A, Ferrada P, Maduekwe U, Maung A, Melo N, Odom S, Olasky J, Reinhorn M, Smink D, Stassen N, Wilson CT, Kaafarani H, King D, Yeh D, Velmahos G, Stefanidis D, Fagenholz P (2016) Needs assessment for a focused radiology curriculum in surgical residency: a multicenter study. Am J Surg 211(1):279–287. https://doi.org/10.1016/j.amjsurg.2015.05.027

Cancer Research UK (2022) What is neuroblastoma? Available: https://www.cancerresearchuk.org/about-cancer/childrens-cancer/neuroblastoma/about [21 Aug 2023]

Chheang V, Saalfeld P, Huber T, Huettl F, Kneist W, Preim B, Hansen C (2019) Collaborative virtual reality for laparoscopic liver surgery training. In: 2019 IEEE international conference on artificial intelligence and virtual reality (AIVR), pp 1–17. https://doi.org/10.1109/AIVR46125.2019.00011

Children's Cancer and Leukaemia Group (CCLG) (2020) Low and intermediate risk neuroblastoma treatment guidelines. Available: https://www.cclg.org.uk/write/MediaUploads/Member%20area/Treatment%20guidelines/LIRNB_Guidelines_Feb_2020_Final.pdf [22 May 2023]

Cohn SL, Pearson ADJ, Mosseri V, Simon T, Garaventa A, Castel V, Matthay KK, London WB, Monclair T, Ambros PF, Brodeur GM, Faldum A, Hero B, Iehara T, Machin D (2009) The International Neuroblastoma Risk Group (INRG) classification system: An INRG Task Force report. J Clin Oncol 27(2):289–297. https://doi.org/10.1200/JCO.2008.16.678

Eid J, Macedo F, Negussie E, Mittal V (2017) Assessing surgical residents' imaging interpretation skills. Am J Surg 213(3):498–501. https://doi.org/10.1016/j.amjsurg.2016.11.029

Eijlers R, Utens EMW, Staals L, de Nijs PF, Berghmans J, Wijnen RM, Hillegers MH, Dierckx B, Legerstee J (2019) Systematic review and meta-analysis of virtual reality in pediatrics: effects on pain and anxiety. Anesth Analg 129(5):1344–1353. https://doi.org/10.1213/ANE.0000000000004165

Fati F, Pulvirenti R, Paraboschi I, Martucciello G (2021) Surgical approaches to neuroblastoma: review of the operative techniques. Children (Basel) 8(6):446. https://doi.org/10.3390/children8060446

Fischer J, Pohl A, Volland R, Hero B, Dübbers M, Cernaianu G, Berthold F, von Schweinitz D, Simon T (2017) Complete surgical resection improves outcome in INRG high-risk patients with localized neuroblastoma older than 18 months. BMC Cancer 17(1):520. https://doi.org/10.1186/S12885-017-3493-0

Glenn-Cox S, Hird K, Sweetman G, Furness E (2019) Radiology teaching for interns: Experiences, current practice and suggestions for improvement. J Med Imaging Radiat Oncol 63(4):454–460. https://doi.org/10.1111/1754-9485.12896

Guerriero L, Quero G, Diana M, Soler L, Agnus V, Marescaux J, Corcione F (2018) Virtual reality exploration and planning for precision colorectal surgery. Dis Colon Rectum 61(6):719–723. https://doi.org/10.1097/DCR.0000000000001077

Karuppiah R, Munusamy T, Bahuri NFA, Waran V (2021) The utilisation of 3D printing in paediatric neurosurgery. Childs Nerv Syst 37(5):1479–1484. https://doi.org/10.1007/s00381-021-05123-w

Krauel L, Fenollosa F, Riaza L, Pérez M, Tarrado X, Morales A, Gomà J, Mora J (2016) Use of 3D prototypes for complex surgical oncologic cases. World J Surg 40(4):889–894. https://doi.org/10.1007/s00268-015-3295-y

Lessiter J, Freeman J, Keogh E, Davidoff J (2001) A cross-media presence questionnaire: the ITC-sense of presence inventory. Presence 10(3):282–297. https://doi.org/10.1162/105474601300343612

Li J, Dai Y, Kuo S (2014) A massive retroperitoneal neuroblastoma with stenosis of the inferior vena cava in a 5-month-old boy. BMJ Case Rep. https://doi.org/10.1136/bcr-2014-203904

Li L, Yu F, Shi D, Shi J, Tian Z, Yang J, Wang X, Jiang Q (2017) Application of virtual reality technology in clinical medicine. Am J Transl Res 9(9):3867–3880

Lundberg KI, Treis D, Johnsen JI, Azim T, Aravindan N (2022) Neuroblastoma heterogeneity, plasticity, and emerging therapies. Curr Oncol Rep 24(8):1053–1062. https://doi.org/10.1007/s11912-022-01270-8

Maris JM (2010) Recent advances in neuroblastoma. N Engl J Med 362(23):2202–2211. https://doi.org/10.1056/NEJMra0804577

Martelli N, Serrano C, van den Brink H, Pineau J, Prognon P, Borget I, El Batti S (2016) Advantages and disadvantages of 3-dimensional printing in surgery: A systematic review. Surgery 159(6):1485–1500. https://doi.org/10.1016/j.surg.2015.12.017

Matthay KK, Maris JM, Schleiermacher G, Nakagawara A, Mackall CL, Diller L, Weiss WA (2016) Neuroblastoma. Nat Rev Dis Primers 2(1):16078. https://doi.org/10.1038/nrdp.2016.78

McKay KG, Ghani MOA, Henry C, Pruthi S, Benedetti DJ, Friedman D, Lovvorn HN, Zamora IJ (2023) 3D printed model aiding in minimally invasive thoracoabdominal ganglioneuroblastoma resection: A case report. J Pediatr Surg Case Rep 93:102630. https://doi.org/10.1016/j.epsc.2023.102630

Monclair T, Brodeur GM, Von Schweinitz D, Simon T, Cohn SL, Pearson ADJ, Ambros PF, Brisse HJ, Cecchetto G, Holmes K, Kaneko M, London WB, Matthay KK, Nuchtern JG (2009) The International Neuroblastoma Risk Group (INRG) staging system: an INRG Task Force report. J Clin Oncol 27(2):298–303. https://doi.org/10.1200/JCO.2008.16.6876

Newman EA, Abdessalam S, Aldrink JH, Austin M, Heaton TE, Bruny J, Ehrlich P, Dasgupta R, Baertschiger RM, Lautz TB, Rhee DS, Langham MR, Malek MM, Meyers RL, Nathan JD, Weil BR, Polites S, Madonna MB (2019) Update on neuroblastoma. J Pediatr Surg 54(3):383–389. https://doi.org/10.1016/j.jpedsurg.2018.09.004

Noecker A, Chen J, Zhou Q, White R, Kopcak M, Arruda M, Duncan B (2006) Development of patient-specific three-dimensional pediatric cardiac models. ASAIO J (1992) 52(3):349–353. https://doi.org/10.1097/01.mat.0000217962.98619.ab

Otte J, Dyberg C, Pepich A, Johnsen JI (2021) MYCN function in neuroblastoma development. Front Oncol 10:624079. https://doi.org/10.3389/fonc.2020.624079

Papaioannou G, McHugh K (2005) Neuroblastoma in childhood: review and radiological findings. Cancer Imaging 5(1):116–127. https://doi.org/10.1102/1470-7330.2005.0104

Park JR, Eggert A, Caron H (2010) Neuroblastoma: biology, prognosis, and treatment. Hematol Oncol Clin N Am 24(1):65–86. https://doi.org/10.1016/j.hoc.2009.11.011

Pears M, Konstantinidis S (2022) The future of immersive technology in global surgery education. Indian J Surg 84(Suppl 1):281–285. https://doi.org/10.1007/s12262-021-02998-6

Pereira HR, Barzegar M, Hamadelseed O, Esteve AV, Munuera J (2022) 3D surgical planning of pediatric tumors: a review. Int J Comput Assist Radiol Surg 17(4):805–816. https://doi.org/10.1007/s11548-022-02557-8

Punyaratabandhu T, Liacouras PC, Pairojboriboon S (2018) Using 3D models in orthopedic oncology: presenting personalized advantages in surgical planning and intraoperative outcomes. 3D Print Med 4(1):12. https://doi.org/10.1186/s41205-018-0035-6

Sampogna G, Pugliese R, Elli M, Vanzulli A, Forgione A (2017) Routine clinical application of virtual reality in abdominal surgery. Minim Invasive Ther Allied Technol 26(3):135–143. https://doi.org/10.1080/13645706.2016.1275016

Sánchez-Sánchez Á, Girón-Vallejo Ó, Ruiz-Pruneda R, Fernandez-Ibieta M, García-Calderon D, Villamil V, Giménez-Aleixandre MC, Montoya-Rangel CA, Hernández Bermejo JP (2018) Three-dimensional printed model and virtual reconstruction: an extra tool for pediatric solid tumors surgery. Eur J Pediatr Surg Rep 6(1):e70–e76. https://doi.org/10.1055/s-0038-1672165

Sokol E, Desai AV (2019) The evolution of risk classification for neuroblastoma. Children 6(2):27. https://doi.org/10.3390/children6020027

Souzaki R, Kinoshita Y, Ieiri S, Kawakubo N, Obata S, Jimbo T, Koga Y, Hashizume M, Taguchi T (2015) Preoperative surgical simulation of laparoscopic adrenalectomy for neuroblastoma using a three-dimensional printed model based on preoperative CT images. J Pediatr Surg 50(12):2112–2115. https://doi.org/10.1016/j.jpedsurg.2015.08.037

Tack P, Victor J, Gemmel P, Annemans L (2016) 3D-printing techniques in a medical setting: a systematic literature review. Biomed Eng Online 15(1):115. https://doi.org/10.1186/s12938-016-0236-4

Tejo A, Castellví A, Lustig P, Fenollosa F, Uceda R, Buj I, Krauel L, Valls A, Munuera J (2021) 3D printed surgical planning prototype manufactured by a hybrid multi-material 3D printer. IOP Conf Ser Mater Sci Eng 1193:01211

Tejo-Otero A, Fenollosa-Artés F, Uceda R, Castellví-Fernández A, Lustig-Gainza P, Valls-Esteve A, Ayats-Soler M, Munuera J, Buj-Corral I, Krauel L (2021) 3D printed prototype of a complex neuroblastoma for preoperative surgical planning. Ann 3D Print Med. 2:100014

Uehara S, Takama Y, Yoshida H, Hashii Y, Oue T, Usui N (2013) Abdominal neuroblastoma with inferior vena cava and right atrial extension. J Pediatr Surg Case Rep 1(6):119–121. https://doi.org/10.1016/j.epsc.2013.05.001

Uruthiralingam U, Rea PM (2020) Augmented and virtual reality in anatomical education—a systematic review. Adv Exp Med Biol 1235:89–101. https://doi.org/10.1007/978-3-030-37639-0_5

Part II

3D Animations

Vertebral Fractures and Juvenile Osteoporosis: Increasing Parent/Carer Awareness with an Interactive Application

7

Georgena Buesnel, Ibrahim Daniel Buksh, Sze Choong Wong, and Matthieu Poyade

Abstract

Glucocorticoids used long-term to treat young people with Duchenne muscular dystrophy (DMD) are toxic to bone and may result in the development of osteoporosis which can lead to vertebral fractures. In addition, vertebral fractures are difficult for families to visualise from two-dimensional lateral radiographs. There is a lack of three-dimensional (3D) resources for families and young people with DMD to understand the morphology of the fractures causing difficulty visualising and understanding them in a clinic. Parents and carers must be able to make informed decisions for treatment plans as well as understand future health implications. Positive results have been seen in numerous studies indicating that interactive applications utilising digital technologies have benefitted knowledge acquisition, motivation and engagement in anatomical, medical and patient education. Therefore, this study aimed to create a web-based interactive application with 3D models and animation to aid awareness of osteoporosis and vertebral fractures in parents or carers of children with DMD. Nine caregivers completed an online questionnaire before and after viewing the application. Awareness of key aspects of the conditions increased for most participants. Additionally, the application scored 80.6 on the System Usability Scale showing that the application was easy to use. Learnability also scored well, suggesting the application was intuitive. As a pilot study, this research suggests that a web-based interactive application with 3D models and animation could benefit the parents and carers of young people with DMD regarding their awareness of osteoporosis and vertebral fractures. This could help parents and carers understand their child's needs better as well as allow more efficient use of time with clinicians. Further research to include a larger and more diverse group of participants could be conducted to include statistical analysis for more reliable results.

Keywords

Interactive application · Duchenne muscular dystrophy · Vertebral fracture cascade · Vertebral fracture

G. Buesnel (✉)
School of Innovation and Technology, The Glasgow School of Art, Glasgow, UK

School of Medicine, Dentistry and Nursing, College of Medical, Veterinary and Life Sciences, University of Glasgow, Glasgow, UK

I. D. Buksh · M. Poyade
School of Innovation and Technology, The Glasgow School of Art, Glasgow, UK

S. C. Wong
Human Nutrition, School of Medicine, Dentistry and Life Sciences, University of Glasgow, Glasgow, UK

Department of Paediatric Endocrinology, Royal Hospital for Children, Glasgow, UK

J. Clancy, M. Poyade (eds.), *Medical Visualization and Applications of Technology – Volume 2*, Biomedical Visualization 5, https://doi.org/10.1007/978-3-031-63463-5_7

7.1 Introduction

Duchenne muscular dystrophy (DMD) is caused by the malfunction of a protein called dystrophin (Crisafulli et al. 2020). Dystrophin maintains muscle fibre strength and protects fibres from damage (Ma et al. 2017). In DMD, the dystrophin produced does not function normally, and consequently, muscle fibres become damaged (Crisafulli et al. 2020). Globally, it affects around 19.8 per 100,000 live male births (Crisafulli et al. 2020).

Young people with DMD usually present with symptoms in early childhood as their muscle fibres are replaced by fat or fibrosis (Gao and McNally 2015). These symptoms include progressive muscle weakness and overall motor delay (Phung et al. 2023). This results in the loss of general everyday movement and a lack of weight-bearing through the lower limbs. Therefore, some patients lose the ability to walk by puberty (Gao and McNally 2015). Not only does DMD affect voluntary actions, but some may suffer from respiratory issues due to the weakening of both respiratory and cardiac muscles (Gao and McNally 2015). Therefore, the diagnosis often comes with a shortened life expectancy (around 27 years) (Ma et al. 2017; Phung et al. 2023).

Clearly, DMD can have a drastic effect on a child's quality of life. The condition is currently incurable but is managed by glucocorticoids. This treatment is used to prevent the progression of DMD by slowing the damage to the muscle fibres which in turn allows patients to carry out normal everyday functions for longer (Phung et al. 2023). As a result, some young people have been able to retain the ability to walk for up to two to three years longer in comparison to those untreated (Ma et al. 2017). Glucocorticoids have been shown to reduce early mortality, improve cardiac and respiratory outcomes and improve the quality of life of patients (Phung et al. 2023). However, the side effects of the treatment can have other negative implications on numerous health outcomes which could significantly impact on quality of life. The prolonged use of glucocorticoids is known to be deleterious to bone as they impair normal bone accrual, reduce trabecular bone density and microarchitecture and lead to abnormal cortical bone geometry (Hartmann et al. 2016; Lui and Baron 2010; Ward 2021b). This, as well as the underlying myopathy, adds to glucocorticoid-induced osteoporosis in DMD (Hartmann et al. 2016; Phung et al. 2023).

7.1.1 Osteoporosis, Vertebral Fractures and Further Treatment

Young people with DMD are highly likely to suffer from fragility fractures (FF) due to ongoing muscle weakness, lack of weight-bearing and the side effects of glucocorticoid treatment (Ma et al. 2017; Phung et al. 2023). Fragility fractures are four times more likely to occur in DMD patients (Phung et al. 2023).

The types of fractures observed in young people with DMD are not only long bone fractures such as femoral fractures, but also vertebral fractures (Ward 2021b). However, it is important to note that these fractures are morphologically different—long bone fractures occur due to breaks in cortical bone, whereas vertebral fractures result in changes to the vertebral body's shape. The change in shape is due to a loss of height either at the anterior, middle, or posterior part of the vertebral body. Anterior compression results in a wedge fracture, compression in the middle of the vertebral body leads to a biconcave fracture and posterior compression results in a crush fracture (Wáng et al. 2017). The Genant semi-quantitative method is used to classify the severity of vertebral fractures (Fig. 7.1).

Generally, anterior wedge and biconcave fractures are most common and usually occur in the lower thoracic or lumbar regions of the spine (Phung et al. 2023). Vertebral fractures can lead to severe back pain or chronic low-grade back pain which impairs quality of life in people who are wheelchair-dependent and can lead to thoracic kyphosis when there are multiple severe vertebral fractures which may compromise lung

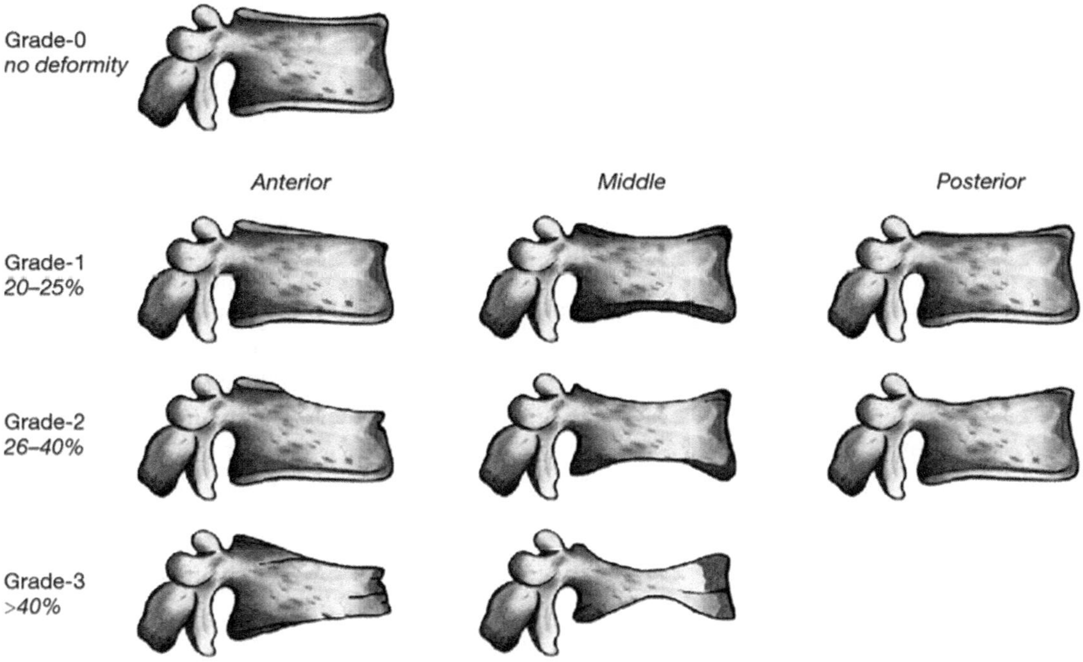

Fig. 7.1 Genant semi-quantitative classification of vertebral fractures (Wáng et al. 2017)

volumes (Ma et al. 2017; Phung et al. 2023; Sakka 2022). Asymptomatic vertebral fractures, however, are common. Phung et al. (2023) reported that half of their cohort ($n = 60$) had at least one moderate (grade 2) to severe (grade 3) vertebral fracture, yet 50% of these were asymptomatic. Likewise, Ma et al. (2017) reported that half of their cohort of DMD patients with vertebral fractures ($n = 30$) were asymptomatic. If left untreated, one vertebral fracture can worsen over time, and surrounding vertebrae may also fracture (Ma et al. 2017). This is known as the vertebral fracture cascade. Since vertebral fractures are likely in DMD patients, it is important to identify and treat vertebral fractures to prevent them from contributing to the vertebral fracture cascade to ensure treatment begins promptly. Routine screening via lateral spine radiographs should begin soon after beginning glucocorticoid treatment to diagnose vertebral fractures as early as possible in accordance with current standards of care (Ma et al. 2017; Phung et al. 2023; Sakka 2022). Both Phung et al. (2023) and Ma et al. (2017) observed that the earliest finding of a vertebral fracture in glucocorticoid-treated patients was within six months to one year of treatment beginning.

When DMD is diagnosed, clinicians can begin bisphosphonate therapy (BPT) which may improve bone mineral density and decrease fracture incidence in adults with osteoporosis (Phung et al. 2023). Bisphosphonates may not completely prevent fractures but can stabilise existing vertebral fractures and slow the progression of the vertebral fracture cascade (Ward 2021a). Bisphosphonate therapy should be implemented at the earliest opportunity to prevent permanent deformity (Ma et al. 2017; Phung et al. 2023; Ward 2020). Therefore, by diagnosing vertebral fractures early and promptly beginning treatment, the quality of life of DMD patients could be improved. Diagnosis can be alarming, especially as 2D lateral radiographs are difficult to understand for the public (Ward 2021b). The images contain many other anatomical structures, and the vertebrae themselves may appear blurry due to the presence of the ribs. Resources able to show the 3D morphology of vertebral fractures may be beneficial in these cases to aid awareness of the condition and its implications.

7.1.2 Patient Communication

It is extremely important that parents and carers of young people with DMD have various resources available to them to aid their understanding of the condition and treatment to allow them to make informed choices when it comes to treatment. The resources given to patients usually comprise traditional leaflets or links to various websites. Evidently, there is a lack of 3D material for parents and carers of young people with DMD.

7.1.2.1 Animation

Animations can provide a succinct, digestible way of explaining complex information to patients to aid their understanding. For example, Aisah et al. (2022) used animation to educate 16-year-old girls on anaemia. They found that knowledge of examination, susceptibility and treatment in those showed that the animation (study group) significantly increased ($p < 0.005$) between their pre-knowledge test and post-video tests. On the other hand, the knowledge of those given traditional leaflets (control group) did not significantly differ (Aisah et al. 2022). Animations have also been used to educate patients about sudden unexpected death in epilepsy. Greenlaw et al. (2021) presented teenage patients and their parents with an animation to aid awareness of the condition. The results concluded that it was beneficial as the patient's knowledge increased very significantly ($p < 0.001$) after watching the animation. All the parents gave feedback that the animation was informative. An interesting finding during this study was that less than 20% of the parents had discussed the condition with medical professionals despite their child having epilepsy, with less than 40% of the patients themselves doing so (Greenlaw et al. 2021). Evidently, this demonstrates the need for patients and parents to be provided with suitable resources to help facilitate important discussions with their healthcare providers.

Despite the promising evidence, not all animations have been shown to be beneficial. Shqaidef et al. (2023) tested an animation, detailing orthodontic treatment to parents of patients, on knowledge retention, and compared it to traditional methods. The results concluded that between the two groups, those shown the animation and those given leaflets, there was no difference in the mean scores in knowledge. Additionally, members in both groups were unable to recall root damage facts and how often their children should brush their teeth. Interestingly, however, despite the lack of knowledge retention in both groups, they discovered that dentists took 9 minutes longer to explain procedures within the control group (Shqaidef et al. 2023). Therefore, this does provide evidence that animation can potentially benefit patients and healthcare providers in terms of time management.

7.1.2.2 Interactive 3D Models and Applications

Despite animations providing positive results in most cases, they are passive. A lack of engagement with animations may lead to dissatisfaction. This is where interactive 3D models could be more effective. Not only could they provide patients and carers with a more detailed picture of anatomy, but an increase in interaction with the resources could foster user engagement, with some studies proving their benefits in medical and anatomical education (Erolin 2019). With a wide variety of software available for creating 3D models from pre-existing data such as CT or MRI scans, these models could be created for a variety of conditions, such as vertebral fractures.

To increase interactivity, these models could be placed within interactive applications to provide a customised user experience. Since applications can be deployed onto a variety of hardware, such as iOS, PC and Android (Erolin 2019), they can be more accessible to patients with scheduled appointments. More often, interactive applications are used within higher education with various applications being produced for this audience. Weldon et al. (2019) performed a pilot study in which they developed an interactive application, containing 3D models and animation, discussing obsessive-compulsive disorder. Out of five participants, four rated the application as 'very useful'. Furthermore, a knowledge test concluded that knowledge increased after the use of their application (Weldon et al. 2019). An application aimed at anatomy students, developed by Khayruddeen et al. (2019), detailed skull anatomy and contained 3D models and animations within the PC application. User testing (n = 12) showed that 92% indicated that it aided their understanding, and 83% found it beneficial for spatial anatomy. The animation within the application was only deemed useful by just over half of the cohort. However, feedback such as including more labels and help with functionality was provided by users to improve this aspect. Lastly, Iannucci et al. (2022) developed a web-based application containing animations and 3D models detailing coronavirus proteins. The application performed well and received 1700 views in the first six months while gaining positive feedback. Therefore, it is evident that applications containing both 3D models and animations can be beneficial for aiding awareness and understanding of complex topics all in one, accessible place.

Healthcare applications are utilised frequently by institutions to provide patients with information outside of appointments. A randomised, control trial by Timmers et al. (2019) found that a study group provided with an application discussing post-operative care after total knee replacement surgery yielded significantly higher increases in their QoL and lower decrease in mobility when compared to a control group who were given basic information. This is promising, but it should be noted that out of all features within the application, the text-only feature was utilised the most. In addition, a study by Oudkerk Pool et al. (2021) concluded that digital resources, including web-based and 3D animated content, had a positive impact on cardiac patient awareness and quality of life, highlighting that improved resources can encourage patient motivation. Furthermore, an application created to increase awareness of the National Health Service's Abdominal Aortic Aneurysm screening programme received positive feedback, with users wishing to attend the screenings after use of the application (Jones et al. 2022), showing that digital resources have a positive impact in at-risk individuals.

7.1.3 A Novel Approach

It is extremely important that parents and carers of young people with DMD have various resources available to them to aid their understanding of the condition and treatment to allow them to make informed choices when it comes to treatment. However, there is a lack of resources aimed at the parents and carers of young people with DMD. Incorporating 3D models and animation within an interactive application may not only make information accessible, but also digestible and engaging for those wishing to educate themselves. Considering the evidence that these all-in-one resources have been beneficial in aiding awareness and improving patient outcomes (Erolin 2019; Iannucci et al. 2022; Khayruddeen et al. 2019; Oudkerk Pool et al. 2021), creating a similar resource for parents and carers of DMD patients may potentially yield similar results. A walkthrough style of the application would provide an active learning experience while using 3D models and animation to communicate information efficiently and effectively. Therefore, this study aims to design and develop an interactive, web-based application for parents and carers of DMD to help increase awareness of osteoporosis and vertebral fractures. In addition, usability will be assessed, and the user's awareness of key points about the conditions before and after the use of the application will be determined.

The aim of this pilot study is to develop an interactive web-based application to aid parent/carer awareness of vertebral fractures in children with DMD.

To achieve these aims, the following objectives were completed:

1. Conduct a literature review to identify gaps in the field and to build upon current knowledge.
2. Create 3D models of bone density and healthy and fractured vertebrae from freely accessible volumetric data using 3D Slicer, and iterate on these models in 3DS Max and ZBrush.
3. Develop an application to be deployed online which is engaging and informative.

4. Use a game hosting platform to host the application which is accessed using a link provided in recruitment posts for the social media pages of patient organisation groups.
5. Gather user feedback to gain insights into changes in the user's awareness of the condition after using the application, and analyse the usability of the application.

7.2 Materials and Methods

An Apple iPad (9th generation) and HP Laptop (14-cf2518na) were used to run the various software and applications throughout the design and development of the application. The design process was mainly conducted on GoodNotes 5 and Canva, while 3DS Max, 3D Slicer and ZBrush were used to create the assets for the application. Inspiration images gathered for textures, assets and overall app design were also gathered using various websites. Unity and Visual Studio Code were used to develop the application's UI functionality and animations. Finally, JISC was used to conduct the survey, and Microsoft Excel was used for analysis (Table 7.1). Sample datasets and data provided by Dr. Jarod Wong were used for inspiration for the design and development of the application (Table 7.2).

The key features of the application were arranged in a MoSCoW prioritisation matrix under the Must have, Should have, Could have and Will not have categories (Hudaib et al. 2018). These identified aspects of the application were most important to ensure the development process was conducted efficiently (Table 7.3).

7.2.1 Design

The initial idea was to develop a walkthrough style application, beginning with osteoporosis and steroid use in DMD patients, to then explaining how vertebral fractures occur and contribute to the vertebral fracture cascade, ending with a brief explanation of treatment used for vertebral

Table 7.1 Software used for application development

Software	Reason	Produced by
Visual Studio Code	C# script creation	Microsoft Corporation https://code.visualstudio.com
Unity 3D	UI development and animation	Unity Technologies https://unity3d.com/unity
Autodesk 3DS Max	3D model retopology, animation and UV map creation	Autodesk https://www.autodesk.co.uk
ZBrush	3D model creation	Pixologic (Maxon) https://www.maxon.net/en
3D Slicer	Indirect volume rendering of sample medical datasets	3D Slicer https://www.slicer.org
Adobe Illustrator 2023	2D sprite creation	Adobe, Inc. https://www.adobe.com/uk/
Adobe Photoshop	3D model texturing	Adobe, Inc. https://www.adobe.com/uk/
Adobe Color	Colour palette creation and test for suitability for colour blindness	Adobe, Inc. https://www.adobe.com/uk/
GoodNotes 5	Storyboard creation	Time Base Technology Limited
Canva	Moodboard and poster creation	Canva https://www.canva.com
Adobe Audition	Editing voiceover clips	Adobe, Inc. https://www.adobe.com/uk/
Jisc	Survey platform	Jisc https://www.jisc.ac.uk
Microsoft Excel	Data analysis	Microsoft Corporation https://www.microsoft.com/en-gb/

Table 7.2 Data used for application development

Data	Reason	Produced by
CTLiver	Sample medical dataset used to obtain data for the vertebrae	3D Slicer https://www.slicer.org
Lateral radiographs of vertebral fractures	Images used as reference images when creating the vertebral fractures for the spine model animation	Dr. Jarod Wong
Lato font	Font used throughout the application	Google Fonts https://fonts.google.com/specimen/Lato?query=lato
Bone texture	Texture used for 3D models	https://www.freepik.com/free-photo/aged-cement-wall-texture_932387.htm#query=bone%20texture&position=3&from_view=keyword&track=ais
Bone density model	Inspiration for bone density models	https://www.turbosquid.com/3d-models/3d-bone-sponge-structure-1758582

Table 7.3 MoSCoW analysis

Must have	Should have	Could have	Will not have
Explanation of osteoporosis regarding bone density	4 3D bone density models	Animated osteoporosis scene	Labels appear when hovering over structures, e.g. 'This is a wedge fracture in L2'
2D medicine bottle and long bone fracture graphics with explanation of link between Duchenne's and osteoporosis	Explanation of functions of buttons	Bone density model in scene 4	Full thoracic and lumbar 3D spine model
3D model of T9-L5 with a vertebral fracture	Voiceover for all animations	Animated bone density models	
Animation showing vertebral fracture cascade (original fracture and progression)	Reset button for 3D models to return them to the original position after being rotated	Captions for all voiceovers	
Treatment scene explaining bisphosphonate treatment	Animated treatment scene	Ability to pause the animation	
Function to rotate 3D models		3D long bone fracture model	
Simple, coherent design			

fractures. A mood board (Fig. 7.2) was created using Canva. The colours were chosen to maintain similarity with current patient information resources such as those provided by the NHS but altered, including analogous colours, for a unique, coherent design (Imtiaz 2017). The font chosen was 'Lato', a sans-serif font, as this is deemed simple and readable in web design (Hojjati and Muniandy 2020). To maintain the accessibility of the application, Adobe Color's (Table 7.2) colour blind simulator was used and deemed the colours chosen suitable for users with any colour blindness. The name 'OP3D' was chosen for the application.

A storyboard (Fig. 7.3) was created on a 9th-generation Apple iPad using GoodNotes5 to detail the user's journey through the application and to detail the animations which would occur throughout. This also highlighted the user interface (UI) layout and described UI functionality.

Adobe Illustrator was used to create UI buttons, and 2D graphics were taken from Pixabay and Lovepik for use throughout the application. Finally, the logo was created with Wix for use within the application and on social media posts for recruitment.

7.2.1.1 Development of 3D Assets

For developing the spine model, it was decided to include only the thoracic and lumbar vertebrae to ensure a simple model suitable for a web-based application. Using evidence from Phung et al.

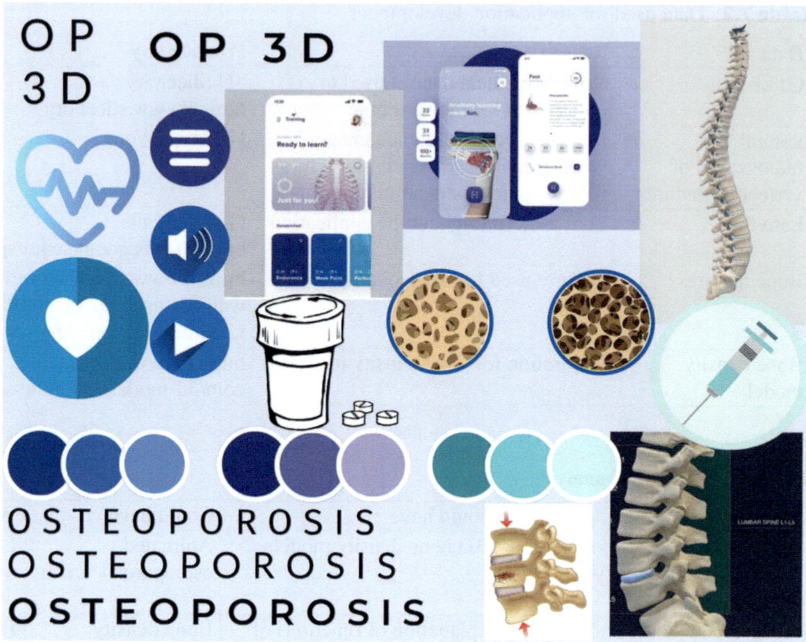

Fig. 7.2 Moodboard

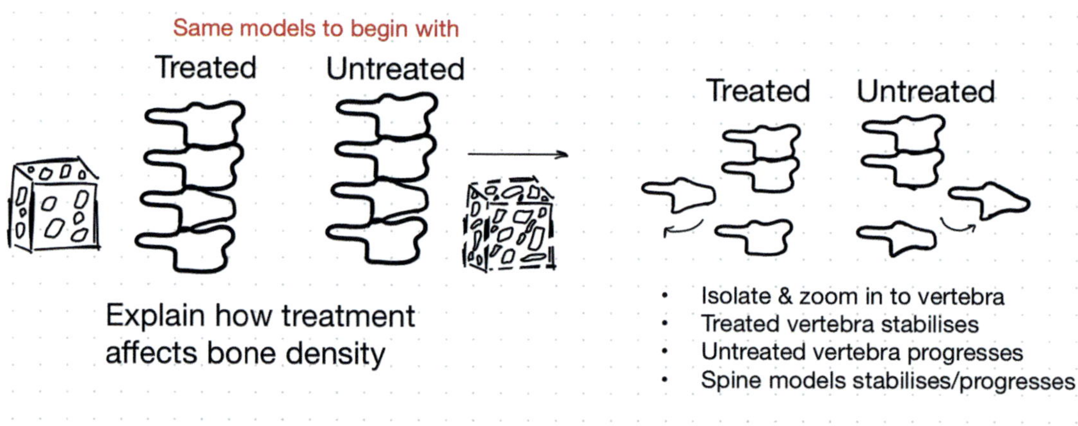

Fig. 7.3 Example of the application's storyboard

(2023), the specific vertebrae chosen were T9-L5 as these are where vertebral fractures are most found in DMD patients.

3D Slicer was used to create one thoracic and one lumbar vertebra using the sample data CTLiver, specifically, L2 and T10. The Laplacian Sharpening Image Filter was used to filter the data, and the contrast was then adjusted to make the boundaries between vertebrae more visible. Then, a region of interest was defined to crop the dataset for accurate segmentation. The Segment Editor module was utilised for the indirect volume rendering of the dataset (Fig. 7.4).

Once created, the segmentations were exported as label maps and developed into models using the Model Maker module, with 30% decimation and smoothing. To reduce the number of vertices, the Surface Toolbox module was used, and Laplacian smoothing was added, both at 30% to produce the models which were exported as .obj files for use in 3DS Max.

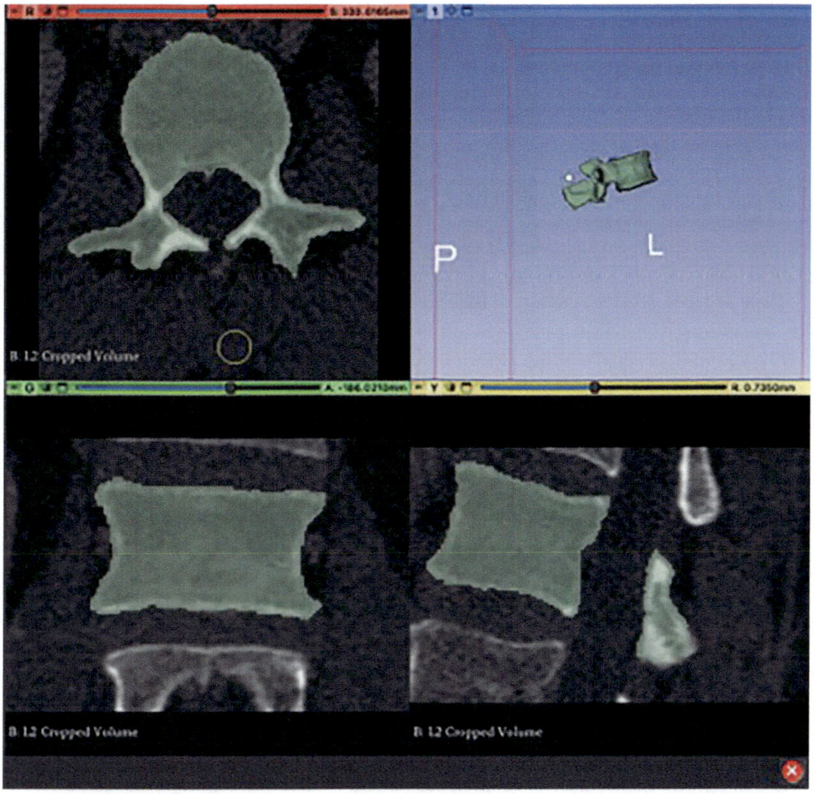

Fig. 7.4 Final L2 segmentation

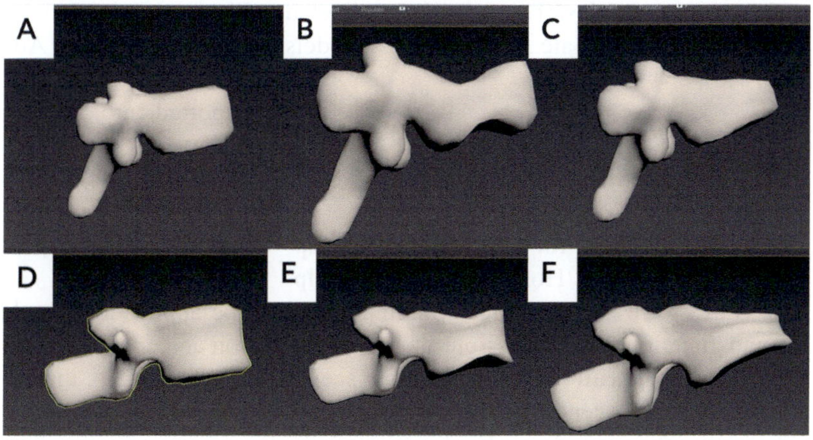

Fig. 7.5 Healthy T10 (**a**) with a grade 2 biconcave fracture (**b**), grade 1 anterior wedge fracture (**c**). Healthy L2 (**d**) with a grade 1 biconcave fracture (**e**) and grade 2 anterior wedge fracture (**f**)

In 3DS Max, the models were simplified using the Retopology modifier where the maximum polygon count was set to 1000 + −10% and anisotropy, adaptivity and regularise set to 1.0. This ensured detail was retained in some areas.

The spine model was animated to have vertebrae fracture over time by creating copies of the vertebra and using the Morpher modifier. The copies were adjusted using Soft Selection, producing models (Fig. 7.5).

Targets for the animation were identified as the corresponding copied, and now fractured, vertebrae. The Auto Key function was used to set the vertebrae to begin as the healthy models and slowly morph into the fractured vertebrae.

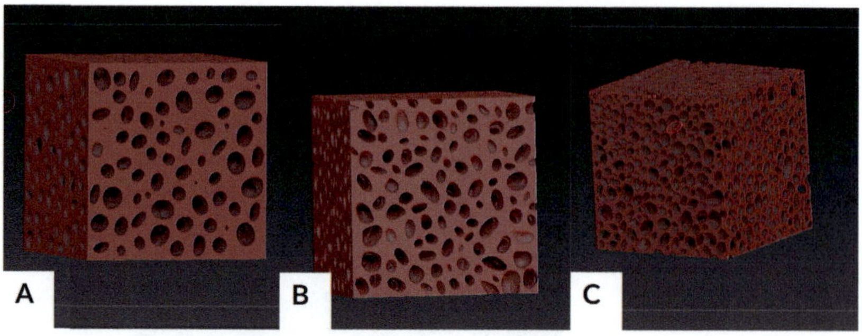

Fig. 7.6 Healthy (**a**), intermediate (**b**) and osteoporotic (**c**) bone models

Texturing the models was also done in 3DS Max using the UVW Unwrap modifier. The UV Maps created were exported into Adobe Photoshop, where the cement wall texture (Table 7.3) was added and then reimported into 3DS Max to be added to the vertebrae.

Bone density models were developed using ZBrush. These models were to show the user the differences in bone microstructure between healthy and osteoporotic bone. For timing purposes, 3 models (healthy, intermediate and osteoporotic) were created. The healthy model was created first, using a simple cube with spheres subtracted from it using the Boolean tool to create cavities. This was then adjusted as necessary to create the other 2 models (Fig. 7.6).

7.2.2 Application Development

Unity 3D was used for application development. Four scenes, 'Home', 'About', 'Help' and 'Quit', were created which contained basic UI and functionality, accessible at the beginning of the application. A further four scenes were developed, scenes 1–4, which were considered as the walkthrough element of the application. A primitive scene was built to block out the design and then filled with the relevant models and UI. For the models, animations were created as per Table 7.4 and implemented by created animations and animation controllers within Unity.

To accompany the animations, a voiceover was created. The script was developed by an expert from the Department of Paediatric Endocrinology, Royal Hospital for Children, Glasgow, and distributed to a parent of a child with DMD to check that it was understandable by a lay audience. Once finalised, the voiceovers were recorded in the dubbing studio at The Glasgow School of Art, School of Simulation and Visualization. Adobe Audition was utilised to edit and save the clips which were then imported into Unity and added to the relevant scenes.

7.2.3 Final Application Deployment

The application was built as a WebGL application and compressed as a ZIP file to be uploaded to www.itch.io, the game hosting platform used. The dimensions were set to 1280 × 720 matching how it was built in Unity.

Table 7.4 Animations in OP3D

Model (scene)	Animation	Reason
UI text/arrows (all scenes)	Enabled and disabled as required	To link the voiceovers with the models
Bone 1 (healthy bone, scene 1)	Rotate 360 degrees	Highlights bone microstructure
Bone 2 (intermediate bone, scene 1)	Enabled and rotated	Portrays progression from healthy bone to beginning of osteoporotic bone
Bone 3 (osteoporotic bone, scene 1)	Enabled and rotated	Portrays progression from healthy bone to osteoporotic bone
Spine final (scene 3)	Rotated 90 degrees	Visualises spine from anterior view and how the spine appears on an X-ray, laterally
L2 of spine final (scene 3)	Enlarged, moved to centre and fractured as time elapses	To show the morphology of a wedge fracture and progression from a mild to severe fracture
T10 of spine final (scene 3)	Enlarged, moved to centre and fractured as time elapses	To show the morphology of a biconcave fracture and progression from a mild to severe fracture
L2, L3, T10 and T11 of spine final (scene 3)	Fracture at different time points at different rates	To portray the vertebral fracture cascade and how one fracture can develop into multiple
Bone 1 (scene 4)	Enabled, transform (position) altered and disabled	To highlight how bone microstructure can stabilise in treated DMD patients
Bone 3 (scene 4)	Enabled, transform (position) altered and disabled	To highlight how bone microstructure can worsen in untreated DMD patients
L2 of mild spine (scene 4)	Enlarged, isolated and fractured as time elapses	To highlight how fractures stabilise in treated DMD patients
L2 of fractured spine (scene 4)	Enlarged, isolated and fractured as time elapses	To highlight how fractures worsen in untreated DMD patients
Mild spine (scene 4)	Fractured as time elapses	To portray a treated spine in a DMD patient
Fractured spine (scene 4)	Fractured as time elapses	To portray an untreated spine in a DMD patient

7.3 Results

Navigation through OP3D, which contains a 'Home', 'About', 'Help' and 'Quit' scenes and four individual walkthrough scenes, is outlined in Fig. 7.7.

The 'Home' (Fig. 7.8) scene acts as an introductory scene, providing quick access to the 'About', 'Help' and 'Quit' scenes.

Walkthrough scene 1 (Fig. 7.9) contains the healthy and osteoporotic interactive 3D models of bone density to help explain osteoporosis and its effect on bone density. These models can be rotated by the user and reset to their original position, and a 3D animation can be triggered via the 'Play' button.

Scene 2 (Fig. 7.10) did not contain 3D models but did contain 2D animation to explain how DMD and osteoporosis are linked via glucocorticoid treatment.

Scene 3 (Fig. 7.11) contains a 3D model of the spine with vertebral fractures and includes an animation which helps explain the types of fractures and fracture progression.

Scene 4 (Fig. 7.12) details bisphosphonate treatment and compares a treated with an untreated spine to aid awareness of how the treatment can help stabilise existing fractures and make clear that it does not prevent vertebral fractures from occurring.

The application was built in a way which told the story of how osteoporosis can affect children with DMD utilising 3D, interactive models and narrated animations and was successfully deployed online in July 2023.

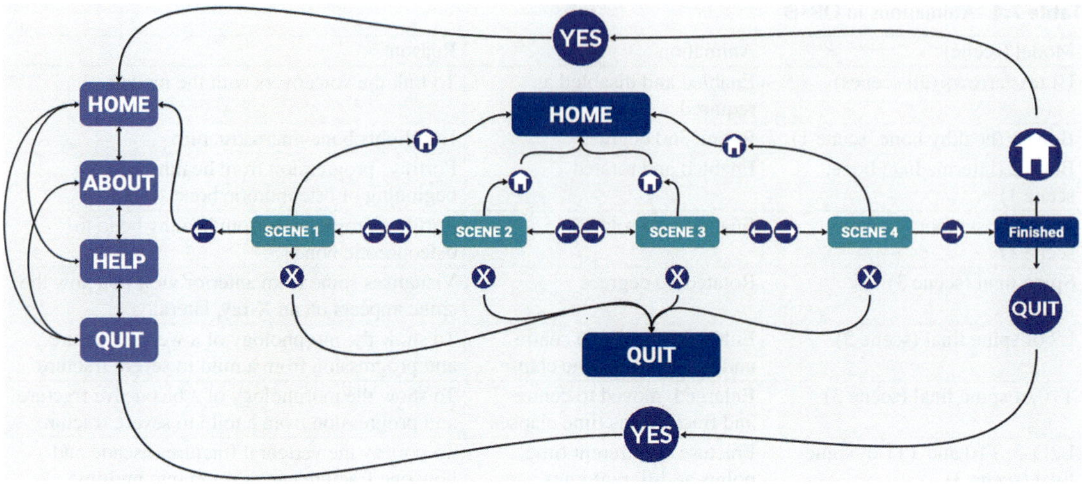

Fig. 7.7 Navigation through OP3D

Fig. 7.8 'Home' scene

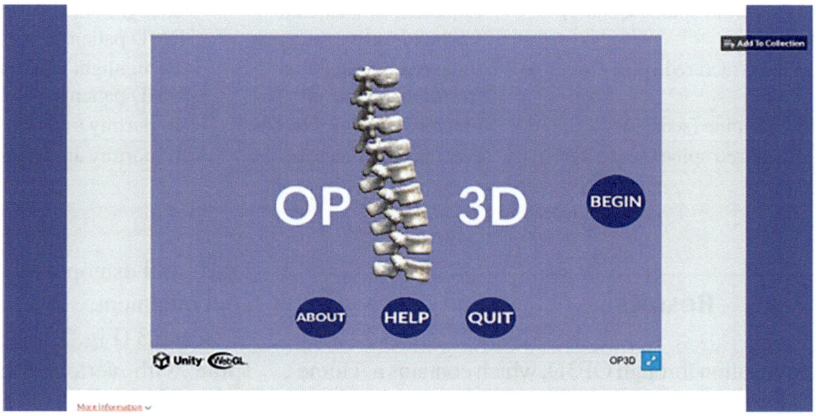

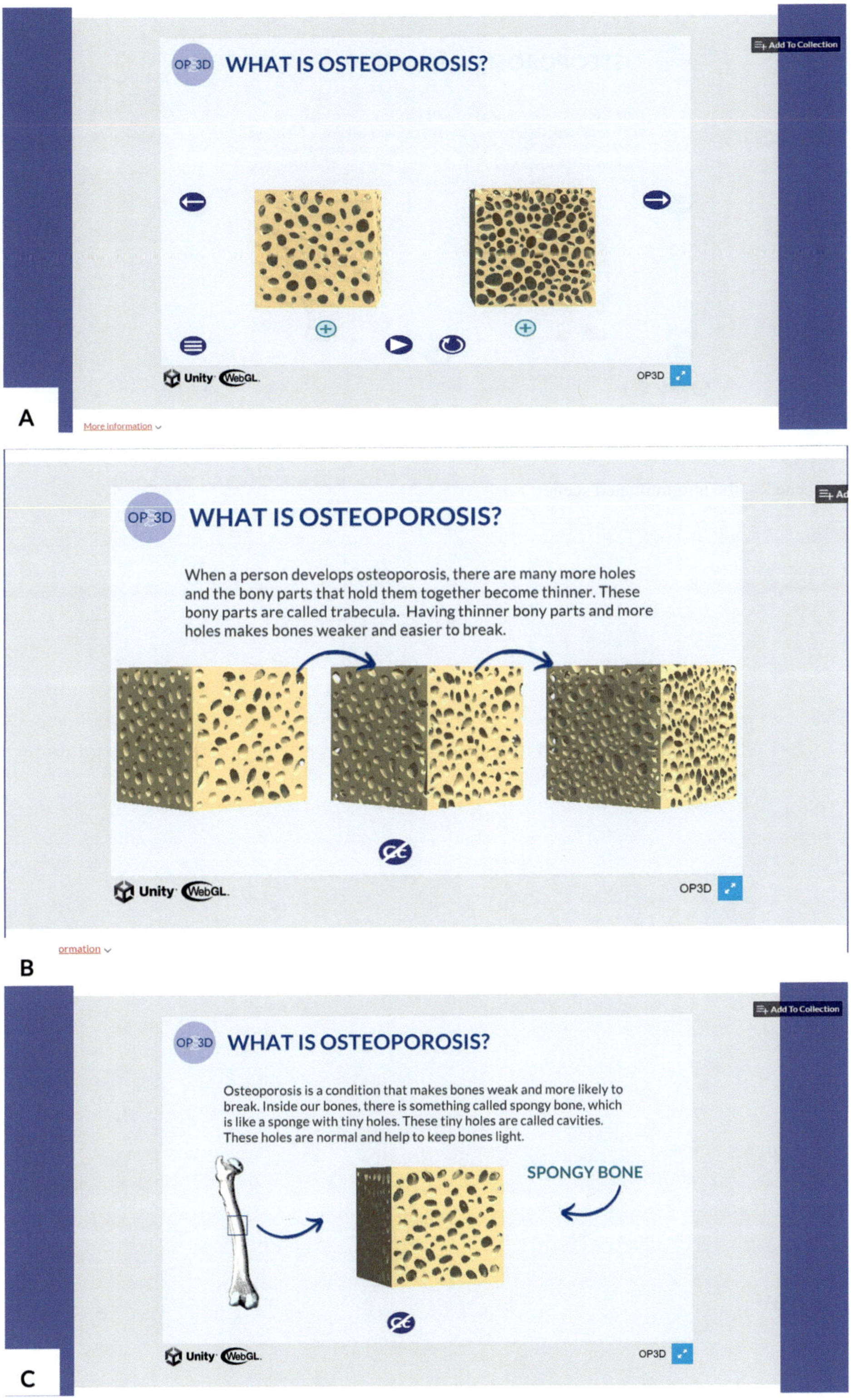

Fig. 7.9 Initial appearance of scene 1 (**a**) and stills from the animation sequence (**b**) and (**c**)

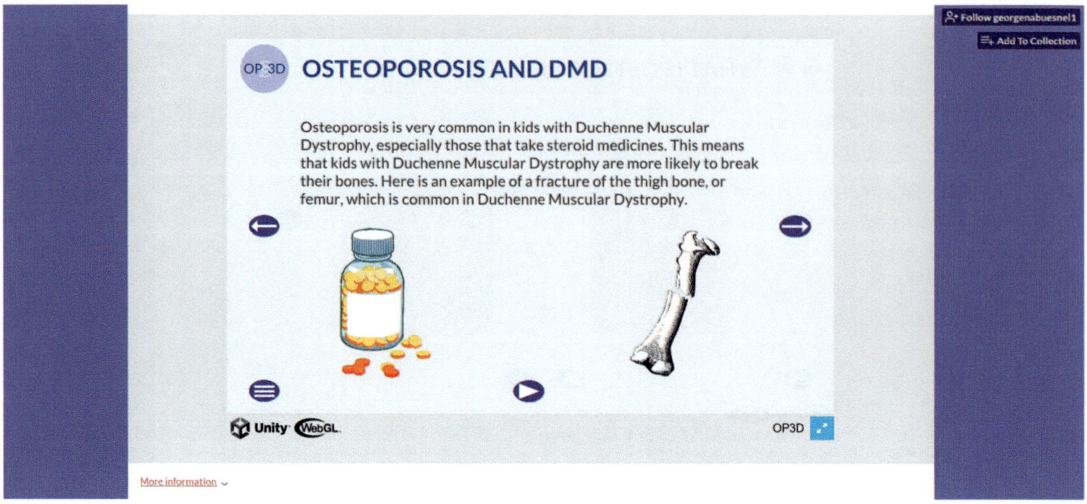

Fig. 7.10 Scene 2—the non-animated scene

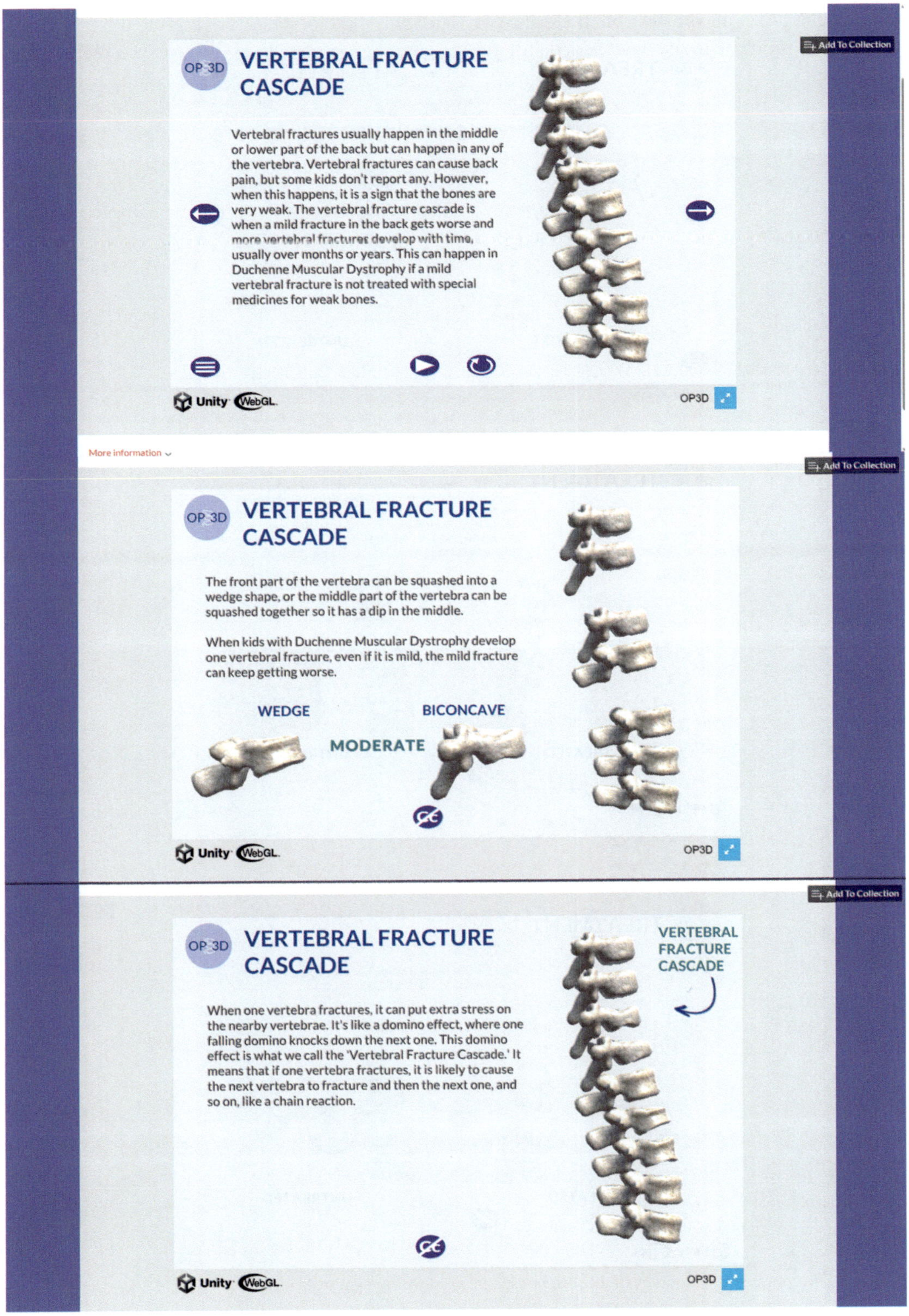

Fig. 7.11 Scene 3 start-up (**a**) and stills from the animation (**b**) and (**c**)

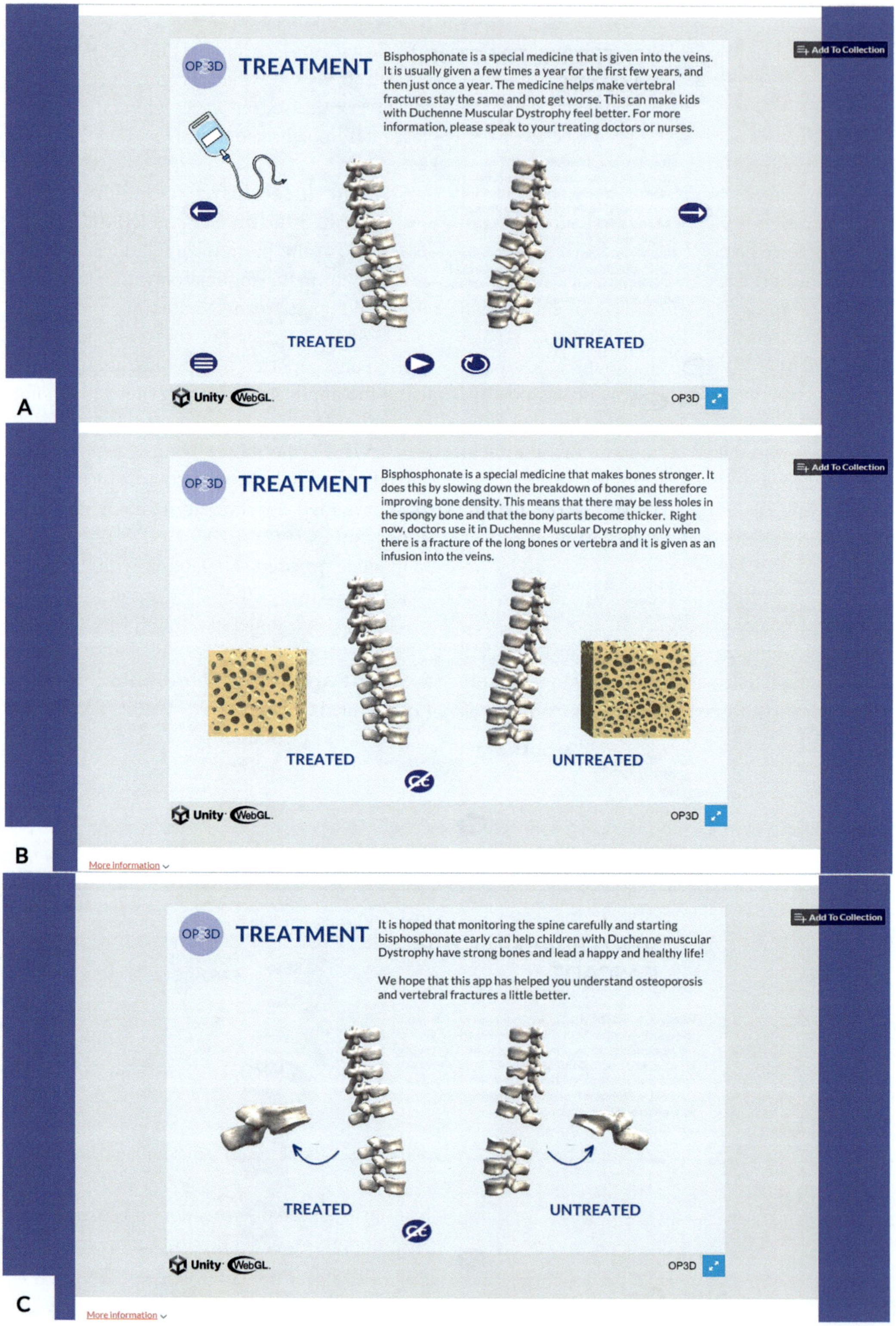

Fig. 7.12 Scene 4 start-up (**a**) and stills from the animation (**b**) and (**c**)

7.4 Evaluation

The online application was evaluated to determine whether it affected the user's awareness of osteoporosis and vertebral fractures, and its usability was assessed to determine how easy the application was to use using the System Usability Scale (SUS) (Brooke 1996).

Currently, there is no resource encompassing interactive 3D models and animation about osteoporosis and vertebral fractures in DMD patients, despite promising evidence from many authors. Hence, this experiment aimed to address the following research question:

Does an interactive application containing 3D models and animation help aid the awareness of osteoporosis and vertebral fractures in the parents or carers of children with DMD?

7.4.1 Participants

The Glasgow School of Art Postgraduate Taught Research Ethics Committee provided ethical approval for this research. Participants were recruited via patient organisation groups Action Duchenne, Muscular Dystrophy UK and Duchenne UK's social media pages such as Facebook, Instagram and Twitter. A poster was developed on Canva, and a written post was developed for the organisations to post.

The criteria for inclusion were as follows:

1. Individuals aged 18 or over
2. Individuals who give consent
3. Individuals who are the parent or carer of a child with DMD

Ten participants (seven females and three males) aged between 30 and 59 years, with the majority falling into the 40–49 age range, were recruited. Of the 10 participants seven responded that they had a child with DMD who had been diagnosed with osteoporosis, with six indicating their child had at least one vertebral fracture.

7.4.2 Apparatus and Procedure

Jisc (https://www.jisc.ac.uk), GSA-approved surveying platform, was used to develop and distribute the survey for testing. The website www.itch.io was used to host the application which could be run on the participant's own device (PC or laptop) at home. A post on social media contained the survey link.

Participants were first provided with information about the rationale, aims and researchers via the participant information sheet and provided consent via the form within the survey. This ensured anonymity. Demographic information, such as age category, highest completed education and whether their child had vertebral fractures, was also gathered. Demographic data was collected via a survey similar to Jones et al. (2022) and Iannucci et al. (2022). The digital literacy of the group was determined through a set of questions to gather information on access to devices at home, time spent on laptops or personal computers and how often they utilise online applications. The pre-application awareness survey assessed the opinions of the user about their awareness of DMD, osteoporosis and vertebral fractures using a unique questionnaire with eight statements. A 7-point Likert scale deemed reliable and easy to use (Taherdoost 2019) was used for both the pre- and post-application questionnaires. After completion, participants were directed towards OP3D via the link. Once finished, participants were asked to return to the survey to complete the post-application questionnaire which was identical to the pre-application questionnaire. This determined whether their opinions had changed before and after viewing OP3D. Next was the SUS survey (Brooke 1996) which determined the usability of OP3D, and finally, participants were given the option to provide open-text feedback in the way of listing three positives and criticisms about the app, as well as how they believed their young person would view OP3D.

7.4.3 Data Analysis

The pre-application questionnaire was used to create a benchmark of the user's responses regarding their awareness and was then compared to their second questionnaire responses. For analysis, responses were converted into numbers from 1 indicating 'strongly disagree' to 7 indicating 'strongly agree'. To establish whether the individual perceived their awareness to increase after the use of OP3D, means, standard deviation (SD) and delta (Δ) values were calculated.

The subjective usability of OP3D was determined using the SUS using the guidelines from Bangor et al. (2009).

It is important to note that participant 1's data was excluded from the analysis. This is because they gave 80% 'undecided' responses for the SUS survey. Furthermore, they stated that their child had not been diagnosed with osteoporosis or vertebral fractures, and they gave no additional comments. The average time spent completing the survey was 11.4 minutes yet participant 1 only dedicated 4 minutes. Statistical analysis was not conducted.

7.4.4 Results

7.4.4.1 Demographics

All participants except for one had completed some form of higher education (Fig. 7.13), with 22% obtaining graduate degrees.

All participants indicated that they had access to at least one type of technological device at home—the majority owned a smartphone (89%) and a laptop (100%). The majority (89%) spent between 2 and 5 hours a day using a laptop or personal computer, and 55% utilised online applications 'very often'. As expected, most of the participants had researched osteoporosis or vertebral fractures using online resources (Fig. 7.14) which suggests despite not all having a child diagnosed with osteoporosis of vertebral fractures, these were terms they had been exposed to.

7.4.4.2 Awareness Questionnaires

Participants perceived their awareness to increase after the use of OP3D (Fig. 7.15) with the most notable differences occurring in response to 'I am aware of the difference between a long bone and a vertebral fracture' (delta difference 1.2) and 'I

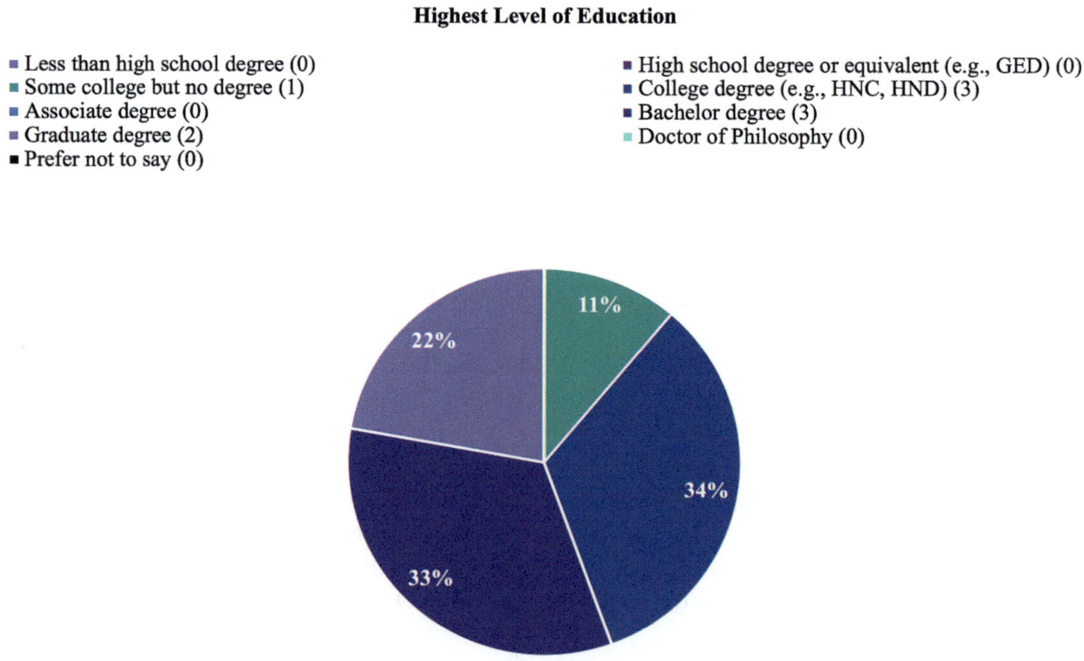

Fig. 7.13 Education levels of the participants

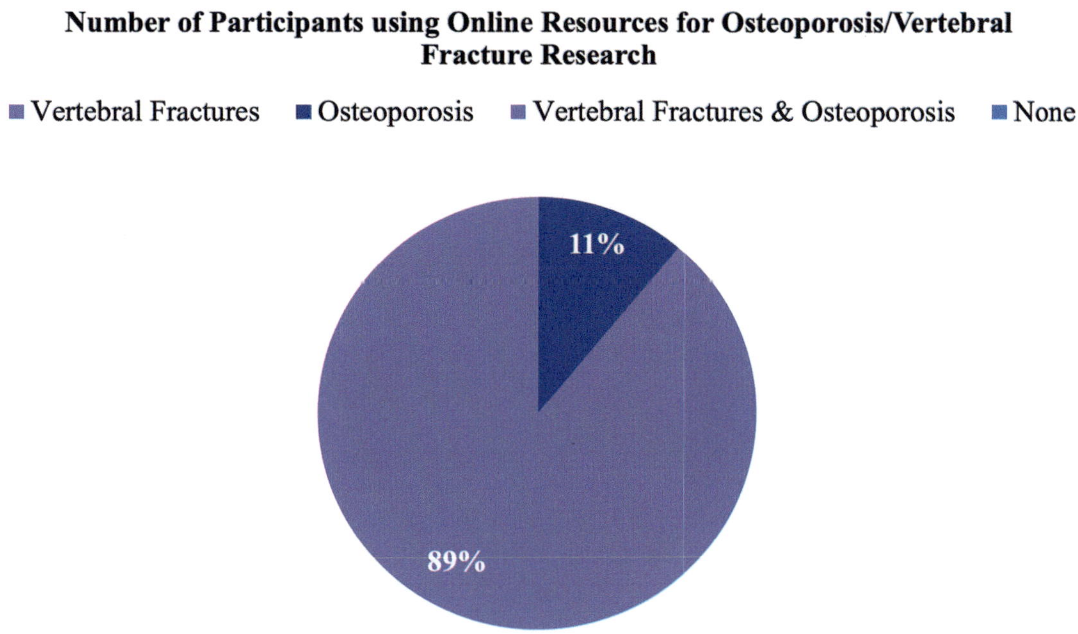

Fig. 7.14 The use of online resources for research related to osteoporosis and vertebral fractures

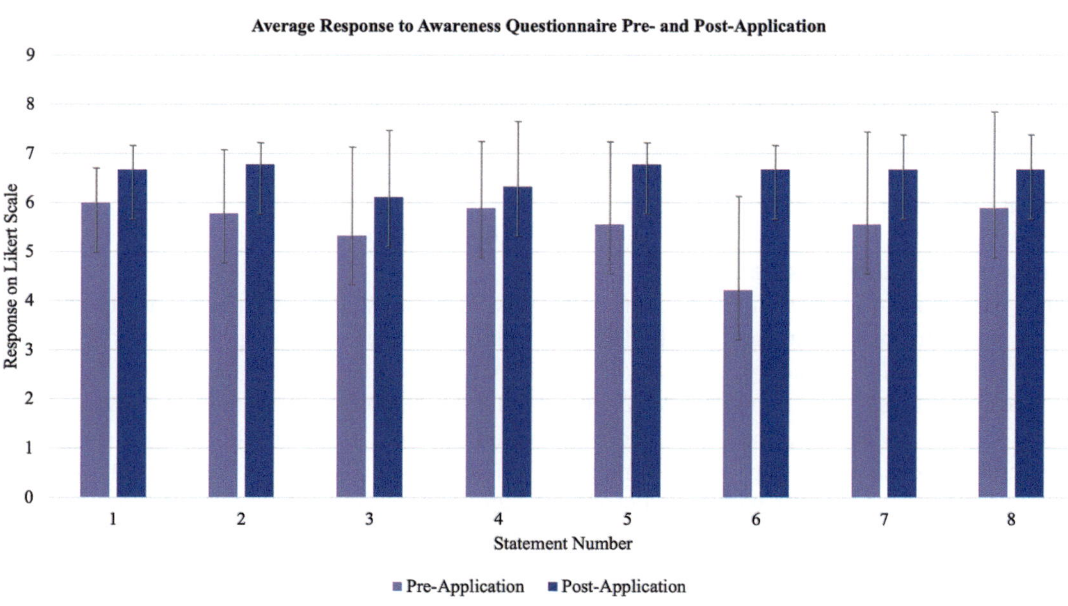

Fig. 7.15 The average responses from each statement in the pre- (purple) and post-application (blue) questionnaire. SD is shown as error bars

am aware of the vertebral fracture cascade' (delta difference 1.11).

7.4.4.3 Usability

OP3D received a SUS score of 80.6, and hence, received a grade A− and could be considered 'Excellent' according to Bangor et al. (2009) (Fig. 7.16).

Learnability of OP3D was established through the responses to SUS item 4, 'I think that I would need the support of a technical person to use this system' and 10 'I needed to learn a lot of things

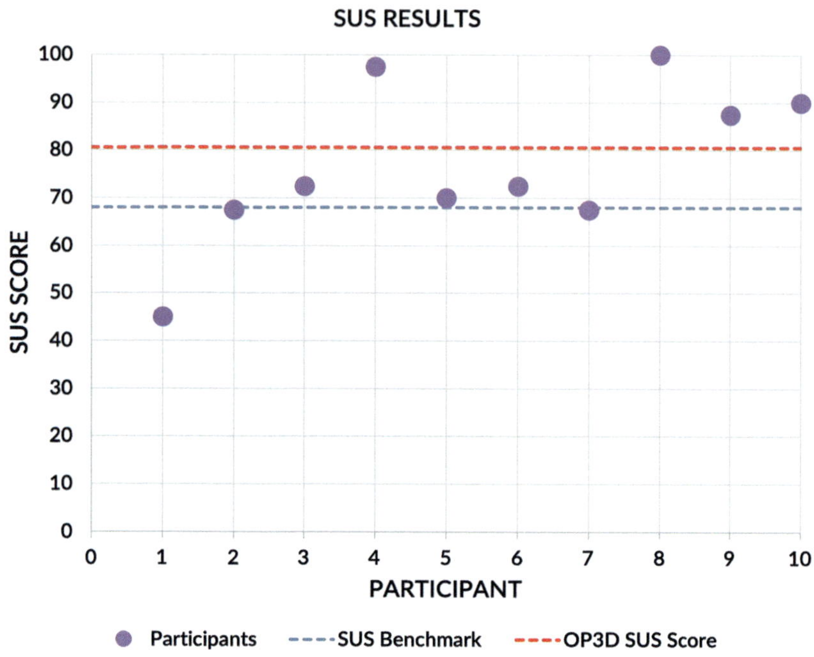

Fig. 7.16 SUS scores plotted on a scatterplot. The dashed, red line represents OP3D's SUS score with the grey dashed line representing the benchmark score for usability (68). Each dot indicates the participants' individual SUS score

before I could get going with this system'. On average, the responses to SUS item 4 were 0.22 ± 0.44 (mean ± SD) and to SUS item 10 was 0.44 ± 0.53. This indicates that OP3D was easy to learn how to use as users did not require support in guiding them through the application before using it themselves.

7.4.4.4 Qualitative Feedback

Nine participants gave additional comments. There were positive comments which deemed OP3D to be '*simple*' (3) and '*easy to use*' (4) and that the content was '*concise*' (1) and '*clear*' (3). One found the visuals to be '*engaging*' (1). Common amongst the group were comments about '*more interactivity*' (3), with one suggesting to '*make interactive with a quiz*' and another suggesting adding a '*zoom in*' feature. Furthermore, navigation throughout OP3D confused some participants with one stating '*needs clearer explanation that you need to press the arrow to move on*' and another '*no contents page or ability to navigate to a certain section*'. Further insightful comments were made about the use of the word 'kids' throughout OP3D, suggesting changing this to 'children' as well as including a form of progress tracker to inform the user of their progress throughout the application. Mixed opinions were observed regarding how their children would perceive OP3D with one stating '*positively*' or '*I think they would like it*' while another stating '*it wouldn't be something they use all the time*'.

7.4.5 Discussion

Overall, this study has shown that the use of a digital resource explaining vertebral fractures in DMD, aimed at parents and carers of children with DMD, positively affected their awareness of the condition. This is beneficial as it shows that implementing 3D, accessible resources could help with patient education, allowing families and clinicians to use appointment times more efficiently. In addition, the families may be able to better prepare for how to support their child.

Evidently, the group of participants who took part in the study were highly educated and digitally literate. The method of recruitment used for this study may have been more appealing to those within scientific fields or interested in technology or both due to advertisement via patient organisation groups on social media which are likely to be followed by those involved with DMD research.

Furthermore, it is evident that the participants were familiar with the terms osteoporosis and vertebral fractures yet somewhat less so with the vertebral fracture cascade. Clearly, this is not a diverse group of participants, and so to include more ages, digital literacies and educational backgrounds, continuing this study on a larger group of participants would be beneficial. Lengthening the recruitment process and including individuals with no prior exposure to DMD or vertebral fractures may result in participants with lower educational backgrounds and/or digital literacy taking part. This would give insightful evidence of the usability of OP3D and its impact on the awareness of a diverse group of individuals.

The results of the pre- and post-application questionnaire indicate that most of the participants perceived their awareness of key points to increase after the use of OP3D. However, the majority ranked their awareness high in the pre-application questionnaire, further cementing the idea that the individuals who took part were already familiar with the conditions before taking part. The notable difference in awareness in statement 6 alludes to the idea that participants were least confident in their awareness of the vertebral fracture cascade but that OP3D has provided them with some clarity on the topic. Lastly, there was a large difference in SD for statements 6, 7 and 8 in the pre-application questionnaire which decreased the most out of all eight statements in the post-application questionnaire. This suggests that there was more varying awareness of these topics before the use of OP3D but that the application allowed them to perceive their awareness as like others after use. The strong educational background of the participants was also made clear as participants 4, 6 and 8 responded 'strongly agree' to most statements in both questionnaires.

OP3D is considered usable as it is within the 90th percentile (Sauro 2018). The application can also be deemed easily learnable due to participants indicating that it would not take long to understand how to use OP3D or require a skilled person to help them use it. This suggests that the design of the application is simple and easy to use.

Responses to various statements in the SUS questionnaire varied. For example, responses to 'I think I would use this system frequently' varied between those stating 'undecided' (participants 2, 5 and 6) and 'disagree' (participant 7). However, consulting the demographic data shows that participant 5 has a bachelor's degree and participants 6 and 7 have a graduate degree, with participant 2 obtaining a college degree. This suggests that the content within OP3D may have been too simple or covered areas they were already familiar with from their own experiences and research which can be confirmed by a comment from participant 7, '*It doesn't actually give a great deal of information, certainly no more than I could find on a Google search*'. An important note is that this participant indicated they had used digital resources to research osteoporosis and vertebral fractures before taking part in the study yet answered both 'somewhat agree' and 'somewhat disagree' to various statements in their pre-application questionnaire. This may show that despite self-directed research, they were still unfamiliar with key points of the conditions. Their post-application responses show that their perceived awareness had improved regarding the difference between a long bone and vertebral fracture and the vertebral fracture cascade, suggesting that OP3D was in fact beneficial in increasing their awareness.

The above-average SUS score suggests that OP3D is not only intuitive but easy to use. Similar studies such as the one conducted by Iannucci et al. (2022) gained a score of 80.6, highlighting the potential for online applications with 3D models and animations to increase knowledge and awareness, particularly of complex medical topics.

The open-text comments show that the content within OP3D was digestible and easily understood. Navigation throughout OP3D should be addressed and made clearer to the user. Despite their being a 'Help' page accessible via the 'Home' page and a 'Help' pop-up panel accessible in each walkthrough page, participants still required clearer instruction. To do this, incorporating a 'Contents' page would provide access to all other pages at any given time but also give an indication of how lengthy the application is. Furthermore, a tutorial video could be embedded into this page to give a visual and narrated explanation of navigation. In addition, the code associated with the 'Play' button should be reviewed to ensure the animation plays once despite multiple clicks. Some comments provided allude to the fact that the system took a short while to adjust to, such as '*took a minute to work out but not too long*', but show that it did not appear to hinder the user experience. These comments, however, were from those who could be considered digitally literate, and so therefore, if OP3D were to be given to those less comfortable with digital technology, these issues should be addressed fully.

The comments regarding interaction within the application made it clear that participants expected a higher level of interactivity with the models in the walkthroughs. Including a zoom function to allow participants to view the vertebral fractures more clearly, as well as adding pop-up labels when hovering over anatomical regions, could add to the interactivity and make the user experience more engaging. Lastly, to allocate more room to the visual aids within OP3D, the captions could be re-coded to have them appear as they are spoken, rather than one block of text.

7.5 Conclusion

Learning with digital resources has been shown to be beneficial across various disciplines, particularly in anatomical and medical education (Erolin 2019: Iannucci et al. 2022; Jones et al. 2022). Increasing evidence that these resources are also beneficial for patient education suggests that providing patients and their families with easily accessible, digestible material with appointments may aid in understanding and awareness of complex medical topics (Oudkerk Pool et al. 2021; Timmers et al. 2019; Aisah et al. 2022). Increasing awareness of vertebral fractures in parents and carers of children with DMD will aid understanding of their child's condition allowing them to make informed decisions about treatment. In addition, they may better understand future health implications as well as ensure the child feels at ease knowing that their guardians are aware of their needs. As such, time during appointments could be more focussed on specific patient requirements.

References

Aisah S, Ismail S, Margawati A (2022) Animated educational video using health belief model on the knowledge of anemia prevention among female adolescents: an intervention study. Malays Fam Physician 17(3):97. https://doi.org/10.51866/oa.136

Bangor A, Kortum P, Miller J (2009) Determining what individual SUS scores mean: adding an adjective rating scale. J Usability Stud 4(3):114–123

Brooke J (1996) SUS: a quick and dirty usability scale. In: Jordan PW, Thomas B, Weerdmeester BA, McClelland IL (eds) Usability evaluation in industry. Taylor & Francis, London, pp 189–194

Crisafulli S, Sultana J, Fontana A, Salvo F, Messina S, Messina S, Trifirò G (2020) Global epidemiology of Duchenne muscular dystrophy: an updated systematic review and meta-analysis. Orphanet J Rare Dis 15(1):141. https://doi.org/10.1186/s13023-020-01430-8

Erolin C (2019) Interactive 3D digital models for anatomy and medical education. In: Rea P (ed) Advances in experimental medicine and biology, vol 1138. Springer, Cham. https://doi.org/10.1007/978-3-030-14227-8_1

Gao QQ, McNally EM (2015) The dystrophin complex: structure, function, and implications for therapy. Compr Physiol 5(3):1223. https://doi.org/10.1002/cphy.c140048

Greenlaw C, Elhefnawy Y, Jonas R, Douglass LM (2021) Using an animated video to promote an informed discussion on SUDEP with adolescents. Epilepsy Behav 122:108182. https://doi.org/10.1016/j.yebeh.2021.108182

Hartmann K, Koenen M, Schauer S, Wittig-Blaich S, Ahmad M, Baschant U, Tuckermann JP (2016) Molecular actions of glucocorticoids in cartilage and bone during health, disease, and steroid therapy. Physiol Rev 96(2). https://doi.org/10.1152/physrev.00011.2015

Hojjati N, Muniandy B (2020) The effects of font type and spacing of text for online readability and performance. Contemp Educ Technol, 5(2). https://doi.org/10.30935/cedtech/6122

Hudaib A, Masadeh R, Qasem MH, Alzaqebah A (2018) Requirements prioritization techniques comparison. Mod Appl Sci 12(2):62. https://doi.org/10.5539/mas.v12n2p62

Iannucci S, Harvey W, Hughes J, Robertson DL, Hutchinson E, Poyade M (2022) Using molecular visualisation techniques to explain the molecular biology of SARS-CoV-2 spike protein mutations to a general audience. In: Rea P (ed) Advances in experimental medicine and biology, vol 1388. Springer, Cham. https://doi.org/10.1007/978-3-031-10889-1_6

Imtiaz S (2017) The psychology behind web design. Researchgate.Net. January

Jones E, Poyade M, Varsou O (2022) Developing and evaluating a prototype public health mobile app on the UK NHS abdominal aortic aneurysm screening programme. J Vis Commun Med 45(3):160. https://doi.org/10.1080/17453054.2022.2037409

Khayruddeen L, Livingstone D, Ferguson E (2019) Creating a 3D learning tool for the growth and development of the craniofacial skeleton. In: Rea P (ed) Advances in experimental medicine and biology, vol 1138. Springer, Cham. https://doi.org/10.1007/978-3-030-14227-8_5

Lui JC, Baron J (2010) Effects of glucocorticoids on the growth plate. Endocr Dev 20:135. https://doi.org/10.1159/000321244

Ma J, McMillan HJ, Karagüzel G, Goodin C, Wasson J, Matzinger MA, DesClouds P, Cram D, Page M, Konji VN, Lentle B, Ward LM (2017) The time to and determinants of first fractures in boys with Duchenne muscular dystrophy. Osteoporos Int 28(2):597. https://doi.org/10.1007/s00198-016-3774-5

Oudkerk Pool MD, Hooglugt JLQ, Schijven MP, Mulder BJM, Bouma BJ, De Winter RJ, Pinto Y, Winter MM (2021) Review of digitalized patient education in cardiology: a future ahead? Cardiology (Switzerland) 146(2):263. https://doi.org/10.1159/000512778

Phung K, McAdam L, Ma J, McMillan HJ, Jackowski S, Scharke M, Matzinger MA, Shenouda N, Koujok K, Jaremko JL, Smit K, Walker S, Hartigan C, Khan N, Konji VN, MacLeay L, Page M, Sykes E, Robinson ME et al (2023) Risk factors associated with prevalent vertebral fractures in Duchenne muscular dystrophy. Osteoporos Int 34(1):147. https://doi.org/10.1007/s00198-022-06578-6

Sakka SD (2022) Osteoporosis in children and young adults. Best Pract Res Clin Rheumatol 36(3):101776. https://doi.org/10.1016/j.berh.2022.101776

Sauro J (2018) 5 ways to interpret a SUS score. Measuring U

Shqaidef AJ, Saleh MYN, Kussad J, Khambay BS (2023) Do parents of adolescent patients undergoing fixed appliance treatment recall more information using written material or an animated video? A randomized controlled trial. Saudi Dent J 35(1):95. https://doi.org/10.1016/j.sdentj.2022.11.011

Taherdoost H (2019) What is the best response scale for survey and questionnaire design; review of different lengths of rating scale/attitude scale/Likert scale. Int J Acad Res Manag (IJARM) 8(1):136

Timmers T, Janssen L, van der Weegen W, Das D, Marijnissen WJ, Hannink G, van der Zwaard BC, Plat A, Thomassen B, Swen JW, Kool RB, Heerspink FOL (2019) The effect of an app for day-to-day postoperative care education on patients with total knee replacement: randomized controlled trial. JMIR Mhealth Uhealth 7(10):e15323. https://doi.org/10.2196/15323

Wáng YXJ, Santiago FR, Deng M, Nogueira-Barbosa MH (2017) Identifying osteoporotic vertebral endplate and cortex fractures. Quant Imaging Med Surg 7(5):555–591. https://doi.org/10.21037/qims.2017.10.05

Ward LM (2020) Glucocorticoid-induced osteoporosis: why kids are different. Front Endocrinol 11:576. https://doi.org/10.3389/fendo.2020.00576

Ward LM (2021a) Part 2: when should bisphosphonates be used in children with chronic illness osteoporosis? Curr Osteoporos Rep 19(3):289–297. https://doi.org/10.1007/s11914-021-00672-0

Ward LM (2021b) Part I: which child with a chronic disease needs bone health monitoring? Curr Osteoporos Rep 19(3):278–288. https://doi.org/10.1007/s11914-021-00667-x

Weldon M, Poyade M, Martin JL, Sharp L, Martin D (2019) Using interactive 3D visualisations in neuropsychiatric education. In: Rea P (ed) Advances in experimental medicine and biology, vol 1138. Springer, Cham. https://doi.org/10.1007/978-3-030-14227-8_2

Cerebral Magnetic Resonance Angiography (MRA) Learning: A Methodological Framework to Develop a Web-Based Interactive 3D Application for Indonesian Medical Education

8

Tara M. Mulyawan, Matthew Poyade, Jenny Clancy, Fathul Huda, and Uti Nilam Sari

Abstract

Cerebral magnetic resonance angiography (MRA) is an economical and minimally invasive imaging method utilised to diagnose various neurological disorders. Nevertheless, MRA images are two-dimensional and require a solid grasp of cerebral vascular anatomy for interpretation. In modern medical education, technology-enhanced learning approaches, such as interactive applications and digital 3D models, have been embraced to improve learning outcomes. However, in Indonesia, conventional 2D illustrations in textbooks, lecture slides and anatomical specimens remain prevalent in the learning process. Recognising this disparity, the research presented here is dedicated to developing a web-based interactive 3D application for learning about cerebral MRA and exploring its potential as a supplementary learning tool for Indonesian medical students.

Patient MRA data were digitally reconstructed into 3D models depicting normal cerebral vascularization, which were subsequently refined and integrated into a game engine platform to produce eight interactive 3D anatomy models. These models were then combined with relevant medical information and made available on itch.io as a web-based application to ensure broad accessibility.

The application's evaluation was completed through an online survey aimed at Indonesian medical professionals. Responses from 23 participants indicated a high usability rating (average SUS score = 72), positive

T. M. Mulyawan (✉)
School of Medicine, Dentistry and Nursing, University of Glasgow, Glasgow, UK

School of Simulation and Visualisation, The Glasgow School of Art, Glasgow, UK
e-mail: tara15001@mail.unpad.ac.id

M. Poyade
School of Simulation and Visualisation, The Glasgow School of Art, Glasgow, UK
e-mail: m.poyade@gsa.ac.uk

J. Clancy
School of Medicine, Dentistry and Nursing, University of Glasgow, Glasgow, UK
e-mail: jenny.clancy@glasgow.ac.uk

F. Huda
Faculty of Medicine, Universitas Padjadjaran, Bandung, Indonesia
e-mail: fathul@unpad.ac.id

U. N. Sari
PT. Teknologi Informasi Medimedi, Depok, Indonesia
e-mail: uti@medimedi.co.id

J. Clancy, M. Poyade (eds.), *Medical Visualization and Applications of Technology – Volume 2*, Biomedical Visualization 5, https://doi.org/10.1007/978-3-031-63463-5_8

comments on its usefulness as a learning aid and a significant learning motivation among the participants. While further enhancements are necessary, this research possesses the potential to serve as a valuable supplementary learning approach for integration into Indonesian medical education. Furthermore, it represents an initial step in fostering awareness towards the implementation of technology-enhanced education in the medical field in Southeast Asian countries.

Keywords

Magnetic resonance angiography (MRA) · Interactive application · 3D reconstruction · Cerebral vascular anatomy

8.1 Introduction

Given the continuous technological advancement and growing demand for non-invasive vascular imaging techniques, cerebral magnetic resonance angiography (MRA) is increasingly gaining popularity as a cost-effective and accurate modality to diagnose various cerebral vascular diseases (Anzalone and Tartaro 2005; G. J. Wang et al. 2010; Vo et al. 2014). The craniocervical vessels, which are highly complex anatomical structures, can be clearly visualised through cerebral MRA for diagnosis purposes. However, the interpretation of these images required extensive spatial knowledge of cerebral vascular anatomy. While extensive learning of cerebral MRA is typically reserved for postgraduate specialties, such as neurology, radiology and neurosurgery, the process of anatomy learning, including cerebral vascular anatomy, begins at the undergraduate level (Cottam 1999). Given the varying timelines of learning across these disciplines, it may be advantageous to have a comprehensive learning tool that combines both the anatomy and clinical implications of cerebral MRA within a single platform. This integrated tool could facilitate a thorough understanding of cerebral MRA.

8.1.1 Interactive Digital 3D Anatomy Learning for Medical Education

As traditional anatomy learning methods are considered 'old-fashioned', the trends in medical education are leaning towards the inclusion of digital technologies within the curriculum (Ellis 2008; Han et al. 2014; Gaur et al. 2020). Cadaveric dissection has been the fundamental base of anatomy learning as it has been proven to increase topological anatomical knowledge and improve learning outcomes (Ramsey-Stewart et al. 2010; Ghosh 2015). However, its reliability has diminished over time. Limitations and challenges, such as shifting social expectations, ethical concerns, rapid technological changes and COVID-19, are encouraging the adoption of new learning paradigms (Robbins et al. 2008; Guze 2015; Rondonuwu et al. 2021). Conversely, 2D illustrations in textbooks and lecture presentation slides are static and require significant mental effort to visualise the 3D structure (Azer and Azer 2016). Consequently, 2D anatomical illustrations and physical 3D models are being complemented and, in some cases, replaced by digital models (Azer and Azer 2016).

Interactive digital 3D anatomy learning, where students are given active control over the 3D models, creates a better spatial understanding, especially the relationship between structures (Stull et al. 2009; De Ribaupierre and Wilson 2012). The 3D anatomy models appeared to be a great supportive self-paced learning resource in addition to the traditional single-use cadaveric dissection teaching method. For instance, Brewer et al. (2012) reported that students enjoyed learning neuroanatomy using 3D models as it 'helped them to visualize inner structure better than plastinated or cadaveric models'. In addition, this aligns with the evolving approach of medical institutions, which are increasingly transitioning from lecture-based teaching to a more self-directed learning format (Ellis 2008; Guze 2015; Erolin 2019; Nugraha et al. 2019).

8.1.2 Web-Based Neuroanatomy Learning

There are multiple ways to display 3D anatomy models (Erolin 2019), one of which involves their integration into a web-based interactive application. Web-based applications offer significant advantages in terms of accessibility and flexibility, as they only require a computer and an Internet connection (John 2007). In addition, while MRA results can only be accessed by limited people, displaying MRA data in the form of a 3D model in a web-based application makes it accessible to wider audiences (Wright et al. 2013).

In comparison to other technology-enhanced medical learning methods, web-based applications offer several advantages. While cadaveric dissection and prosection allow students to gain spatial knowledge, both have limitations in restricted learning time, high cost and limited accessibility. Two-dimensional learning tools, such as textbooks, in-class or online presentation slides and videos, are limited in terms of exploring the three-dimensional relationship between anatomical structures (Azer and Azer 2016). On the other hand, virtual reality, although offering interactive and self-paced spatial learning, requires specific devices that may not be widely available, especially in Indonesia (X. Wang et al. 2017). Hence, web-based learning applications displaying 3D anatomy model features 'can be available any time and from any PC connected to the internet' serving as an ideal complementary medical learning method (John 2007).

Additionally, research has explored the usage of 3D neuroanatomy models alongside traditional anatomy learning techniques, such as cadaveric dissections and 2D diagrams. Medical data, such as MRA, serves as a valuable reference to build anatomically accurate 3D anatomy models to be later post-processed and implemented in different platforms, including websites, for educational purposes (John 2007; Nowinski et al. 2009; Adams and Wilson 2011; Kim 2012; Erolin 2019). While freehand modelling of anatomical structures is often based on artistic idealizations, segmentation of real medical image slices allows for achieving anatomically correct 3D models (Adams and Wilson 2011; John 2007; Kim 2012). Nowinski et al. (2009) developed a 3D model of cerebrovasculature based on MRA data, noting that using an automatic segmentation technique on MRA data requires 'checking and correcting' the pre-segmented volume, especially for small and medium vessels. In addition, Erolin (2019) mentioned that freehand modelling can be used to add small anatomical details that may not be clearly visualised through the segmentation process. Moreover, using 3D software for retopology aids the texturing (colour addition) process.

Regarding the user interface, Nowinski et al. (2009) used a unique colour in addition to labels to identify different vessels. In addition, interactions using the mouse, such as rotating and zooming, aid users in orientating and viewing the models from different perspectives (Hamza-Lup and Thompson 2009; Yang et al. 2020). Adding other user interfaces to control the visibility of the models and labels allows user guidance as well as controls to avoid information overload (Adams and Wilson 2011). Furthermore, models of surrounding anatomical structures act as landmarks to show spatial relationships among the anatomical structures (Adams and Wilson 2011; Hamza-Lup and Thompson 2009). In conclusion, achieving a high level of usability in developing a web-based interactive 3D anatomy application requires extensive planning, from creating the 3D anatomy model to developing user interactions.

8.1.3 Anatomy Learning in Indonesia: Where Are We?

Despite its growing popularity, the use of digital 3D anatomical models in Asia, especially Indonesia, is not as common as in the US and Europe. Most medical faculties still maintain the traditional anatomy learning approach, such as cadaveric dissection and PowerPoint-based lectures (Singal et al. 2021). The anatomy learning system in Indonesia has gone through major changes. In the past, anatomy was taught as a standalone fundamental basic science during the first and second years of medical school. Today, the curriculum in Indonesian medical schools has shifted towards problem-based learning (PBL), which integrates anatomy learning with clinical subjects. As a result, less study time is dedicated to learning in the anatomy laboratory. Furthermore, PBL also encourages students to undertake independent learning activities rather than teacher-centred learning (Nugraha et al. 2019). The integrated curriculum also results in reduced knowledge outcomes caused by students focusing more on the clinical part rather than the basic science. Given this situation, and other limitations, such as expensive costs, the need for a specific location to perform the dissection, the need for professionals and ethical issues, cadaveric dissection–based learning seems to fall short of achieving the desired outcome (McLachlan et al. 2004; Saputra and Lisiswanti 2015).

As a response to these challenges, many medical schools in Indonesia are now recognising the need for supplementary learning methods to teach anatomy. Digital 3D anatomy models are emerging as a convenient and effective solution. For example, the Faculty of Medicine at Universitas Indonesia uses a 3D anatomical table to teach neuroanatomy to first-year medical students, yielding positive results despite limited flexibility in terms of time and location (Kusumaningtyas et al. 2021; Universitas Indonesia 2022).

In addition, the pandemic of COVID-19 further encouraged technology usage in distance medical learning. Several studies regarding students' perception of digital 3D models in anatomy learning have been completed in Indonesia and resulted in positive outcomes (Kristiaji et al. 2022; Nugroho and Rachmi 2022). Although digital 3D anatomy models may not have been officially added to the national curriculum in Indonesian medical schools, the potential of this learning method has attracted the initial efforts and interests of medical practitioners in Indonesia.

8.1.4 Aims and Objectives

This research aims to devise a practical methodological framework for the implementation of a web-based interactive 3D application targeting Indonesian medical education and explore the potential usage of a web-based interactive 3D application of cerebral MRA as a supportive learning tool for medical education in Indonesia. This will be achieved by developing a web-based interactive 3D application of cerebral MRA, conducting user testing and gathering data through standardised questionnaires to assess the potential usage of the application.

8.2 Methods

The design and development of the application followed the methodological framework presented in Fig. 8.1.

8.2.1 Planning and Pre-production

A focus group discussion (FGD) was undertaken at the beginning of this project to gather input from potential users towards the initial concept and achieve a better understanding of the user's expectations towards the application (Stalmeijer et al. 2014; Brown 2022). The discussion was conducted using a semi-structured interview method with a total of five participants, all of whom were medical practitioners in Indonesia. The participant group included a radiology consultant, a neurology consultant, a final-year neurology resident, a first-year neurology resident and a medical student.

Responses from the participants were then used as a benchmark to improve the plan. All inputs received from FGD's participants were translated as a series of requirements and prioritised using the MoSCoW method (Fig. 8.2), which classifies requirements into four categories: Must Have, Should Have, Could Have, Won't Have (Interaction Design Foundation 2016; Brush 2020). This was done to set a realistic goal by focusing on the assets and functionality in the 'Must Have' and 'Should Have' categories.

Requirements were integrated into a well-structured plan for the development process, which translated as a moodboard, a storyboard (Fig. 8.3) and the list of assets needed in the application (2D and 3D).

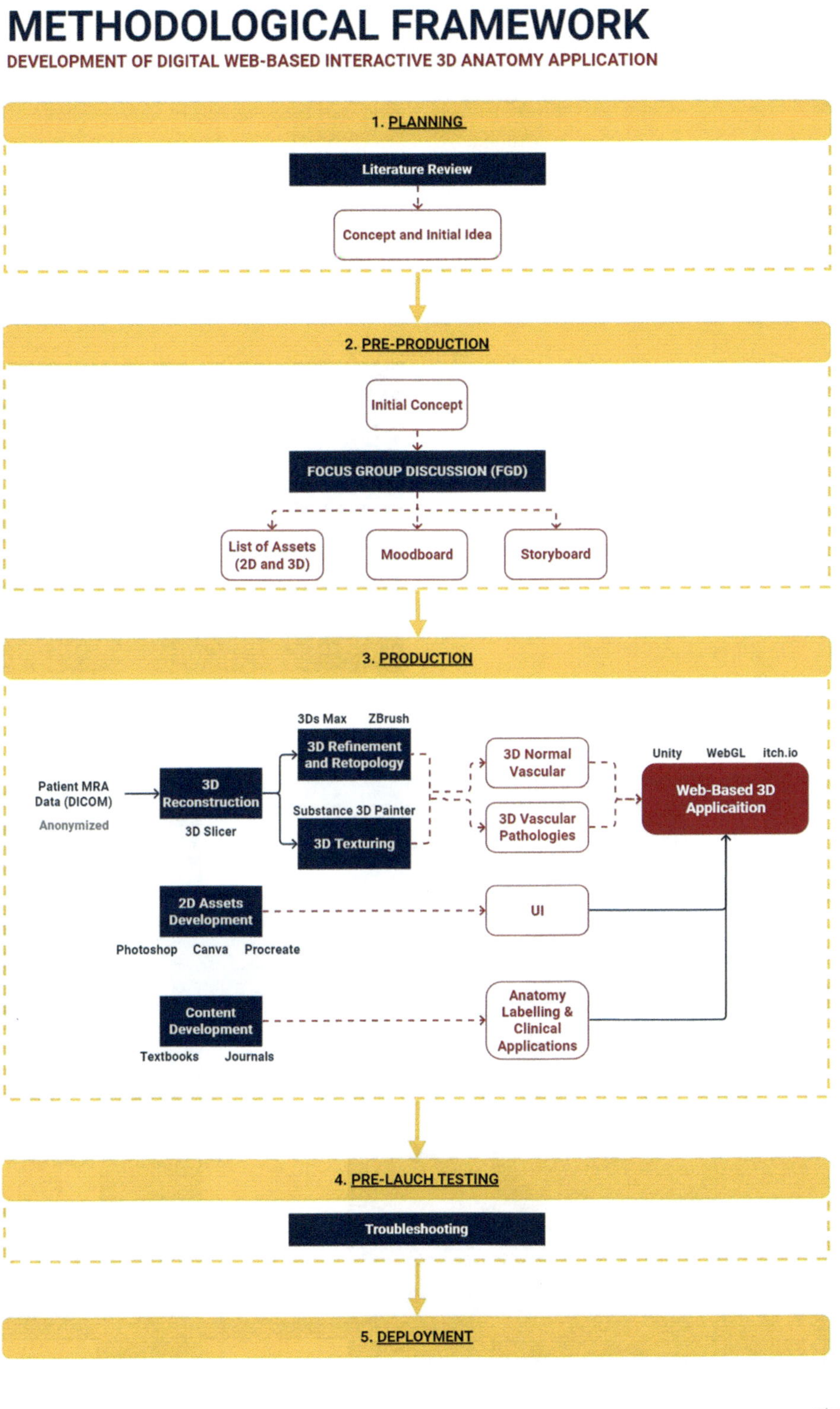

Fig. 8.1 Methodological framework

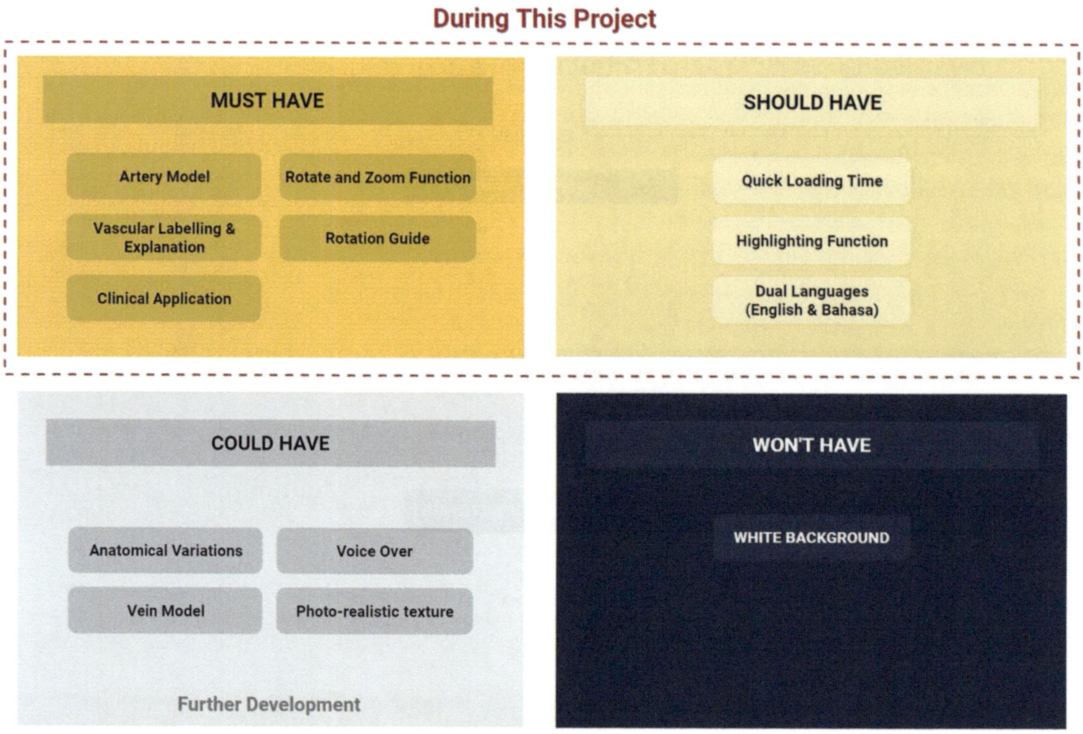

Fig. 8.2 MoSCoW development planning

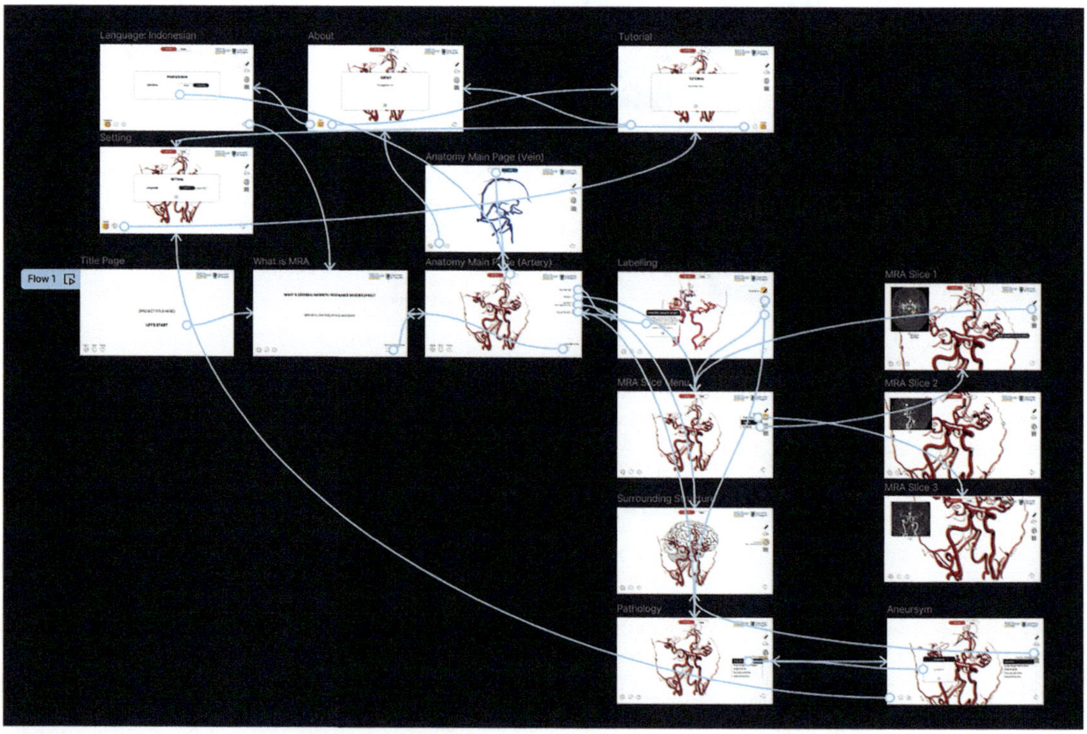

Fig. 8.3 Storyboard and UI prototyping in Figma

The final conceptual design was composed of two main sections: (1) the MRA section, which provided information on the imaging techniques, and (2) the anatomy section, which showcased the cerebral arterial system with labelling, descriptions and its MRA slices. Moreover, a 3D transparent brain model was added as an anatomical landmark. Additionally, five pathology models were developed to demonstrate clinical applications.

8.2.2 Production

8.2.2.1 The Development of 3D Models

The workflow to create a typical cerebral vascularization 3D model from DICOM data was summarised in Fig. 8.4.

The segmentation and 3D reconstruction of the patient's MRA data were completed in 3D Slicer. At first, contrast and brightness adjustment allowed the creation of a clearer definition

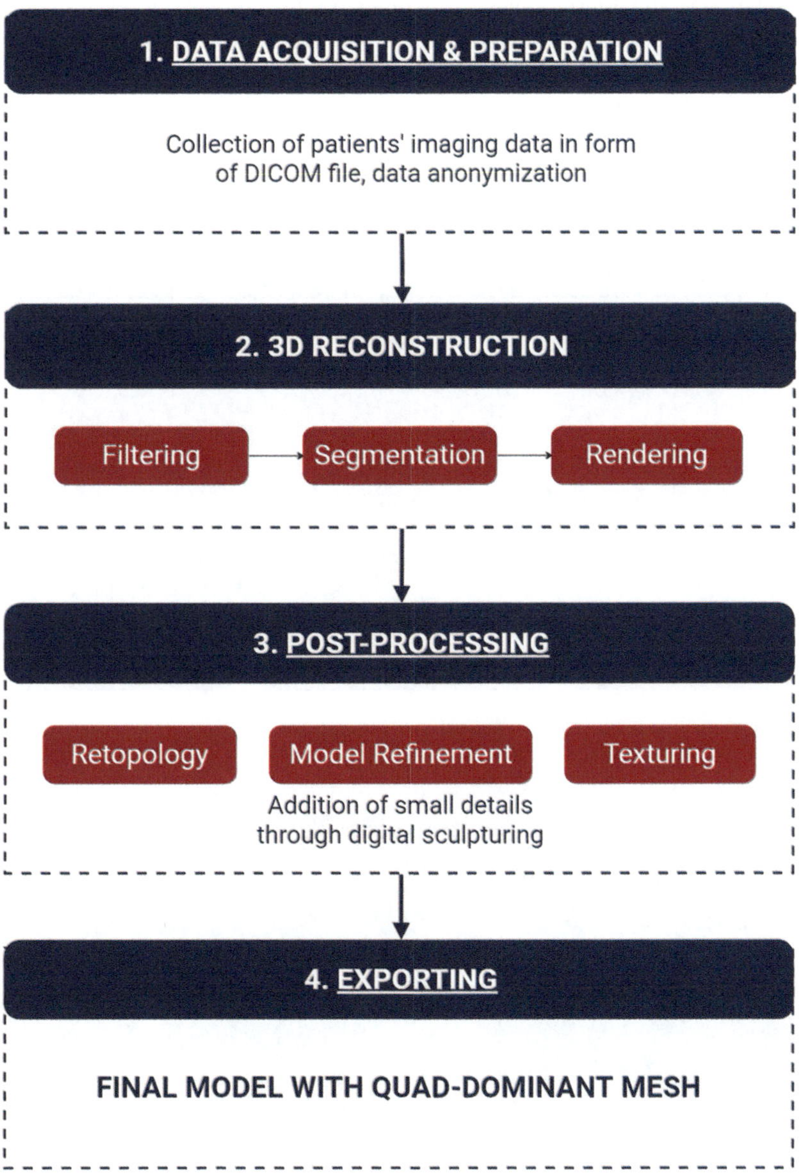

Fig. 8.4 3D modelling framework

between structures. Then, the segmentation process was mainly done using the 'threshold effect' (Fig. 8.5).

The threshold effect, with the range between 157.25 and 1022, worked well to segment the vessels from MRA data because the vessels in MRA data have the highest voxel value compared to the surrounding structures (Passat et al. 2006). The segmentation process revealed that the MRI data used in this project were missing both posterior communicating arteries. Consequently, the segmentation of the arterial system was divided into anterior and posterior circulation and remained separated throughout the segmentation process. Following this, the 'Scissors Effect' and 'Island Selection' were used to clean up the segments while maintaining the important vessels. The segmentation was then exported as a 3D model. Later, the 'Surface Toolbox' module was used to refine the model (Fig. 8.6).

The final model was then exported as OBJ and imported 3DS Max for the retopology process as part of the asset optimization process (Autodesk 2022). The retopology process was aimed to create a more uniform, quad-dominant mesh of the models to lower the polycount as well as make manipulation of the model easier (Bommes et al. 2012). The artery model, which was divided into two separate models, anterior and posterior circulation, and processed separately using automatic

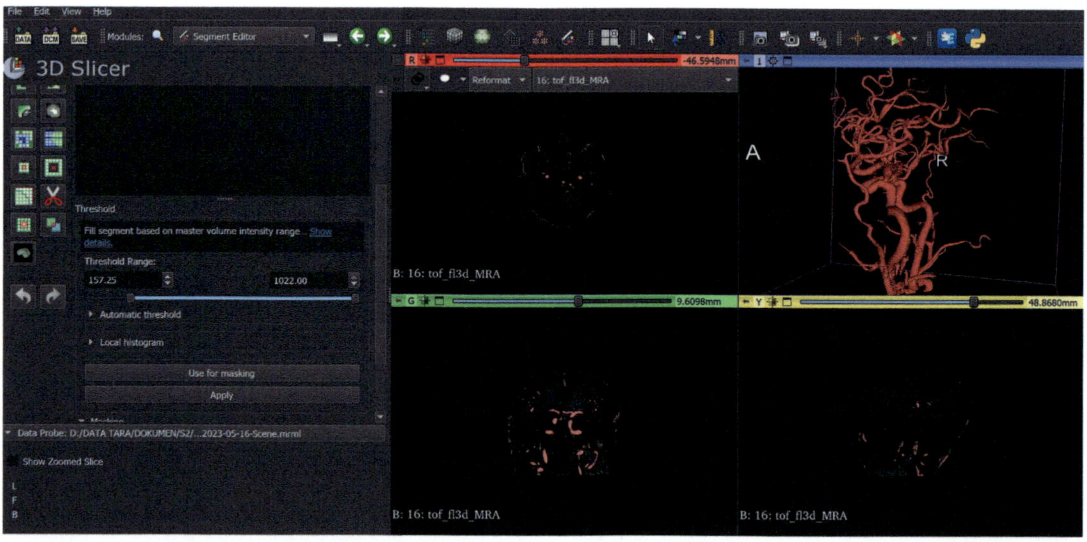

Fig. 8.5 Segmentation using threshold

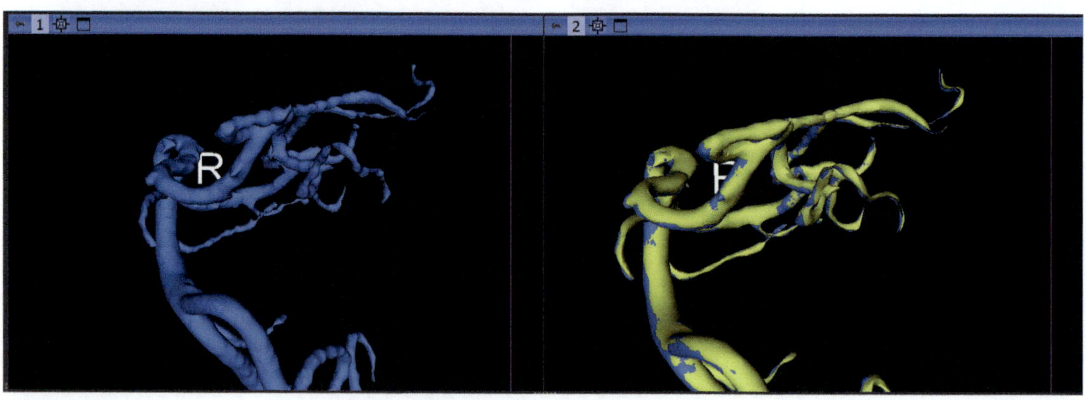

Fig. 8.6 Before and after model refinement using Surface Toolbox

retopology, resulted in quad-dominant models (Fig. 8.7, Table 8.1). Processing anterior and posterior circulation separately for the artery model resulted in less time consumed during the retopology process.

Subsequently, ZBrush played a pivotal role in refining the model's mesh. Features used to refine

Table 8.1 Summary of polycount before and after retopology

Artery	Before retopology	After retopology
Anterior circulation	75.286 polygons	27.571 polygons
Posterior circulation	23.574 polygons	7.325 polygons

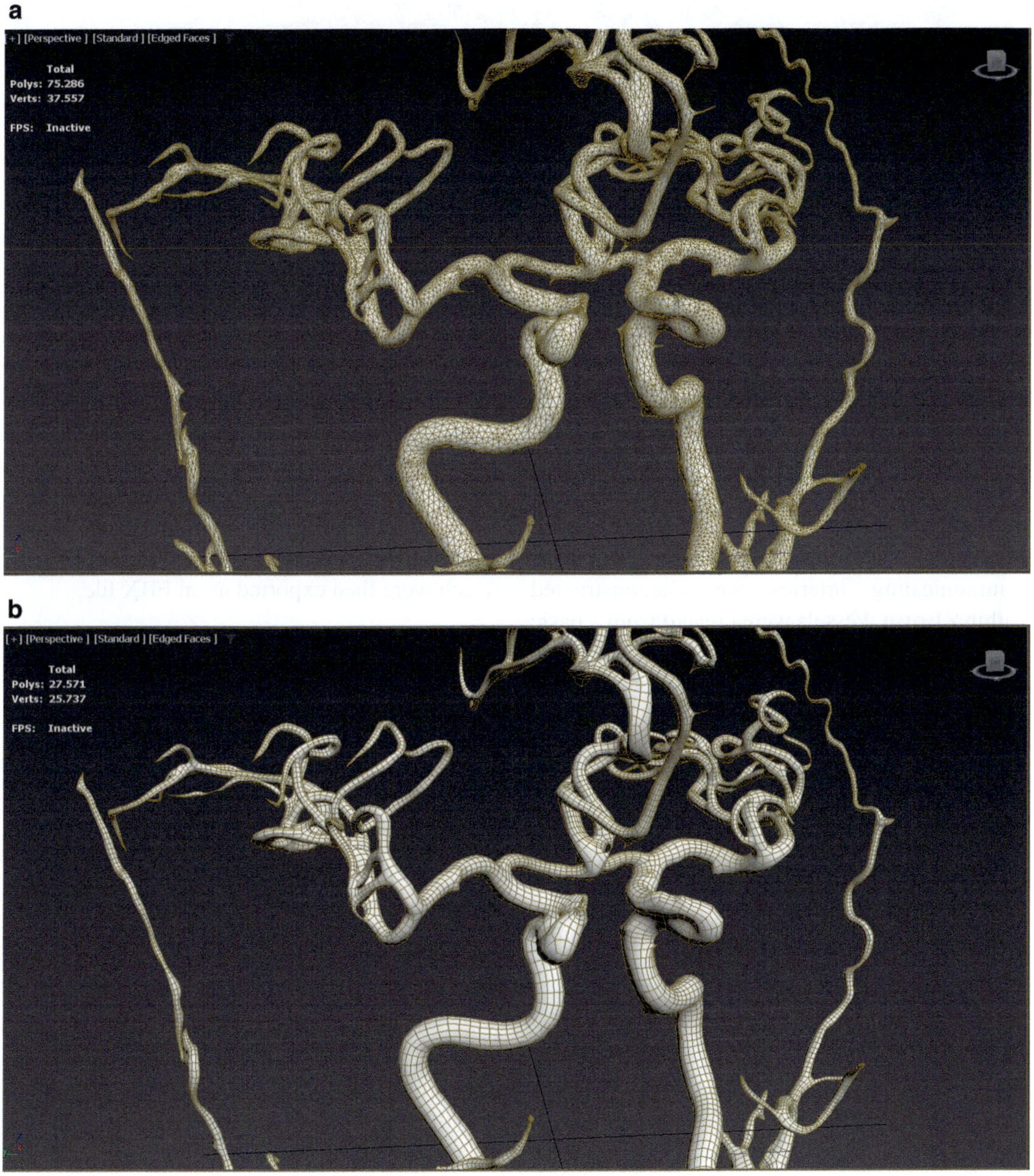

Fig. 8.7 Anterior circulation: before and after retopology

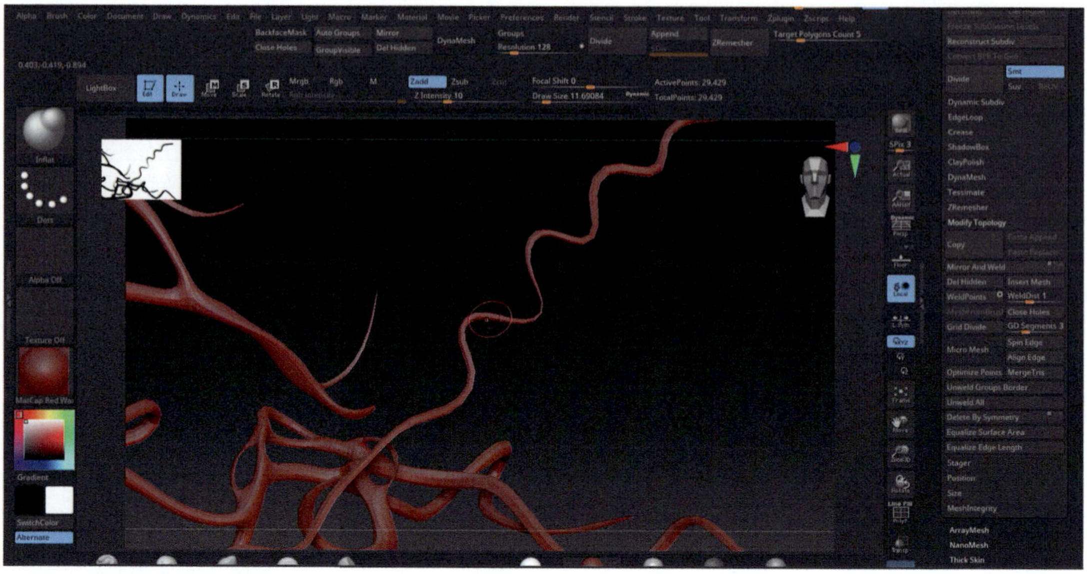

Fig. 8.8 Using 'Inflate' brush to create details in ZBrush

the model included 'Close Holes' to clear any hole's imperfections and 'Inflate' brush to ensure the continuation of the mesh (Fig. 8.8). Furthermore, attention was directed towards smaller vessels that had become detached from the main model during the retopology process in 3DS Max. Additionally, the missing posterior communicating arteries were reconstructed within ZBrush. Vessels were created from a basic cylinder and then shaped according to the main model as reference using a combination of brushes, including 'Move', 'Smooth', 'Inflate' and 'Trim Dynamic'. After achieving the desired shape, the new vessels were merged into the main model. To create a smoother fusion between vessels, a manual hand-modelling approach was adopted, alternating between brushes such as 'ClayBuildup', 'Trim Dynamic' and 'Smooth', with a specific focus on refining the junction between vessels. The tool 'DynaMesh' and 'ZRemesher' were used to regenerate a workable topology. This process resulted in a more uniform quad-based mesh of the models. Subsequently, the models were exported in the OBJ file format.

Later, the refined model was re-imported to 3DS Max. The automatic retopology was performed once again to recalculate the mesh of the model. After getting the desired final topology with a relatively even mesh, the model was then segmented into separate objects based on its anatomical structures. This was achieved by selecting the targeted polygons and detaching them into individual objects. The end result was an artery model composed of 26 different objects, which were then exported as an FBX file.

8.2.2.1.1 Surrounding Structure: Brain

The process of developing the brain model closely adhered to a workflow akin to that of the artery model. However, a notable addition was the integration of an AI-based 3D Slicer extension, HDBrainExtraction, which proved instrumental in separating the brain from its adjacent structures (Lasso 2022).

8.2.2.1.2 Pathological Models

A total of six models were created to depict common pathological MRA findings. These models of pathological vascular conditions were developed by manipulating the normal vascular model using a hand-free modelling technique in ZBrush, guided by reference images. The texturing process was done in Substance 3D Painter by first baking a high poly model's texture as a normal map. This normal map was then applied to the low poly models as shown in Fig. 8.9. By utilising the normal map, the way light is calculated on the model's surface was altered without modifying its topology (Webster 2017). This approach allowed the creation of low poly models with the illusion of details on their surface (Table 8.2).

8.2.2.2 Application Development

The development of the application was performed in Unity version 2021.3.10f1 based on the flowchart in Fig. 8.10. The whole application was built within a single scene to optimise scene loading time (French 2020). Additionally, the

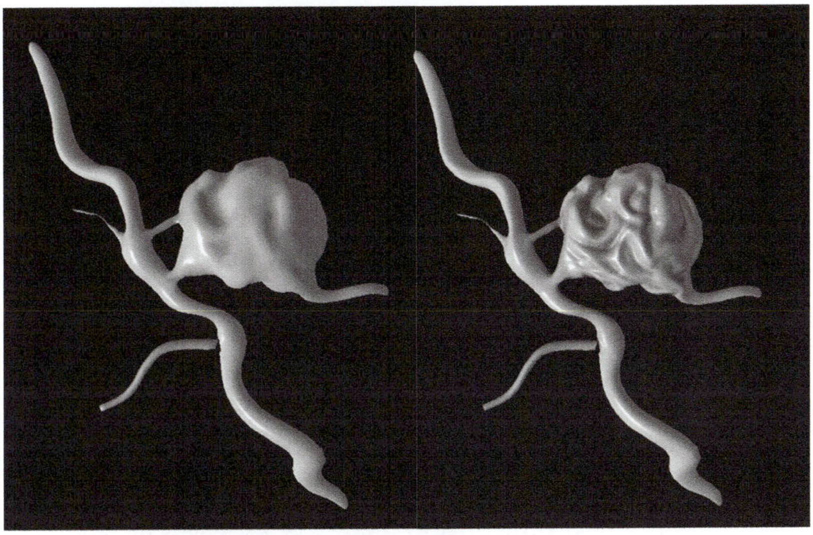

Fig. 8.9 Low poly model without and with normal map

Table 8.2 Summary of the final models' polycount

	Final model	Polycount
Arterial system	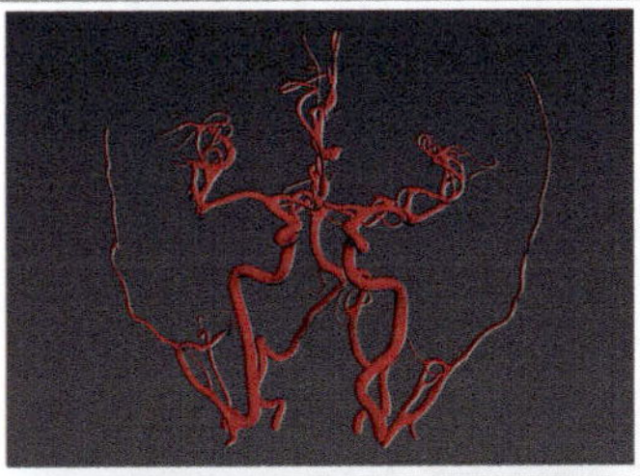	35.199 polygons
Brain	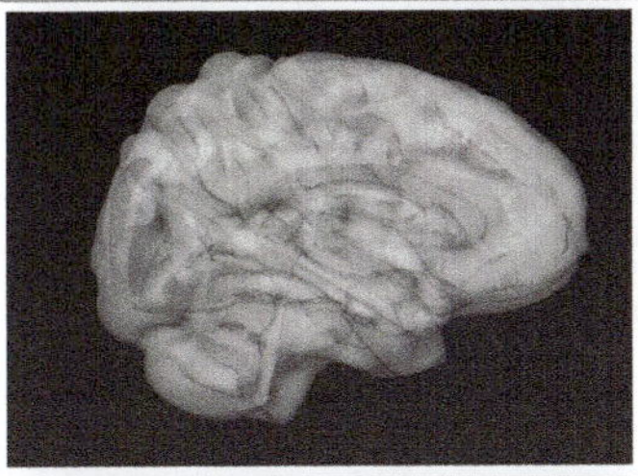	10.025 polygons
Aneurysm (saccular & fusiform)	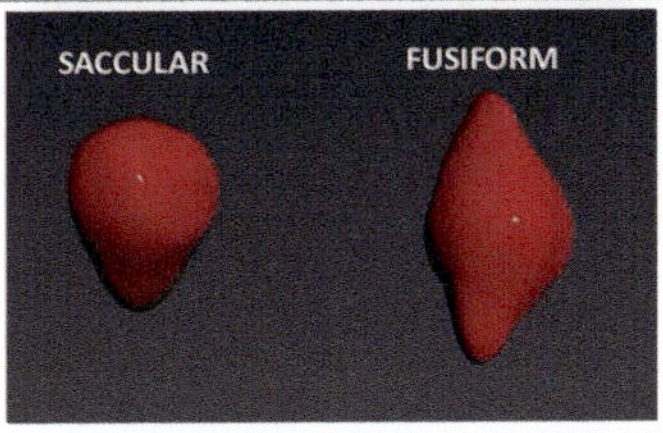	1.045 polygons (saccular) 1.013 polygons (fusiform)

(continued)

Table 8.2 (continued)

	Final model	Polycount
Arteriovenous malformation (AVM)	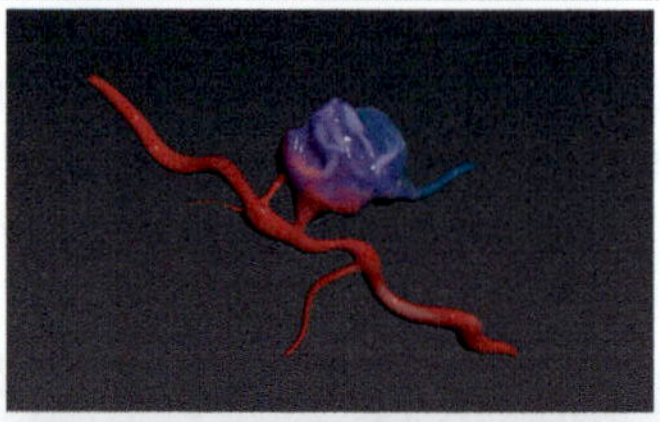	4.430 polygons
	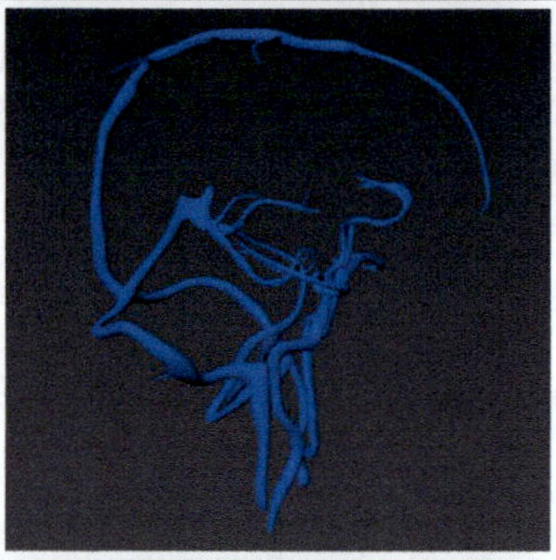	25.648 polygons
Arteriovenous fistulas (AVF)	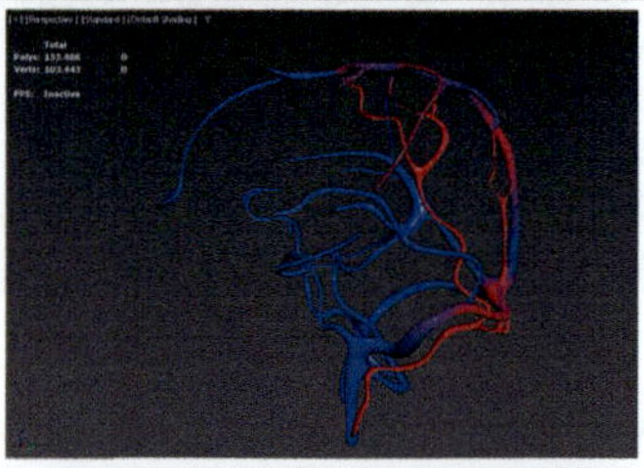	12.048 polygons
Arterial stenosis	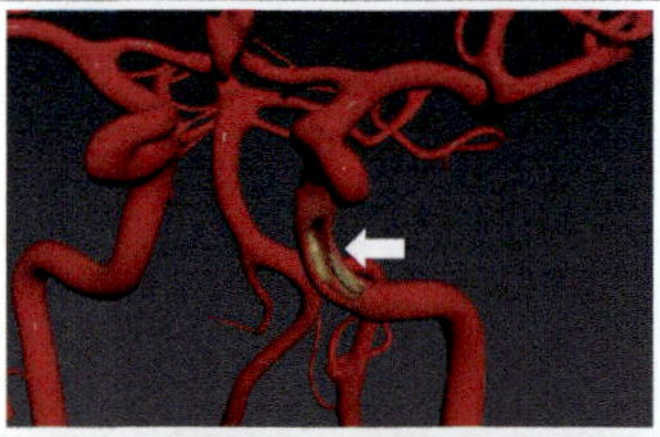	45.432 polygons
Arterial dissection	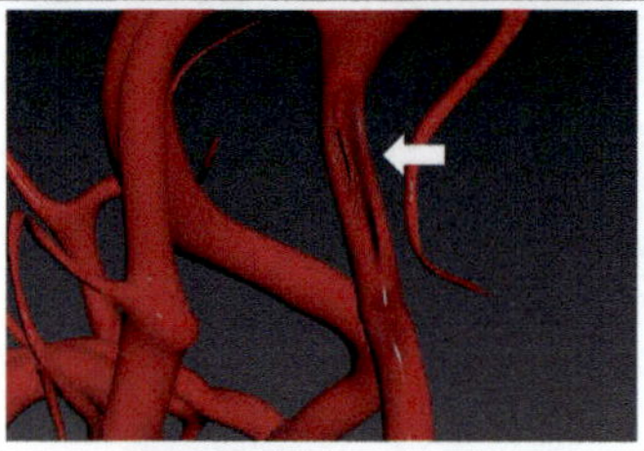	40.676 polygons

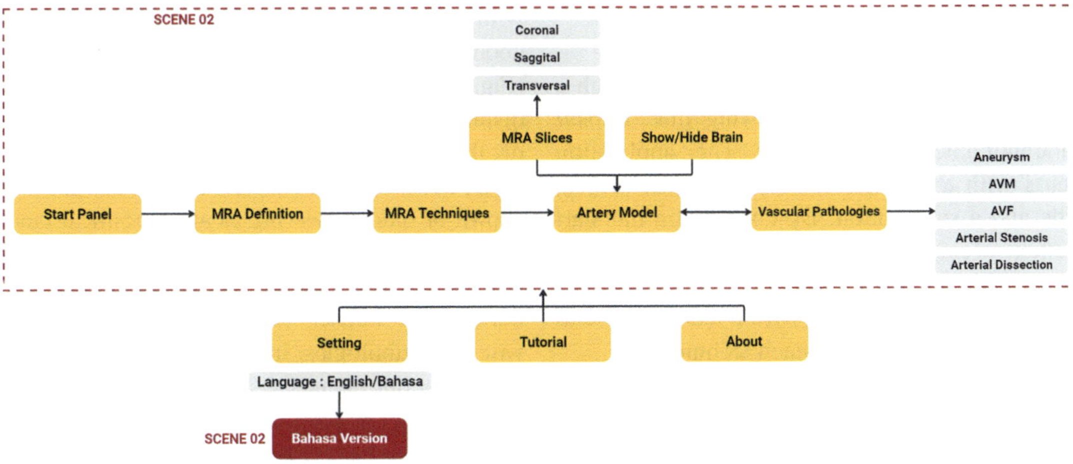

Fig. 8.10 Unity development flow

Bahasa (Indonesian language) version of the application was built in the second scene.

All the assets, both 3D and 2D, were imported into Unity. The 3D models were positioned within the same location in the 3D world. Textures from Substance Painter, including base colour map and normal map, were assigned to the albedo map and normal map, respectively. Meanwhile, the 2D assets were arranged on a single canvas featuring multiple panels.

To create a rotating cube that indicates the orientation of the models, a second camera was placed in the scene focusing on the rotating cube. A new render texture was set as the second camera's target texture and applied to a raw image on the canvas. This approach created an illusion of a 'second screen' displaying the rotating cube on the 2D canvas.

Subsequently, several scripts were developed to implement various functionalities within the application. These scripts included controls for camera movement, the ability to highlight specific structures and the management of information panels.

The final development, which consisted of two scenes (English and Bahasa version), was built as a WebGL application with a resolution of 1280 × 720 pixels.

8.2.2.3 Pre-launch Testing and Deployment

Pre-launch testing was conducted multiple times on the application to ensure its functionality and usability before the final deployment. After implementing the necessary improvements, the final version of the application was compressed and uploaded to www.itch.io/ for hosting.

8.3 Result

The final application can be accessed through a web browser using the following link: https://taramudita.itch.io/mraleaning. The application starts with a start panel, displaying the project title and a start button. By clicking on the start button, users will be directed to the MRA sections, which contain information about the definition of MRA, various MRA techniques and accompanying images of each technique.

The subsequent section is the anatomy section (Fig. 8.11), where users can explore and interact with the 3D models. Users can access information about specific vessels by clicking on the models (Fig. 8.12). In addition, users have the option to display MRA slices along with the labelled names of the vessels using the MRA slices button (Fig. 8.13). A 3D transparent brain can also be shown or hidden, serving as an anatomical landmark for the artery model (Fig. 8.14). This section not on provides a typical cerebral artery model, but also allows users to explore various common vascular pathologies, including aneurysm, AVM, AVF, arterial stenosis and arterial dissection (Fig. 8.15).

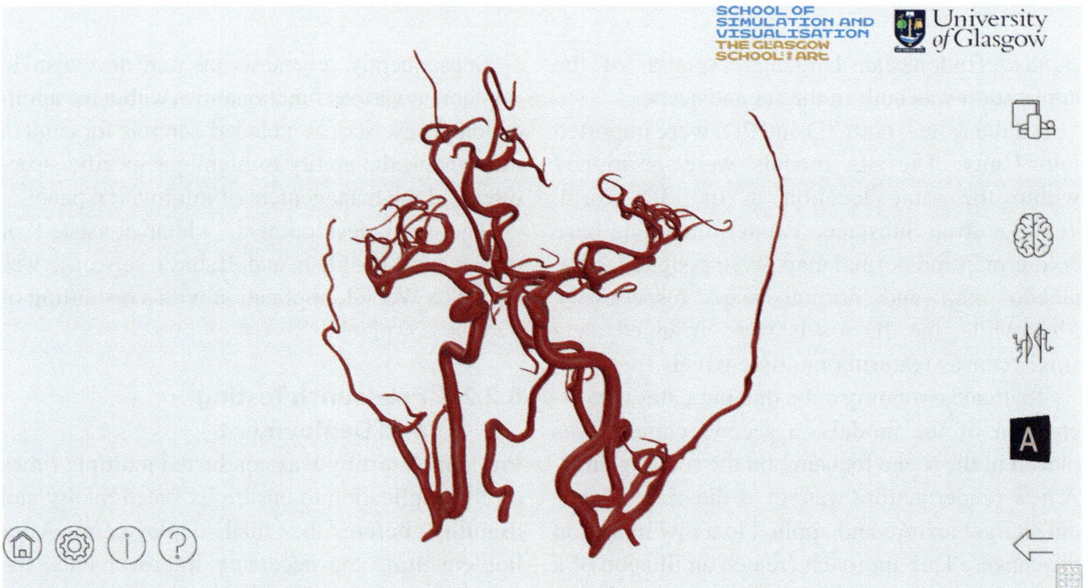

Fig. 8.11 Anatomy section

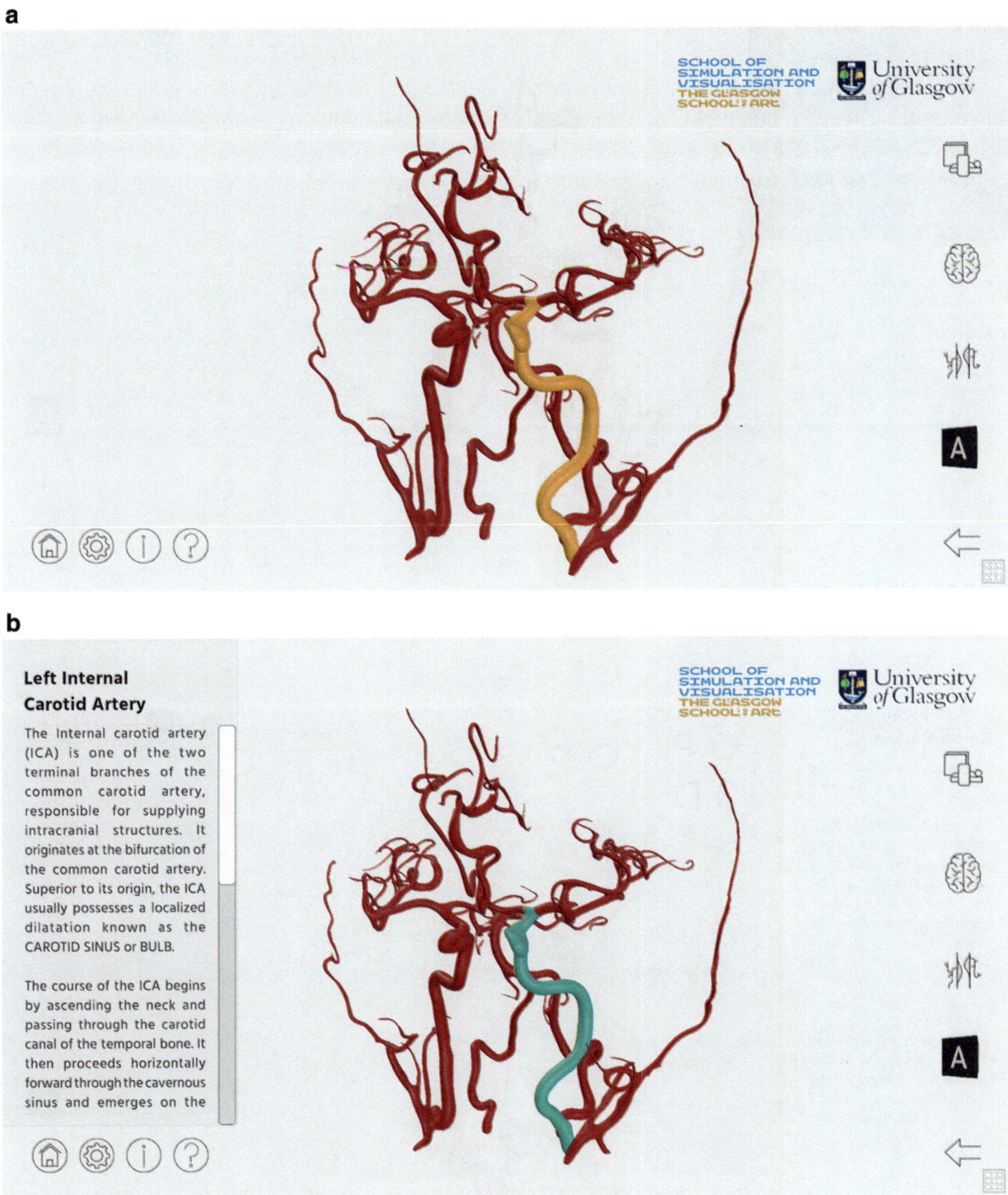

Fig. 8.12 Highlighting and selecting vessels

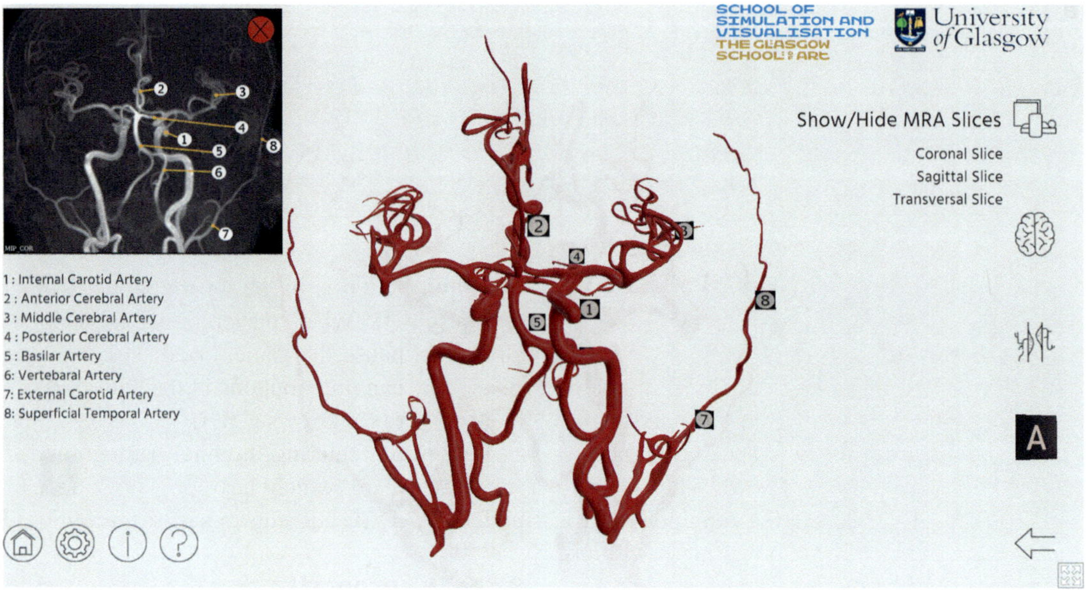

Fig. 8.13 MRA slice interface

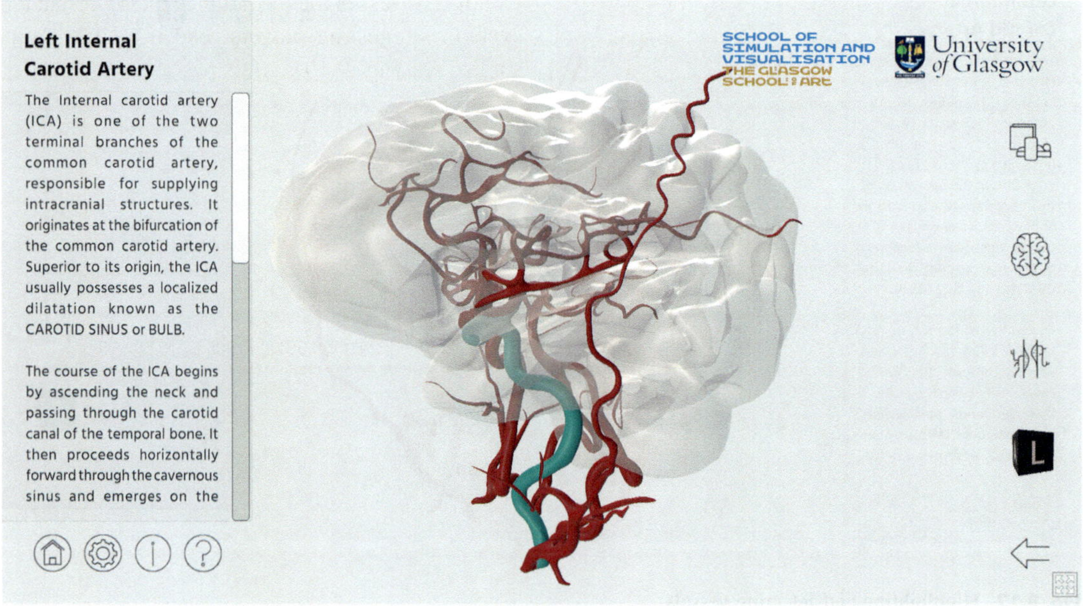

Fig. 8.14 Show/hide the brain

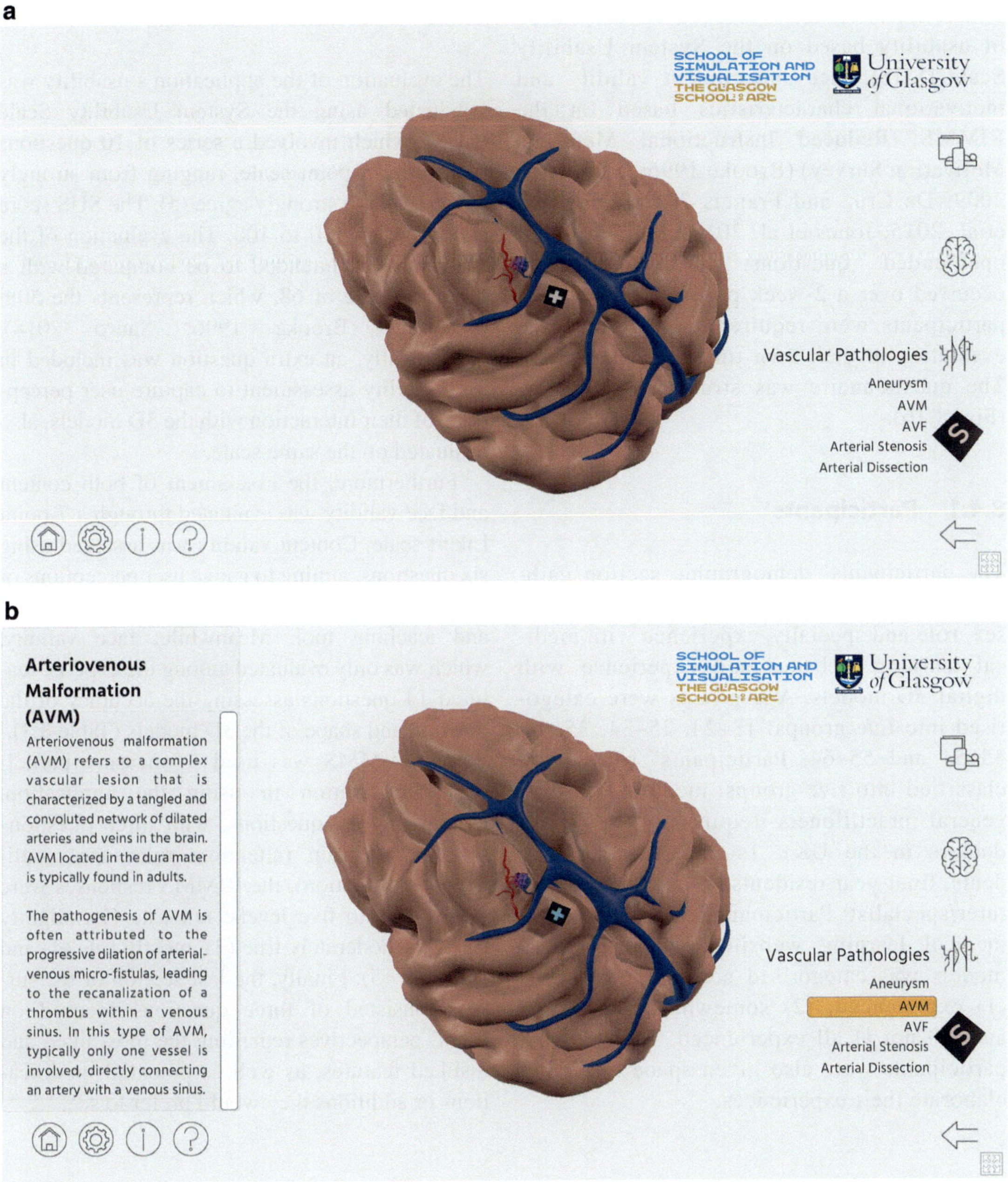

Fig. 8.15 Vascular pathologies

8.4 Evaluation

The evaluation of the application aimed to assess the potential usage of the application in supporting the learning of cerebral MRA within the context of Indonesian medical education, drawing insights from both educators and students. An online questionnaire was used to gather perspectives from both experts and non-experts after using the application. Participants were recruited through outreach messages along with the link to the questionnaire.

The questionnaire included an evaluation of usability based on the System Usability Scale (SUS), face and content validity and motivational characteristics based on the RIMMS (Reduced Instructional Materials Motivation Survey) (Brooke 1996; Cook et al. 2009; Da Cruz and Francis 2015; Loorbach et al. 2015; Jones et al. 2016) and additional open-ended questions. Data collection occurred over a 2-week period during which participants were required to undertake the evaluation in their own time and equipment. The questionnaire was structured as below (Fig. 8.16).

8.4.1 Participants

The participants' demographic section gathered information regarding participants' age, sex, role and specialty, experience with medical learning websites and experience with digital 3D models. Age groups were categorised into five groups: 18–24, 25–34, 35–44, 45–54 and 55–64. Participants' roles were classified into five groups: medical students, general practitioners (equivalent to junior doctors in the UK), 1st/2nd/3rd-year residents, final-year residents and consultant/lecturer/specialist. Participants' familiarity with medical learning websites and digital 3D models was categorised across three levels: (1) experienced, (2) somewhat experienced and (3) not at all experienced. Additionally, participants were also given space to further elaborate their experiences.

8.4.2 Evaluation Methods

The evaluation of the application's usability was conducted using the System Usability Scale (SUS), which involved a series of 10 questions rated on a 5-point scale, ranging from strongly disagree (1) to strongly agree (5). The SUS score can range from 0 to 100. The evaluation of the SUS score is intended to be compared with a baseline score of 68, which represents the 50th percentile (Brooke 1996; Sauro 2018). Additionally, an extra question was included in the usability assessment to capture user perceptions of their interaction with the 3D models, also evaluated on the same scale.

Furthermore, the assessment of both content and face validity was evaluated through a 7-point Likert scale. Content validity was assessed using six questions, aiming to gauge user perceptions of the application's content as an effective learning and teaching tool. Meanwhile, face validity, which was only evaluated among the experts, featured 14 questions assessing the accuracy of the position and shape of the 3D models (Table 8.3).

The RIMMS was used to measure participants' motivation in using the application. Comprising 12 questions, with three questions for each domain (attention, relevance, confidence, satisfaction), the RIMMS responses were classified into five levels: not true (1), slightly true (2), moderately true (3), mostly true (4) and very true (5). Finally, the last section of the survey consisted of three questions focused on users' perspectives regarding the most liked and disliked features, as well as potential modifications or additions they would prefer to see.

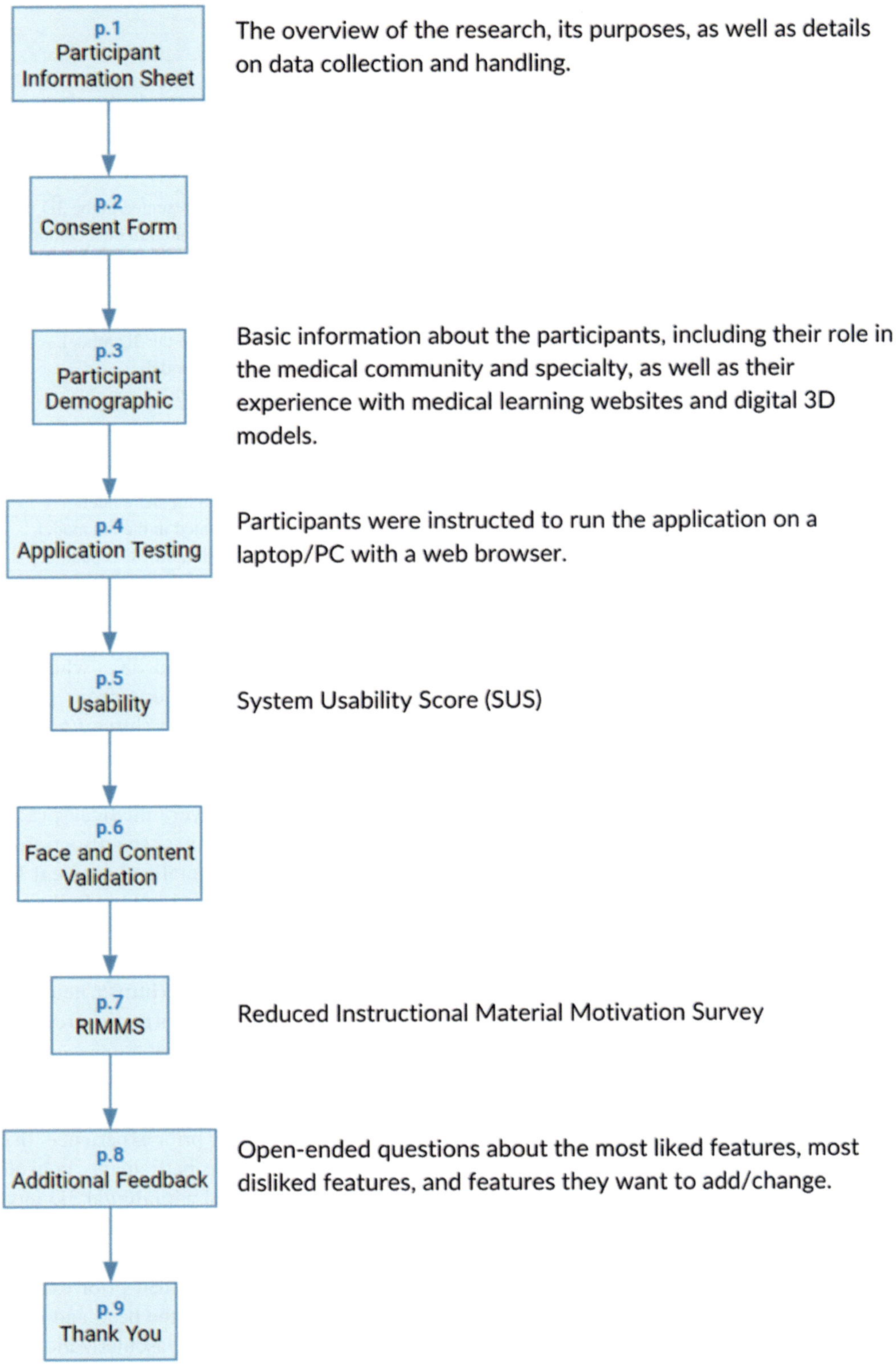

Fig. 8.16 Survey structure

Table 8.3 Face and content validation questions

Question 18	a	This website is useful for learning cerebral vascular anatomy.
	b	This website is useful for learning cerebral MRA.
	c	This website is useful for explaining cerebral vascular anatomy to medical students.
	d	This website is useful for explaining cerebral MRA to medical students.
	e	This website is useful to explain pathological vascular conditions to medical students.
	f	Overall, the website consists of a useful teaching tool.
Question 19	a	The POSITION of the *normal cerebral arteries* is accurately represented in the 3D model.
	b	The SHAPE of the *normal cerebral arteries* is accurately represented in the 3D model.
Question 20	a	The POSITION of the *saccular aneurysm* is accurately represented in the 3D model.
	b	The SHAPE of the *saccular aneurysm* is accurately represented in the 3D model.
Question 21	a	The POSITION of the *fusiform aneurysm* is accurately represented in the 3D model.
	b	The SHAPE of the *fusiform aneurysm* is accurately represented in the 3D model.
Question 22	a	The POSITION of the *AVM* is accurately represented in the 3D model.
	b	The SHAPE of the *AVM* is accurately represented in the 3D model.
Question 23	a	The POSITION of the *AVF* is accurately represented in the 3D model.
	b	The SHAPE of the *AVF* is accurately represented in the 3D model.
Question 24	a	The POSITION of the *arterial stenosis* is accurately represented in the 3D model.
	b	The SHAPE of the *arterial stenosis* is accurately represented in the 3D model.
Question 25	a	The POSITION of the *arterial dissection* is accurately represented in the 3D model.
	b	The SHAPE of the *arterial dissection* is accurately represented in the 3D model.

8.5 Results

8.5.1 Participant Demographic

A total of 23 Indonesian medical practitioners took part in the evaluation, comprising 15 males and eight females. A significant portion of the participants fell within the 25–34 age group. Most of the participants identified as general practitioners (N = 11), followed by consultant/lecturer/specialist (N = 5), 1st/2nd/3rd-year residents (N = 3), final-year residents (N = 2) and medical students (N = 2) (Fig. 8.17). While medical students and general practitioners were not specialised in a specific field, other participants' roles encompassed various specialties, including neurology, radiology and neurosurgery. Additionally, one final-year resident was identified as an OB-GYN resident.

Moreover, concerning participants' experiences with medical learning websites, almost half of the participants (N = 11) claimed to be experienced, while the remaining were evenly distributed between somewhat experienced and experienced (N = 6). These included websites containing 2D illustrations, such as Medscape (https://www.medscape.com/) and online journals, as well as social media platforms like YouTube and X, where they accessed medical animations from channels like Armando Hasudungan (https://www.youtube.com/user/armandohasudungan) and the Khan Academy (https://www.youtube.com/@khanacademy). Moreover, medical practitioners who specialised in a specific field had experience in more specialised medical learning websites. For example, Radiopaedia (https://radiopaedia.org/) was mentioned as a valuable resource for radiology-related content, while Neuroangio (https://neuroangio.org/) contained useful information relevant to neurology and neurosurgery.

When it came to experiences with digital 3D models, most of the participants (N = 11) reported not having any prior experience. In contrast, only three of the participants considered themselves experienced with digital 3D models, and nine of them described their experience as somewhat experienced (Fig. 8.18). Some participants mentioned that they had prior experience with digital 3D models of the head and neck, as well as the brain and its vascularization. They found these 3D models helpful in enhancing their understanding of anatomy, as they could explore the structures layer by layer. On the

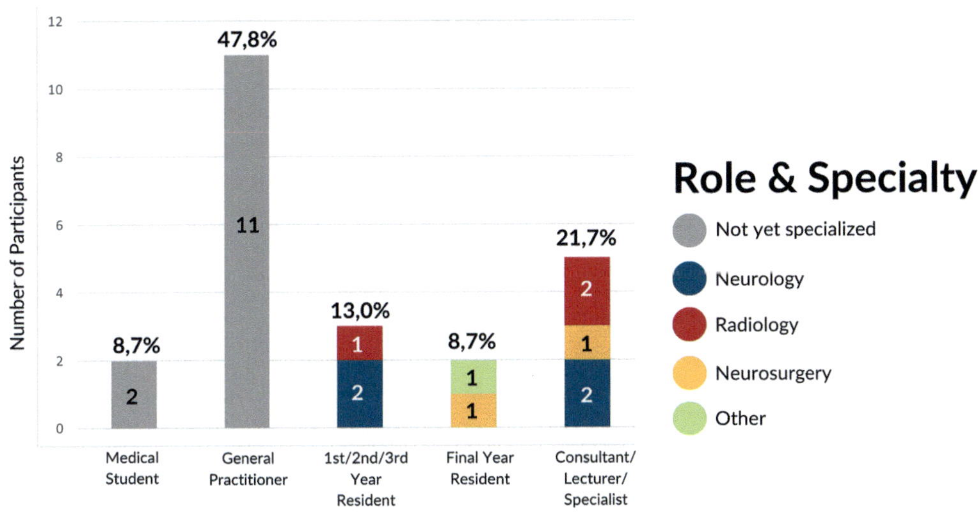

Fig. 8.17 Participants' role and specialty

Fig. 8.18 Participants' experiences with medical learning websites and digital 3D models

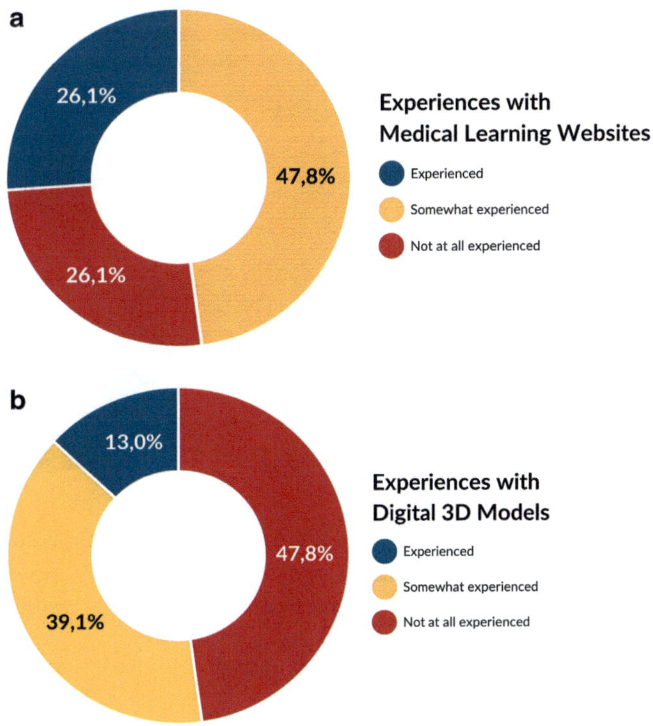

other hand, several participants expressed that they had no prior knowledge of digital 3D models and had a limited understanding of their implementation in medical anatomy education. These highlight the varying levels of familiarity and exposure to digital 3D models among the participants.

8.5.1.1 Usability

Based on the System Usability Scale (SUS), the application received an average SUS score of 72 (Fig. 8.19).

In addition to the SUS, participants were asked about the interaction with the 3D models within the application (Fig. 8.20). While a small

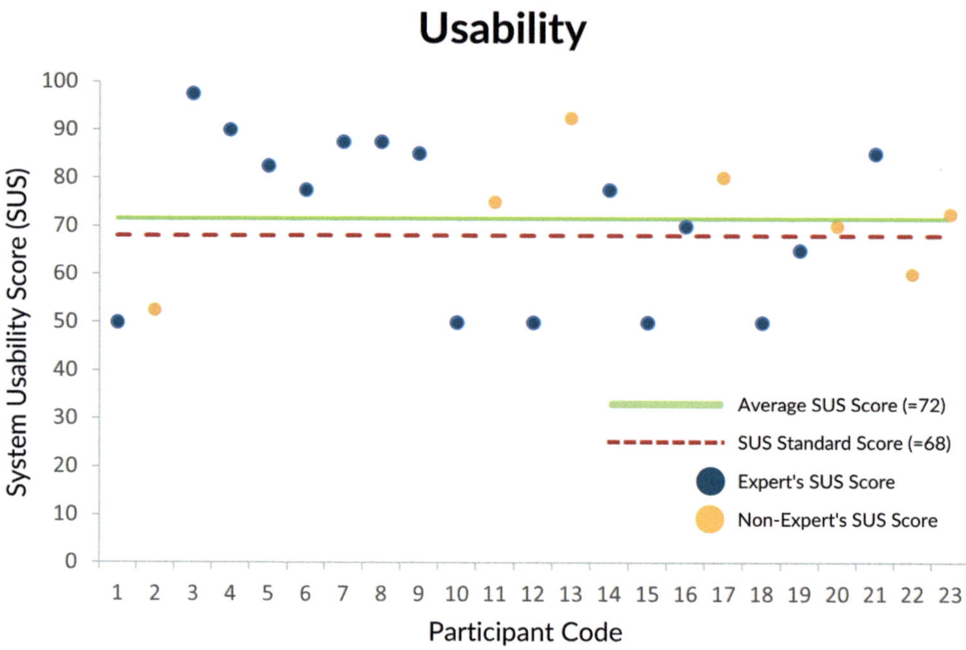

Fig. 8.19 Application's SUS score

Fig. 8.20 Interaction with 3D model usability

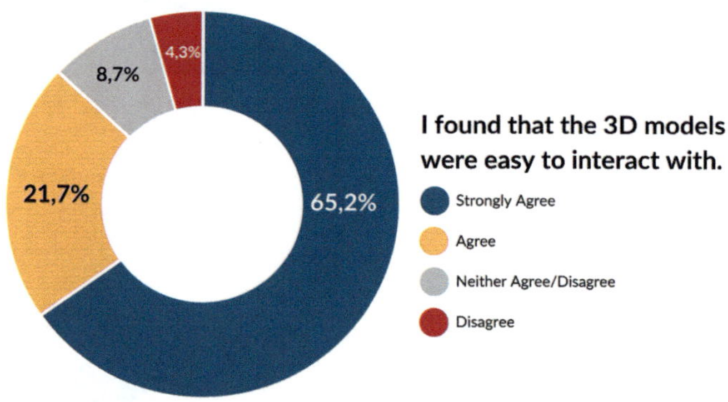

percentage of participants disagreed ($N = 1$) and neither agreed nor disagreed ($N = 2$) that the interaction was easy, most participants agreed that the interaction with the 3D models was easy, with an average score of 4.48 ($\sigma = 0.85$).

8.5.1.2 Face and Content Validation

A total of six questions measured on a 7-point Likert scale were used to assess the content validation (Fig. 8.21). Participant responses were categorised into two groups:

1. Experts, including consultant/lecturer/specialist and final-year residents, specialised in neurology, radiology, or neurosurgery
2. Non-experts, including 1st, 2nd and 3rd-year residents, general practitioners and medical students

Both groups found the application to be useful for learning both cerebral vascular anatomy (question 18a) and cerebral MRA (question 18b). The mean among the experts was $M = 6.17$ ($\sigma = 0.75$) and $M = 5.83$ ($\sigma = 0.75$) out of 7, respectively. Correspondingly, the non-experts reported a mean of $M = 6.47$ ($\sigma = 0.62$) and $M = 5.94$ ($\sigma = 0.83$) for these questions. However, more diverse responses were collected regarding the application's usefulness in explaining cerebral vascular anatomy (question 18c) (experts

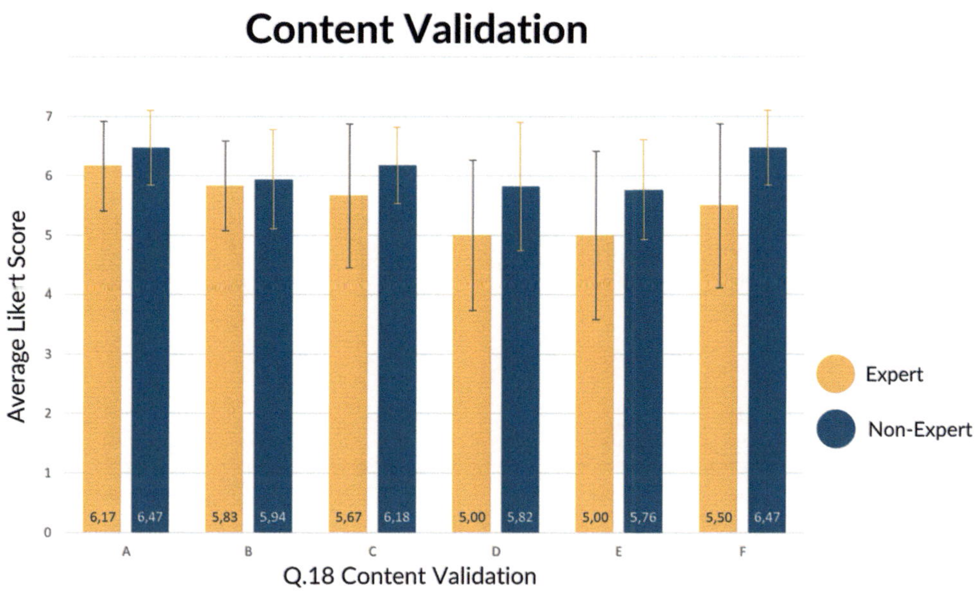

Fig. 8.21 Content validation of the application (see Table 8.3)

M = 5.67; σ = 1.21/non-experts *M* = 6.18; σ = 0.64), cerebral MRA (question 18d) (experts *M* = 5.00; σ = 1.26/non-experts *M* = 5.82; σ = 1.07) and pathological vascular conditions (question 18e) (experts *M* = 5.00; σ = 1.47/non-experts *M* = 5.76; σ = 0.8) to medical students. Experts' feedback in these areas tended to be less positive compared to non-experts. This contrast was accompanied by a broader spectrum of responses, ranging from somewhat agree to neutral and somewhat disagree (σ > 1.00).

Furthermore, varying feedback was also received regarding the usefulness of the overall website as a teaching tool. While non-experts tended to agree with the statement (M = 6.47; σ = 0.62), experts' feedback was not as positive (*M* = 5.50; σ = 1.38). This indicates that non-experts perceived the website more favourably as a teaching tool compared to experts.

Meanwhile, to validate the position and the shape of the 3D anatomy models, only feedback from experts was considered for face validation. Overall, the feedback regarding the representation of anatomical structures in the 3D models was positive, with the agreement that they were accurately depicted, with the mean ranging from 5.5 to 6 out of 7. However, there were more diverse responses concerning the position of the normal cerebral arteries (*M* = 5.50; σ = 1.64) (question 19a) and the position (*M* = 5.50; σ = 1.38) and shape (*M* = 5.17; σ = 1.47) of the AVM (question 22a and b) (Fig. 8.22). One expert expressed a 'somewhat disagree' response, indicating that these structures were not perceived as accurately positioned and shaped.

8.5.1.3 Reduced Instructional Materials Motivation Survey (RIMMS)

Feedback from participants indicated that the content within the application was able to capture and hold participants' attention (*M* = 4.14; σ = 0.8; Fig. 8.23). For the relevance domain, participants reported that the learning experience using the application was relevant and connected to familiar learning experiences before (*M* = 4.32; σ = 0.57). Furthermore, the application was perceived to not undermine participants' confidence, as it provided appropriate challenging learning opportunities (*M* = 4.10; σ = 0.74). Finally, participants expressed satisfaction with the learning experience using the application (*M* = 4.19; σ = 0.77) (S. Wang et al. 2020).

8.5.1.4 Participant Comments

Open-ended questions were included in the survey to gather more comprehensive responses from the

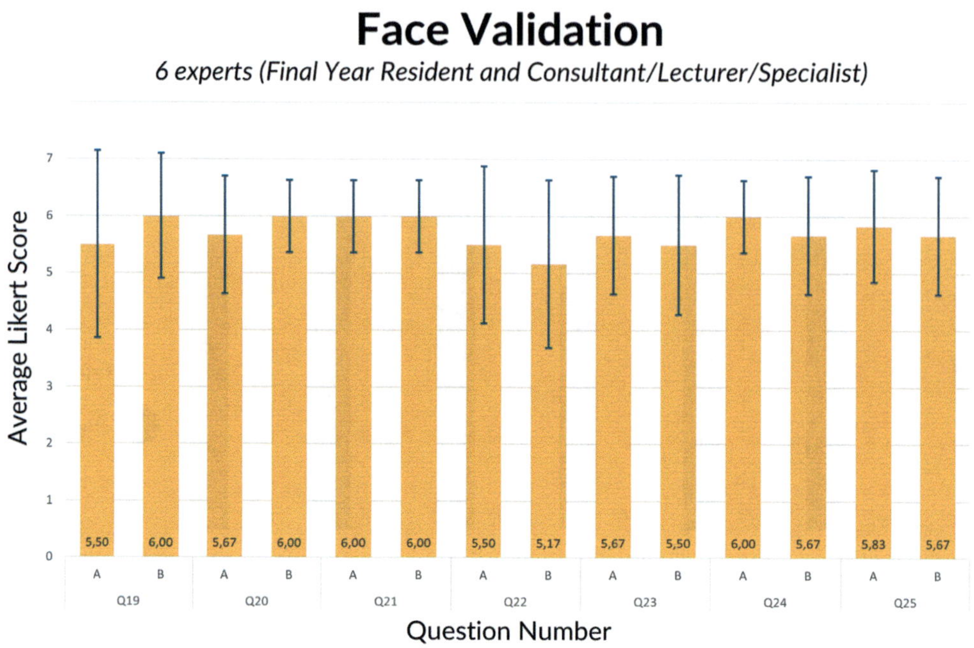

Fig. 8.22 Face validation of the 3D models within the application (see Table 8.3)

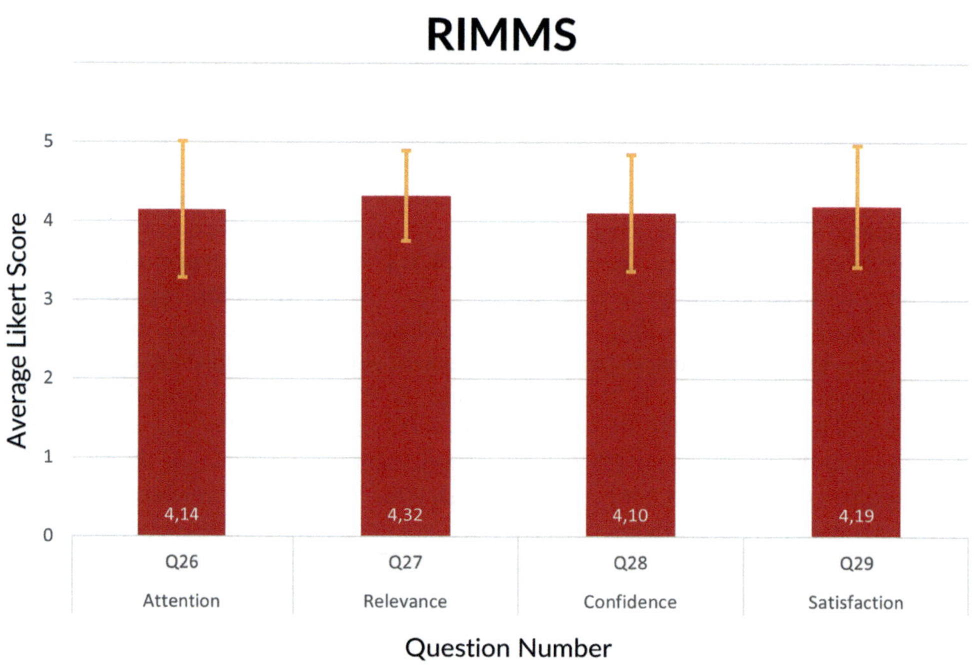

Fig. 8.23 Reduced Instructional Materials Motivation Survey (RIMMS)

participants. Regarding the most liked features of the application, participants emphasised the usefulness of the 3D models and the interactive nature of the application. They also appreciated the clear and straightforward information presented in an easy-to-use interface. One participant commented, 'the descriptions are very clear and detailed, making it easy for people to grasp the anatomy'.

Conversely, participants expressed diverse feedback about features they disliked and areas they believed required improvement. Some participants, particularly those with a deeper understanding of the subject matter, raised concerns about the need for '*further explanation*' within the application. Suggestions included adding MRA images of the vascular pathologies, providing percentages of the pathology locations represented in the 3D models and including comparisons of different MRA techniques.

Regarding the 3D models, participants recommended adding more surrounding structures, such as bones, to serve as anatomical landmarks. One expert also suggested adjusting the brain's transparency to create better visualisation of the relationship between vessels and surrounding structures. Additionally, participants requested a more realistic approach to the texture of the 3D models, especially for the arterial dissection model, where distinct textures for the vessel wall layers were deemed important for representative visuals.

Participants also provided feedback on the UI design, specifically pointing out that the information text appeared too dense. Some participants also noted that certain UI elements were too small. Additional inputs from participants included a request for audio features and the addition of a 3D model of the vein. Moreover, some participants expressed interest in having a mobile version of the application.

8.6 Discussion

8.6.1 Challenges in 3D Model Development

The process of reconstructing the 3D brain arterial system was relatively straightforward, mainly due to the high contrast between the vessels and the surrounding background. This prominent contrast allowed for efficient segmentation using a threshold-based method. However, the asset conditioning process, which involved tasks such as remeshing and decimating the number of polygons, consumed a significant portion of the development time. While several sources provided different suggestions regarding the ideal number of polygons for 3D models, the specific recommendation for web-based applications was not available. Unity (2017) suggested limiting the polycount to 1500–4000 while proposing handling up to 12,000–15,000 polygons for more advanced devices. However, the newer recommendation from Unity (2023) does not mention any specific polygon number limitation. Instead, it advised considering polygon numbers based on the target platform and detail requirement, also suggesting the use of fewer materials for more optimal performance.

This project experimented with different software, including 3DS Max, Blender, ZBrush and Maya, during a trial-and-error period to achieve the lowest number of vertices for faster browser loading. Moreover, efforts were made to improve performance by using limited materials and shaders (Unity 2023). Addressing this issue was a primary focus during the initial phase of the development, prompted by feedback received during the FGD regarding the problem of web-based application loading time and Internet speed in Indonesia, where the average speed is 43.35 Mbps, compared to 145.33 Mbps in the UK (Wisevoter 2023). Although the end number of polygons in the models did not reach as low as suggested in the literature, users' evaluations did not encounter any issues with loading times.

In terms of the materials used for the 3D models, single solid vivid colours were used to enhance performance and create significant contrast, sacrificing realism. While these vibrant colours aided in better recognition and distinction of the anatomical structures, their absence of photorealism resulted in less accurate representation and loss of authenticity of the real human anatomy (Koh et al. 2023). To address this limitation, it is recommended to consider the implementation of more realistic textures, displayed in tandem with colour-coded models.

Furthermore, the creation of the 3D pathological models was based on the modification of the normal arterial system model, relying on 2D reference images. The alterations were primarily carried out through freehand sculpturing in

ZBrush, which consequently relied more on observation, anatomy knowledge and artistic judgement of the modeller.

8.6.2 Evaluation Results

The application's overall usability received an average SUS score of 72, which falls within the 'good' and 'acceptable' range, equivalent to a C+ grade (Sauro 2018). This indicated that the application's usability was satisfactory and generally well received by participants. This aligns with participants' feedback in the open-ended questions, highlighting that the application is easy to use. Most participants also agreed that the interactive nature of the 3D models is easy to navigate, which was one of the most liked features of the application. Additionally, the overall learning motivation of participants towards the application was positive based on the RIMMS results.

In contrast, individuals who reported lower SUS scores tended to also report a lack of experience with digital 3D models. In future research, conducting a correlation analysis between one's familiarity with digital models and their SUS scores would be a valuable endeavour. Moreover, additional feedback revealed that the information within the application lacked enough visual cues, which may also contribute to a lower overall usability score. While the overall information within the application was deemed to be simple, the absence of contrasting colours and different font types to highlight important information through visual hierarchy increased the risk of cognitive overload for users (Yazdi 2023). For further development, additional content should be provided together with enhanced visual cues, such as more contrasting colours and/or bold and italic texts, to improve the overall presentation of information and avoid cognitive overload (Zhou et al. 2022).

Regarding the content validation, while non-experts tended to express more positive responses, experts' responses highlighted the need for refinement in certain areas. Specifically, experts indicated that improvements should be undertaken to enhance the application's ability to explain the anatomy of cerebral vascularization, cerebral MRA and pathological vascular conditions.

Furthermore, the preference of participants towards the application as a learning tool rather than a teaching tool could be attributed to its desktop nature. Since a significant portion of medical teaching, especially during clinical years, occurs outside the traditional classroom setting, a mobile version of the application might offer a more convenient teaching tool for experts to utilise in bedside or hospital teaching situations (Wong and Chan 2023).

Regarding the feedback on the position and shape of the 3D models, although the overall feedback was positive, one expert argued that the normal cerebral artery models lacked arterial segmentations. For example, while the model highlighted the overall structure of the internal carotid artery (ICA), the segments of the ICA, which are crucial anatomical landmarks in the course of the blood vessel, were only described in the application information and not represented in the 3D models (Sheikh 2022). Moreover, the absence of surrounding structures, such as the brain and the skull, in the application led to a less clear position of the normal cerebral artery, contributing to the uncertainty of its position and shape.

Meanwhile, participants also suggested improvements to the application's design, especially in terms of the UI. Recommendations to address these issues included changing the font type, using more engaging colours and employing different approaches to organise and present information. For instance, one participant suggested, 'I would add underline/bold/italic to the text', and another mentioned, 'I would recommend changing the font type as the current font appears quite thin'.

Lastly, during the FGD, participants expressed concerns about the loading time of the web-based application. However, no specific feedback relating to the loading time was received during the final evaluation, indicating that the application development was successful in terms of loading time for accessibility in Indonesia.

In conclusion, this application received overall positive feedback as a valuable supportive learning tool for understanding MRA and the anatomy of cerebral vascularization. Moreover, the feedback from participants has provided valuable directions for further enhancing the application content, 3D models, UI design, functionality and potential features. By incorporating these improvements, the application holds the potential to evolve into an even more valuable resource for medical education in Indonesia.

8.6.3 Research Limitations

The decision to undertake this research remotely, targeting the medical community in Indonesia while operating from Glasgow, presented a set of challenges. First, while opting for a web-based application was pragmatic to ensure broader accessibility to the target audience in Indonesia, it does not provide the same level of user engagement and immersion as more advanced technologies like AR and VR (Coban et al. 2022). In addition, the long-distance evaluation resulted in a less controlled environment where participants conducted the evaluation at their convenience, without direct oversight by the researchers. Given the absence of experimental control, it is essential to thoroughly weigh the evaluation results, and their generalizability is currently limited. To obtain more dependable findings, further research should aim to conduct controlled evaluations.

8.7 Further Directions and Conclusion

The evaluation of the final application yielded promising results, including a high usability score, positive feedback regarding its potential usage as a learning tool and indications of heightened learning motivation among participants. In addition, valuable suggestions were gathered from potential users and experts, providing valuable insights for further development and improvements. To deepen our understanding, a more extensive evaluation, involving a larger number of experts and incorporating statistical analysis to compare expert and non-expert responses, could provide more profound insights. Additionally, broadening the survey to a population engaged directly in medical education will facilitate the collection of specialised feedback from both teacher and student perspectives, ensuring a more comprehensive evaluation of the application's effectiveness as a learning tool.

Moreover, to ensure the application's relevance and integration into medical education, further direction includes adjusting its content with the existing curriculum or, ideally, specific modules within the medical programme. While this project serves as a foundation for technology-enhanced learning in medical education, it is essential to continue its development to meet the specific needs and requirements of Indonesian medical education.

Although further improvements are necessary, the application received positive support from participants. Beyond its immediate impact, this project serves as an important catalyst in increasing awareness of technology-enhanced learning methods in medical education. With continued development and integration, this project can contribute to the broader adoption of technology-enhanced learning methods and contribute to the shaping of medical education in Indonesia.

References

Adams CM, Wilson TD (2011) Virtual cerebral ventricular system: an MR-based three-dimensional computer model. Anat Sci Educ 4(6):340–347. https://doi.org/10.1002/ase.256

Anzalone N, Tartaro A (2005) Intracranial MR angiography. In: Schneider G, Prince MR, Meaney JFM, Ho VB (eds) Magnetic resonance angiography. Springer, Milano, pp 103–138

Autodesk (2022) Retopology Tools for 3ds Max. https://help.autodesk.com/view/3DSMAX/2022/ENU/?guid=GUID-57B77A00-5300-47CB-99E1-22B9C536B060

Azer SA, Azer S (2016) 3D anatomy models and impact on learning: a review of the quality of the literature. Health Prof Educ 2(2):80–98. https://doi.org/10.1016/j.hpe.2016.05.002

Bommes D, Lévy B, Pietroni N, Puppo E, Silva C, Tarini M, Zorin D (2012) State of the art in quad meshing. Vol. xx

Brewer DN, Wilson TD, Eagleson R, De Ribaupierre S (2012) Evaluation of neuroanatomical train-

ing using a 3D visual reality model. Stud Health Technol Inform 173:85–91. https://doi.org/10.3233/978-1-61499-022-2-85
Brooke J (1996) SUS-a quick and dirty usability scale Usable systems view project decision making in general practice view project. https://www.researchgate.net/publication/319394819
Brown R (2022) Best practices for conducting virtual focus groups. https://source.sheridancollege.ca/ctl_publ/6
Brush K (2020) MoSCoW method. TechTarget. https://www.techtarget.com/searchsoftwarequality/definition/MoSCoW-method#:~:text=The%20MoSCoW%20method%20is%20a,make%20the%20acronym%20more%20pronounceable
Coban M, Bolat YI, Goksu I (2022) The potential of immersive virtual reality to enhance learning: a meta-analysis. Educ Res Rev 36:100452. https://doi.org/10.1016/j.edurev.2022.100452
Cook DA, Beckman TJ, Thomas KG, Thompson WG (2009) Measuring motivational characteristics of courses: applying Keller's instructional materials motivation survey to a web-based course. http://journals.lww.com/academicmedicine
Cottam WW (1999) Adequacy of medical school gross anatomy education as perceived by certain postgraduate residency programs and anatomy course directors. Clin Anat 12(1):55–65. https://doi.org/10.1002/(SICI)1098-2353(1999)12:1<55::AID--CA8>3.0.CO;2-O
Da Cruz MJ, Francis HW (2015) Face and content validation of a novel three-dimensional printed temporal bone for surgical skills development. J Laryngol Otol 129(S3):S23–S29. https://doi.org/10.1017/S0022215115001346
De Ribaupierre S, Wilson TD (2012) Construction of a 3-D anatomical model for teaching temporal lobectomy. Comput Biol Med 42(6):692–696. https://doi.org/10.1016/j.compbiomed.2012.03.005
Ellis C (2008) 'You Can't Do That in a Classroom!': how distributed learning can assist in the widespread adoption of hybrid learning strategies. In: Fong J, Kwan R, Wang FL (eds) First International Conference. ICHL 2008
Erolin C (2019) Interactive 3D models for anatomy and medical education. Adv Exp Med Biol 1138:1–16. http://www.springer.com/series/5584
French JL (2020) How to load a scene in unity. Gamedevbeginner. https://gamedevbeginner.com/how-to-load-a-new-scene-in-unity-with-a-loading-screen/
Gaur U, Majumder MAA, Sa B, Sarkar S, Williams A, Singh K (2020) Challenges and opportunities of preclinical medical education: COVID-19 crisis and beyond. SN Compr Clin Med 2(11):1992–1997. https://doi.org/10.1007/s42399-020-00528-1
Ghosh SK (2015) Human cadaveric dissection: a historical account from ancient Greece to the modern era. Anat Cell Biol (ACB) 48(3):153–169. https://doi.org/10.5115/acb.2015.48.3.153
Guze PA (2015) Using technology to meet the challenges of medical education. Trans Am Clin Climatol Assoc 126
Hamza-Lup FG, Thompson T (2009) Interactive 3D user interfaces for neuroanatomy exploration. WEBIST 2009 - Proceedings of the 5th International Conference on Web Information Systems and Technologies, pp 130–134. https://doi.org/10.5220/0001823201300134
Han H, Nelson E, Wetter N (2014) Medical students' online learning technology needs. Clin Teach 11(1):15–19. https://doi.org/10.1111/tct.12092
Interaction Design Foundation (2016) Making your UX life easier with the MoSCoW. Interaction Design Foundation. https://www.interaction-design.org/literature/article/making-your-ux-life-easier-with-the-moscow
John NW (2007) The impact of Web3D technologies on medical education and training. Comput Educ 49(1):19–31. https://doi.org/10.1016/j.compedu.2005.06.003
Jones DB, Sung R, Weinberg C, Korelitz T, Andrews R (2016) Three-dimensional modeling may improve surgical education and clinical practice. Surg Innov 23(2):189–195. https://doi.org/10.1177/1553350615607641
Kim D-Y (2012) 3D volume extraction of cerebrovascular structure on brain magnetic resonance angiography data sets. J Biomed Sci Eng 05(10):574–579. https://doi.org/10.4236/jbise.2012.510070
Koh MY, Tan GJS, Mogali SR (2023) Spatial ability and 3D model colour-coding affect anatomy performance: a cross-sectional and randomized trial. Sci Rep 13(1):7879. https://doi.org/10.1038/s41598-023-35046-2
Kristiaji A, Yunus JMMS, Kurniawati NMMS (2022) Persepsi Mahasiswa Terhadap Penggunaan Aplikasi Virtual 3D Osteologi Manusia Sebagai Media Ajar Pendamping Dalam Pembelajaran Anatomi. Universitas Gadjah Mada. http://etd.repository.ugm.ac.id/penelitian/detail/211532
Kusumaningtyas S, Ramadhan MIA, Margiana R, Wiyarta E, Sutanto R, Liem IK (2021) Anatomy visual learning: a new modality to enhance neuroanatomy learning in first-year medical students. Jurnal Pendidikan Kedokteran Indonesia: Indones J Med Educ 10(1):27. https://doi.org/10.22146/jpki.53276
Lasso A (2022) New extension: HDBrainExtraction for AI-based skull stripping. 3D Slicer. https://discourse.slicer.org/t/new-extension-hdbrainextraction-for-ai-based-skull-stripping/24420
Loorbach N, Peters O, Karreman J, Steehouder M (2015) Validation of the Instructional Materials Motivation Survey (IMMS) in a self-directed instructional setting aimed at working with technology. Br J Educ Technol 46(1):204–218. https://doi.org/10.1111/bjet.12138
McLachlan JC, Bligh J, Bradley P, Searle J (2004) Teaching anatomy without cadavers. Med Educ 38(4):418–424. https://doi.org/10.1046/j.1365-2923.2004.01795.x
Nowinski WL, Volkau I, Marchenko Y, Thirunavuukarasuu A, Ng TT, Runge VM (2009) A 3D model of human

cerebrovasculature derived from 3T magnetic resonance angiography. Neuroinformatics 7(1):23–36. https://doi.org/10.1007/s12021-008-9028-8

Nugraha ZS, Khadafianto F, Fidianingsih I (2019) Refleksi Pembelajaran Anatomi pada Mahasiswa Kedokteran Fase Ketiga melalui Applied and Clinical Question. Refleksi Pembelajaran Inovatif 1(1):21–27. https://doi.org/10.20885/rpi.vol1.iss1.art3

Nugroho H, Rachmi E (2022) Analisis Penggunaan Atlas Elektronik Anatomi Tubuh Manusia 3d Di Fakultas Kedokteran Universitas Mulawarman Samarinda. Jurnal Verdure 4(1):273–282. www.visiblebody.com

Passat N, Ronse C, Baruthio J, Armspach JP, Maillot C (2006) Magnetic resonance angiography: from anatomical knowledge modeling to vessel segmentation. Med Image Anal 10(2):259–274. https://doi.org/10.1016/j.media.2005.11.002

Ramsey-Stewart G, Burgess AW, Hill DA (2010) Back to the future: teaching anatomy by whole-body dissection. Med J Aust 193(11–12):668–671. https://doi.org/10.5694/j.1326-5377.2010.tb04099.x

Robbins BD, Tomaka A, Innus C, Patterson J, Styn G (2008) Lessons from the dead: The experiences of undergraduates working with cadavers. Omega J Death Dying 58(3):177–192. https://doi.org/10.2190/OM.58.3.b

Rondonuwu VWK, Mewo YM, Wungow HIS (2021) Pendidikan Kedokteran di Masa Pandemi COVID-19 Dampak Pembelajaran Daring Bagi Mahasiswa Fakultas Kedokteran Angkatan 2017 Unsrat. JURNAL BIOMEDIK (JBM) 13(1):67. https://doi.org/10.35790/jbm.13.1.2021.31764

Saputra O, Lisiswanti R (2015) Faktor-Faktor yang Mempengaruhi Keberhasilan Pembelajaran Keterampilan Klinik di Institusi Pendidikan Kedokteran. Juke Universitas, Lampung

Sauro J (2018, September). 5 ways to interpret a SUS score. MeasuringU. https://measuringu.com/interpret-sus-score/

Sheikh Y (2022) Internal carotid artery. Radiopaedia. https://radiopaedia.org/articles/internal-carotid-artery-1?lang=gb

Singal A, Bansal A, Chaudhary P, Singh H, Patra A (2021) Anatomy education of medical and dental students during COVID-19 pandemic: a reality check. Surg Radiol Anat 43(4):515–521. https://doi.org/10.1007/s00276-020-02615-3

Stalmeijer RE, McNaughton N, Van Mook WNKA (2014) Using focus groups in medical education research: AMEE Guide No. 91. Med Teach 36(11):923–939. https://doi.org/10.3109/0142159X.2014.917165

Stull AT, Hegarty M, Mayer RE (2009) Getting a Handle on Learning Anatomy With Interactive Three-Dimensional Graphics. J Educ Psychol 101(4):803–816. https://doi.org/10.1037/a0016849

Unity (2017) Modeling characters for optimal performance. Unity Documentation. https://docs.unity3d.com/560/Documentation/Manual/ModelingOptimizedCharacters.html

Unity (2023) Creating models for optimal performance. Unity Documentation. https://docs.unity3d.com/Manual/ModelingOptimizedCharacters.html

Universitas Indonesia F. of M (2022) IMERI: Indonesian Medical Education and Research Institute

Vo KD, Jeck D, McKinstry R (2014) Magnetic resonance angiography of cervical and intracranial vessels. In: Encyclopedia of the neurological sciences. Elsevier Inc., pp 959–963. https://doi.org/10.1016/B978-0-12-385157-4.00196-2

Wang GJ, Litt H, Carpenter JP (2010) Magnetic resonance imaging and angiography. Endovasc Surg 4:195–208

Wang X, Bai H, Cui Y (2017) Virtual reality to read MR angiograhpy. Society for MR Radiographers & Technologists 26th annual meeting

Wang S, Christensen C, Xu Y, Cui W, Tong R, Shear L (2020) Measuring Chinese middle school students' motivation using the reduced instructional materials motivation survey (RIMMS): a validation study in the adaptive learning setting. Front Psychol 11. https://doi.org/10.3389/fpsyg.2020.01803

Webster NL (2017) High poly to low poly workflows for real-time rendering. J Vis Commun Med 40(1):40–47. https://doi.org/10.1080/17453054.2017.1313682

Wisevoter (2023) Internet speed by country. Wisevoter. https://wisevoter.com/country-rankings/internet-speed-by-country/#indonesia

Wong HM, Chan S (2023) Effective bedside teaching as a foundation doctor. Clin Med (London, England) 23(3):264–266. https://doi.org/10.7861/clinmed2022-0422

Wright SN, Kochunov P, Mut F, Bergamino M, Brown KM, Mazziotta JC, Toga AW, Cebral JR, Ascoli GA (2013) Digital reconstruction and morphometric analysis of human brain arterial vasculature from magnetic resonance angiography. NeuroImage 82:170–181. https://doi.org/10.1016/j.neuroimage.2013.05.089

Yang C, Yang X, Yang H, Fan Y (2020) Flipped classroom combined with human anatomy web-based learning system shows promising effects in anatomy education. Medicine 99(46):e23096. https://doi.org/10.1097/MD.0000000000023096

Yazdi S (2023) What is cognitive overload in UX? 3 tips to minimize it in your designs! Bootcamp. https://bootcamp.uxdesign.cc/what-is-cognitive-overload-in-ux-3-tips-to-minimize-it-in-your-designs-f56caba66fe5

Zhou J, Miao X, He F, Miao Y (2022) Effects of font style and font color in news on user cognitive load in intelligent user interfaces. IEEE Access 10:10719–10730. https://doi.org/10.1109/ACCESS.2022.3151915

Part III

Serious Games

An Educational Game to Teach Immune Evasion of the Schistosome and Validation of Its Impact

9

Junlong Dai, Daisy Abbott, and Hannah Bialic

Abstract

The adoption of serious games (SGs) is rapidly growing with new applications emerging in medical education. SGs refer to games whose main content is to teach knowledge and skills, providing professional training and simulation. However, there are limited instances of applying such a paradigm to learning about parasite immunology. This study aimed to create a game to aid understanding of the principles of schistosomes' immune evasion for a wide range of audiences and validated its effectiveness.

The game 'Schistosome: The Escape' was developed in *Unity* using original and third-party assets. This game, 'Schistosome: the Escape', is played in the first person. Players are cast as parasites aiming to achieve victory by evading attacks from immune cells. The game consists of three levels corresponding to the migratory path of schistosomes in the human body. As each level is completed, the parasite undergoes morphological changes. All game mechanics correlate with underlying immunology principles. After development, 27 individuals were recruited and divided into a game-based learning (test) group ($N = 12$) and a text-based learning (control) group ($N = 15$). The inclusion criteria were as follows: (1) age over 18 years old, (2) educational level higher than high school and (3) willingness to be contacted in a follow-up. These two learning methods were assessed by conducting a quiz before and after each experimental condition.

Results showed that the game-based learning group exhibited significant improvements in understanding schistosome immunology. Compared to the reading-based learning group, the test group achieved higher average knowledge acquisition, and 100% of players acknowledged the potential value of SGs for learning parasitology. This study suggested

Supplementary Information The online version contains supplementary material available at https://doi.org/10.1007/978-3-031-63463-5_9.

J. Dai (✉)
Division of Liver Surgery, Department of General Surgery, West China Hospital, Sichuan University, Chengdu, Sichuan, China

School of Medicine, Dentistry and Nursing, College of Medical, Veterinary and Life Sciences, University of Glasgow, Glasgow, UK

School of Innovation and Technology, Glasgow, UK

D. Abbott
School of Innovation and Technology, Glasgow, UK
e-mail: d.abbott@gsa.ac.uk

H. Bialic
Wellcome Centre for Integrative Parasitology, School of Infection & Immunity, College of Medical, Veterinary and Life Sciences, University of Glasgow, Glasgow, UK
e-mail: Hannah.Bialic@glasgow.ac.uk

J. Clancy, M. Poyade (eds.), *Medical Visualization and Applications of Technology – Volume 2*, Biomedical Visualization 5, https://doi.org/10.1007/978-3-031-63463-5_9

that the developed game is comprehensive, visually appealing and effective. Through gameplay, players could successfully grasp schistosome immunology knowledge at a level comparable to reading materials. SGs are a robust complement to and potential replacement for conventional learning patterns.

Keywords

Serious games · Schistosome · Immune evasion · Medical education · Immunology · Parasitology · Game-based learning

9.1 Introduction

Serious games (SGs) are defined as '*games with an application purpose*' (Wilkinson 2016) that primarily focus on teaching knowledge, skills, providing professional training and simulations. Since proposed in the 1970s, SGs have been widely utilised in various fields such as medicine, industry and education (Olgers et al. 2021; Leitao et al. 2021; Tori et al. 2022).

This study aimed to develop and explore a game-based approach to medical education, visualising obscure parasitological knowledge in an easy-play 3-dimensional (3D) game which conveys, through gameplay, the immune rationale behind parasitic prevention.

9.1.1 Medical Serious Game

The combination of medical education and SGs is not new. As teaching and learning within medicine have evolved, many medical educationalists began to study SGs' application in medical education. In 2020, Tsopra et al. developed a multifunctional game teaching antibiotic use and used rigorous statistical methods to measure its acceptance and effect (Tsopra et al. 2020). Results highly recommended game-based learning, especially in teaching intricate content. With respect to immunology, Lima et al. (2022) achieved an ideal effect in teaching nurses the rationale of vaccination through an assistive serious game in class. Medical SGs could also improve medical students' learning attitude and reduce remembering difficulty (García-Redondo et al. 2019). All these findings showed that SGs play an incentive role in medical education and formed the theoretical basis of this project.

Besides, SGs have also addressed public awareness of medical issues. During the global coronavirus pandemic, Suppan et al. (2021) developed a game called *Escape COVID-19* to promote preventative means. This consisted of a scene adventure game with four levels (at home, on the road, in communal areas and in the ward) educating the public towards effective informed decision-making. Adequate infection prevention and control behaviours were rewarded. Researchers translated it into four languages and published it online. Over 1000 people played this game, with 86.1% passing the ending quiz and expressing an inclination to follow the guidelines they learned. For this study, public awareness was an important outcome. Therefore, the target population was the public, necessitating an accessible approach for both parasitology content and gameplay to promote parasite prevention.

9.1.2 Schistosome

A schistosome is a type of parasitic trematode with two genders that resides in blood vessels. The pairing of male and female worms is necessary for the proper maturity of their larvae (cercariae) (see Fig. 9.1). Infected by only a male or female worm, the cercariae cannot develop normally (Nation et al. 2020).

Schistosomiasis is a parasitic disease caused by the presence of schistosomes in the human body. Infection only occurs when the human skin comes into contact with contaminated water containing cercariae. The primary pathological changes are caused by granulomas formed due to the accumulation of schistosome eggs in the portal and mesenteric veins.

According to the World Health Organization (WHO) statistics, schistosomiasis is prevalent in 75 countries and regions worldwide, threatening

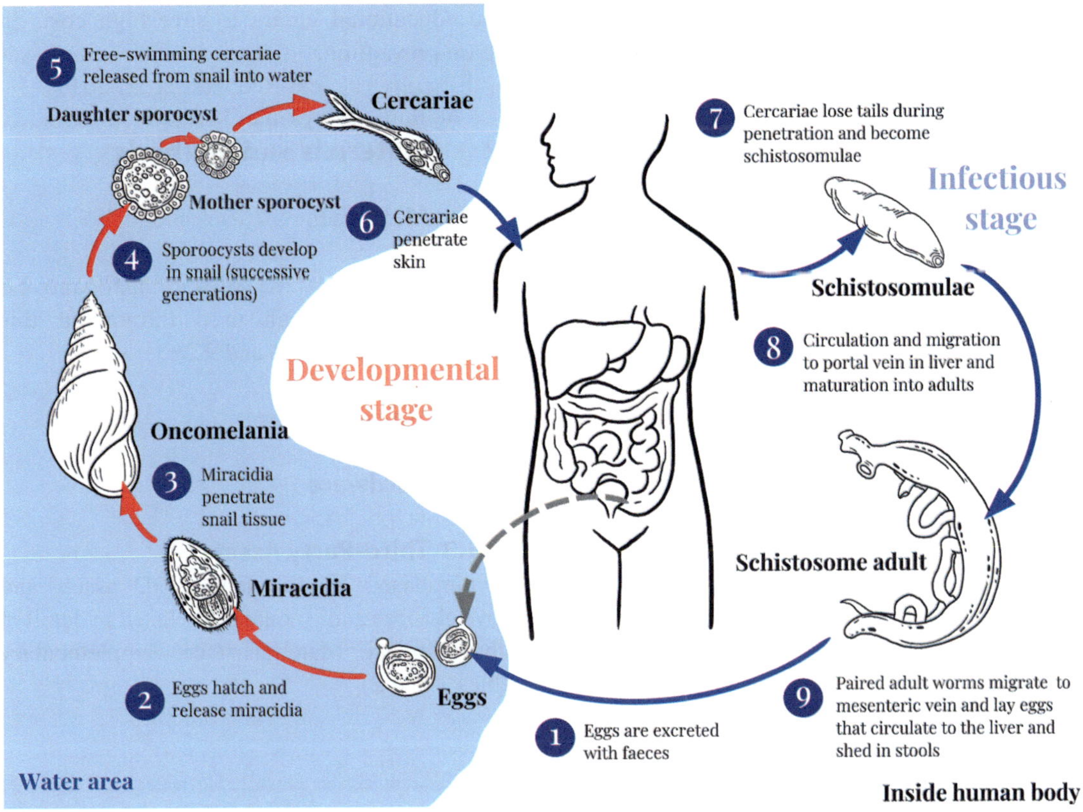

Fig. 9.1 Schistosome life circle

approximately 600 million people (Mcmanus et al. 2018). Two thousand years ago, a body discovered in China found the eggs of schistosomes, which means the history of human battle with this parasite is an ancient one.

The clinical manifestations and severity of the disease vary depending on the type of infection (Gryseels et al. 2006). There may be no obvious clinical symptoms in the early stage of schistosome infection, only some local skin manifestations, such as allergies, rashes and swelling. In the later stage, patients may experience hepatosplenomegaly, bloody diarrhoea, digestive tract obstruction and bleeding caused by portal hypertension. Liver failure, hypoalbuminemia and massive ascites lead to a typical appearance of an enlarged abdomen and skinny skeletal limbs in its terminal stage. It is one of the most dangerous infectious diseases in the world and should be of great concern. It is currently the target of vast educational programmes, especially for residents in endemic areas (Hu et al. 2005).

Scientists have researched schistosomes profoundly (Costain et al. 2018). Some good news is that the principles for primary prevention are not hard to follow. So-called primary prevention is defined as intervening before health effects occur, which is believed to be the most effective and economical way to prevent any disease. Having a better understanding of the immune knowledge of schistosomes could make it easier to know why we should take measures to increase compliance. In addition, it could help people to establish the confidence to confront the parasitic disease.

Therefore, as proposed in this study, the schistosome would make an appropriate case study for exploring the effectiveness of a game-based approach to medical approach.

9.1.3 Groups of Interest

This study may be of interest to several groups. This game has a unique advantage in popularising knowledge. The first intended audience is medical educators. Educational games have been shown to possess specific learning advantages. New generations of medical teachers and students are more likely to accept this new learning modality as they have strong skills in using multimedia platforms and know how to make good use of these e-tools. Furthermore, the positive effect of game-based learning on students' motivation has been well documented throughout serious game literature.

Another group that may be interested in this study is public health organisations or governmental disease control departments. The officials could use this research to raise public awareness and as an exemplar case to develop more educational games to save high costs in disease prevention.

9.2 Materials and Methods

9.2.1 Materials

This section presents the software, hardware and assets that have been used throughout this research (see Tables 9.1 and 9.2).

9.2.1.1 Software

9.2.1.2 Hardware

9.2.1.3 Third-Party Assets

All purchased or downloaded 3D assets and copyright-free audio sources are listed in detail in Supplementary Materials (see Supplementary Tables 1 and 2).

Table 9.1 Software used for development and testing

Logo	Software	Description	Use
Ps	Adobe Premiere Pro CC (2022)	Image-editing software	Edit flat images required in the game development process; modify/create some UI elements
Pr	Adobe Photoshop CC (2021)	Video-editing software	Create a promotional video
Unity	Unity (version 2022.3.0f1)	3D game development engine	Design game levels
Office W X P	Microsoft Office (Word, PowerPoint, Excel)	Daily office software	Dissertation and other paper material writing; data recording
	Microsoft Visual Studio (2022)	Integrated development environment (IDE)	C# scripting

Table 9.1 (continued)

Logo	Software	Description	Use
	Procreate (version 5.3.5) (2023)	Drawing application software	Design relevant art materials
	Statistical Package for the Social Sciences, SPSS (2019)	Mathematical processing software	Statistically analysis
	GraphPad Prism 9	Data visualisation software	Generate statistical tables and images
	Xmind	Mind mapping software	Storyboard drawing
	EndNote 21	Literature management application	Reference management
	Blender	3D model building software	Purchased 3D model modification

Table 9.2 Hardware used for development and testing

Logo	Hardware	Description	Use
	Apple MacBook Pro (13 inch, 2019)	Laptop	Dissertation writing, art designing
	Apple iPad Pro (12.9 inch. 2021)	Tablet computer	Art designing
	HUAWEI MateBook D 15 (15.6 inch, 2023)	Laptop	Game development and testing

9.2.2 Game Development

The design and development approach for this research was established through discussions with game professionals (see Fig. 9.2). The theme and genre were determined to be an atypical escaping game by referring to relevant literature and cases.

In the game, the player will play a kind of parasite. Choosing the immune cells as the protagonist was abandoned at the design stage. Firstly, many different types of immune cells were involved in this game, which means frequent role-switching could lead to a confusing game logic; secondly, the parasite should overcome given obstacles to show the integral infection procedures accompanying the failure of the immune system. So it would be difficult to provide players who control the immune cells with enough sense of achievement within the game.

Based on the considerations above, the guiding concept, Dark Play theory (Buijs-Spanjers et al. 2019), was followed. Dark play refers to games where players are allowed to make unacceptable choices or engage in morally ambiguous behaviours. Dark Play effectively enables players to understand parasites' immune evasion strategies. Such a new gameplay perspective would foster players' sustained enthusiasm for continuous exploration within the game, and as the game's goals align with the parasite's goals, these procedures become memorable to players.

The game's goals are surviving (as a parasite) in the human body, avoiding being detected or harmed by the immune system, finding another gender (female) schistosome in the liver to produce offspring, laying eggs and collecting enough antigens to ensure long-term existence. All the game goals reflect the schistosome's real parasitic behaviours and the course of the disease.

9.2.2.1 Development Tool

Procreate was used to create original 2D materials. For gameplay a personal computer (PC) is preferred; however, considering wider use, the compatibility for a mobile app will remain.

The game engine used for developing this game was Unity, so the programming language foundation is C#. Game programming is the core part of game development, as it transforms the game's design ideas and concepts into an actual playable game (see Fig. 9.3).

This figure listed all involved scripts and arranged its location by function and running goals. For better information, it was further categorized using colours by functional groups. The two most important scripts are *GameManager*, which controls overall game events, and *MoveLogic*, which controls schistosomiasis actions and environmental interactions. The other scripts ultimately control the game operation by changing the specific parameters in the above two scripts. The logical sequence is the direction of the arrow, and new values are generally assigned in the frame update and physics update. Some of these parameters are also passed

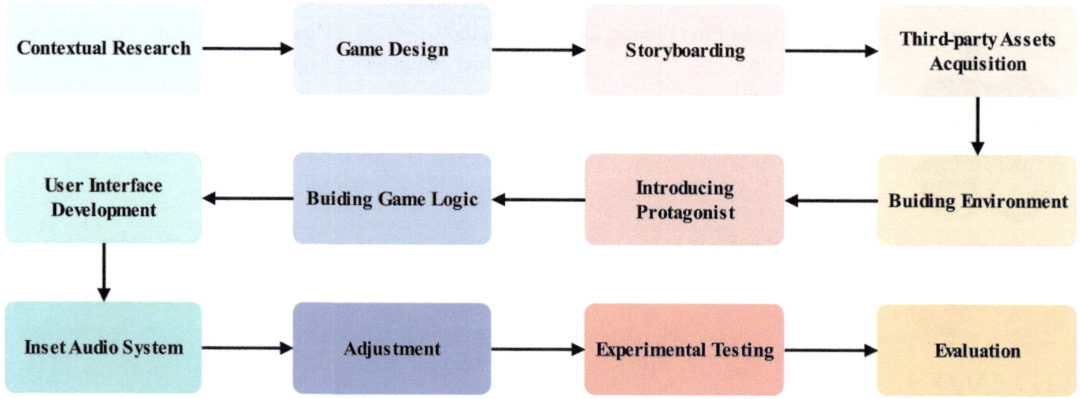

Fig. 9.2 Diagram depicting the design and development method

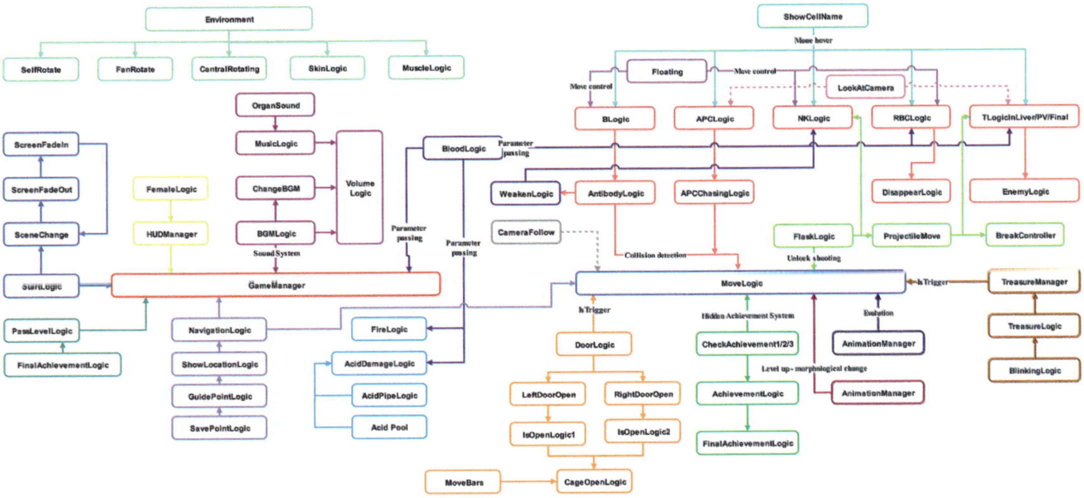

Fig. 9.3 How scripts drive game to run

to the animation state machine to make the role react to environmental events properly.

9.2.2.2 Storyboard

In game development or animation production, a storyboard is a visual tool used to plan and showcase the story plot, scenes and actions. It typically consists of a series of drawings or sketches, aiding creators and teams in visualising the story's progression and the arrangement of scenes. The storyboard for this game was created using Procreate. As designed, it will be a single-player, three-level game (see Fig. 9.4).

9.2.2.3 Scene Creation

The game consists of three levels, simulating the trajectory of schistosomes moving inside the human body. The creation of the environment also revolves mainly around this concept.

The first level simulates the journey of a cercariae as it breaks through the skin, travels through the peripheral circulation to reach the heart and then passes through the lungs (see Fig. 9.5).

The second level simulates the schistosomulum returning to the heart through the lungs and reaching the digestive system via the arteries (see Fig. 9.6). At the far end of the scene, the player needs to pass through an acid pool, which is quite challenging, so a save point is implemented.

The third level has a more intricate map. This level simulates the process of a mature schistosome travelling from the intestines to the liver, finding a mate and then returning to the mesenteric veins to lay eggs and collect human antigens (see Fig. 9.7). A save point is placed in front of the final battlefield to prevent players from becoming fatigued due to repeatedly starting at the same level too many times.

In terms of aesthetic style, the confined and dark realistic internal body scenes, like vessels, are problematic for navigation and may trigger psychological conditions such as claustrophobia for some users. Therefore, the entire scene has been artistically reimagined as futuristic corridors and environments to represent anatomical structures. This symbolism is a mature technique and common in a large number of SGs.

9.2.2.4 Game Protagonist

The players control a tropical parasite called schistosome. Its most notable physical feature is a cephalic sucking disc which was taken into account when searching for a proper 3D model (see Fig. 9.8).

Schistosome undergoes three shape changes inside the human body. So the asset called 'Queen Worm Earthworm Evolution Pack Cute Series' was selected for the protagonist model due to its appropriate look for each stage and the same evo-

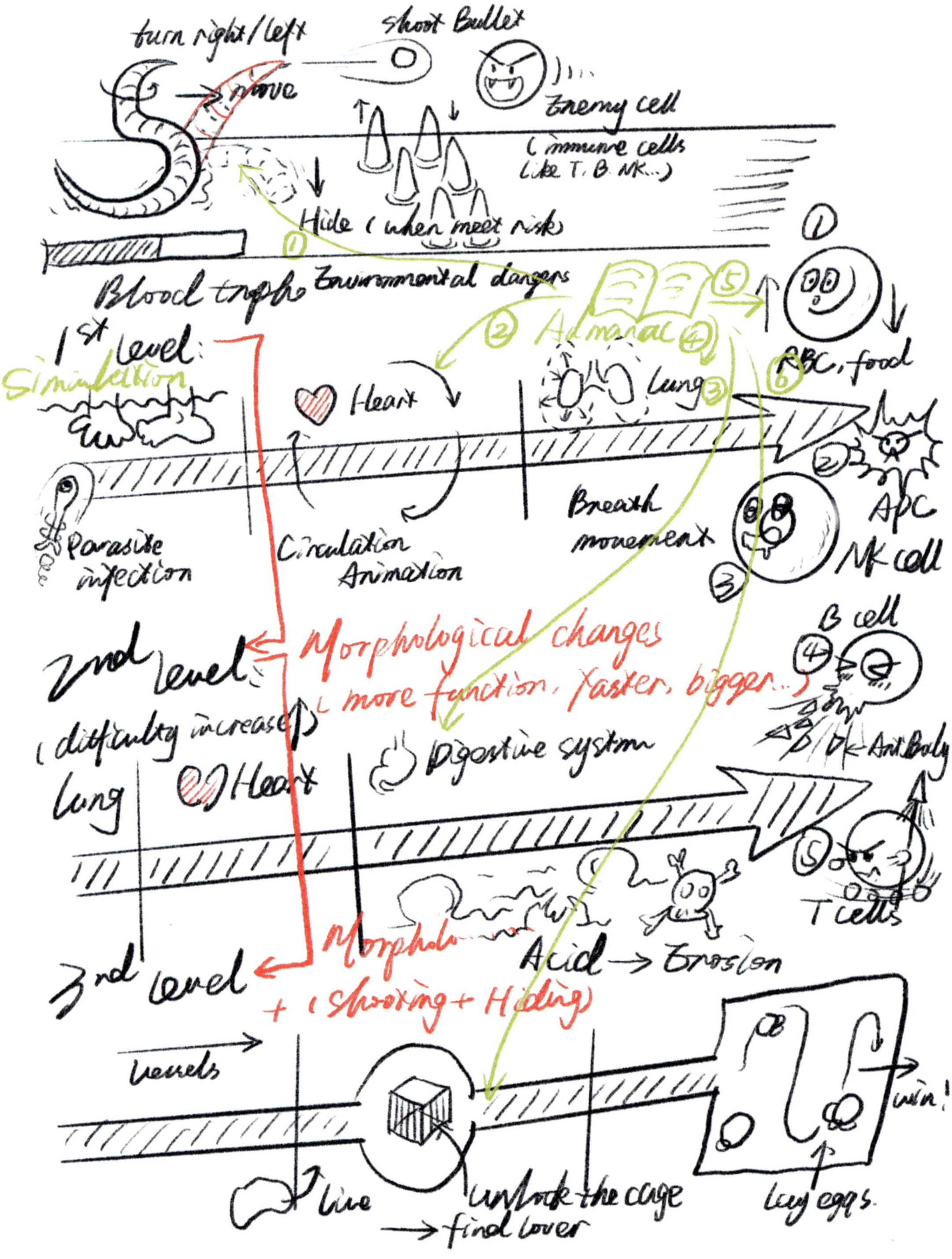

Fig. 9.4 Rough storyboard depicting the whole process of the game

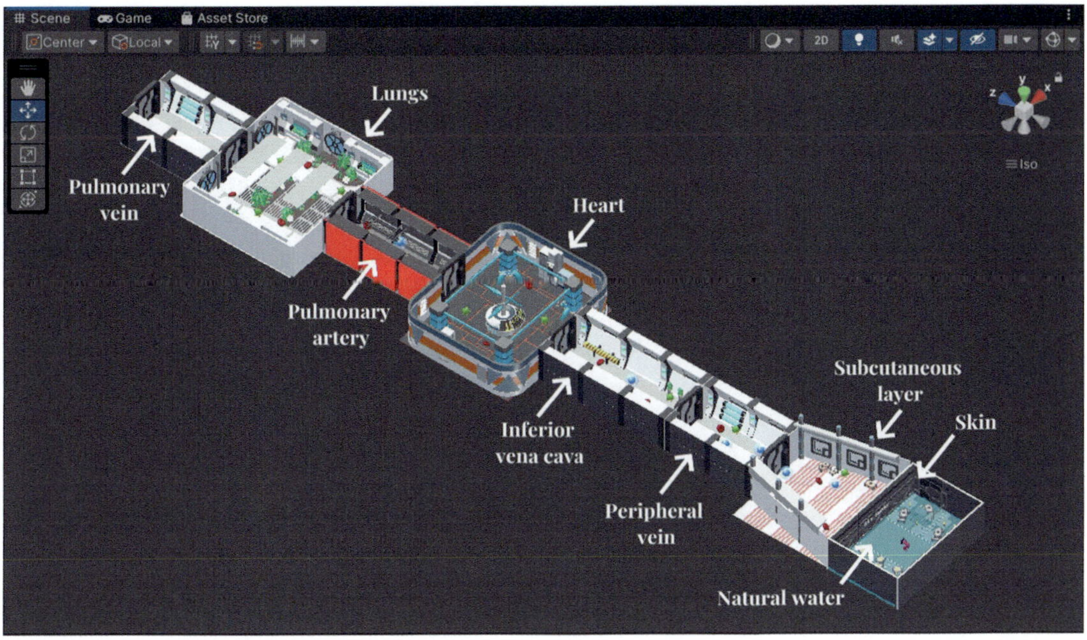

Fig. 9.5 Level 1 panorama

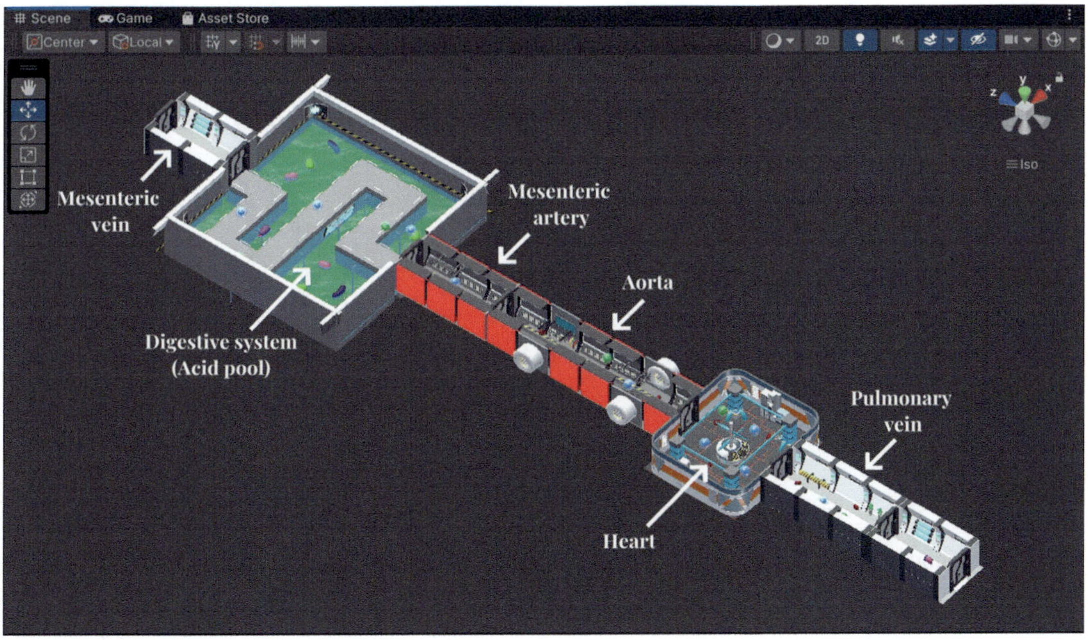

Fig. 9.6 Level 2 panorama

lution times (see Fig. 9.9). A scene was specially designed between levels to show the parasite's evolution. As the parasite grows, not only does its physical size enlarge, but its movement speed also increases.

The keyboard and mouse are essential for controlling the character (see Fig. 9.9). The 'W' key is used to move forward, while the 'A' and 'D' keys are used to turn left and right, respectively. Pressing the 'S' key allows the fluke to burrow

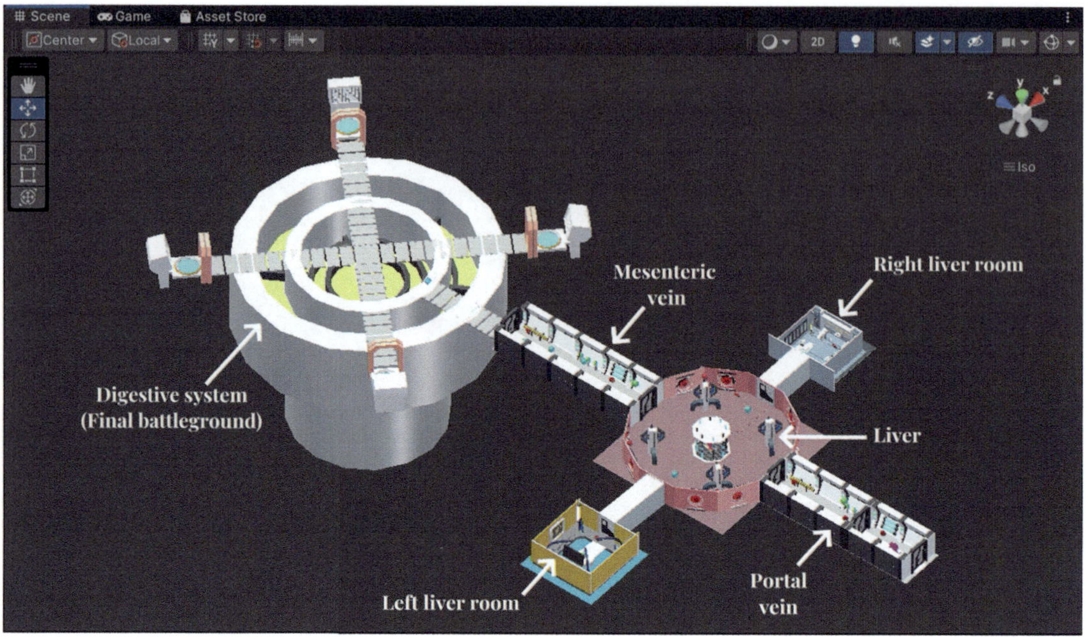

Fig. 9.7 Level 3 panorama

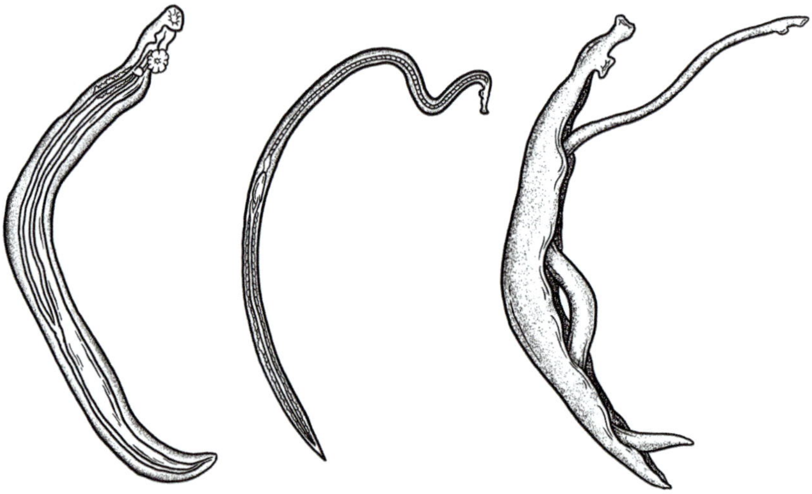

Fig. 9.8 The prototype of schistosome

into the ground (blood vessel wall) and hide. Clicking the left mouse button allows performing interactions with pop-ups.

Two types of bullets are to be unlocked in the second and third stages of the schistosome. There is no fixed conclusion as to how schistosomes engage in immune evasion. The main views include blocking antibody-induced immune reactions, secreting parasite-derived molecules interfering with normal immune cells' function, mimicking human surface antigens to camouflage shunning immune surveillance, etc. All these hypotheses could be found or experienced in game playing, which means the relevant obscure immune knowledge has permeated into the game's basic logic. To be more specific, players could either click on the right or middle mouse button to shoot accordingly. The first type of bullet is the 'Freeze Bullet', which, upon hitting immune cells, freezes them in place for

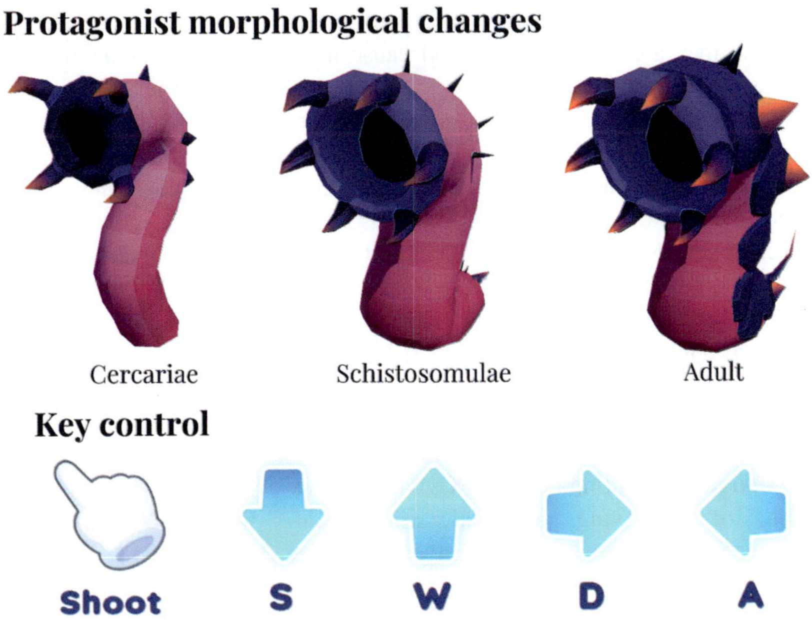

Fig. 9.9 Three stages of schistosome undergoing in the game

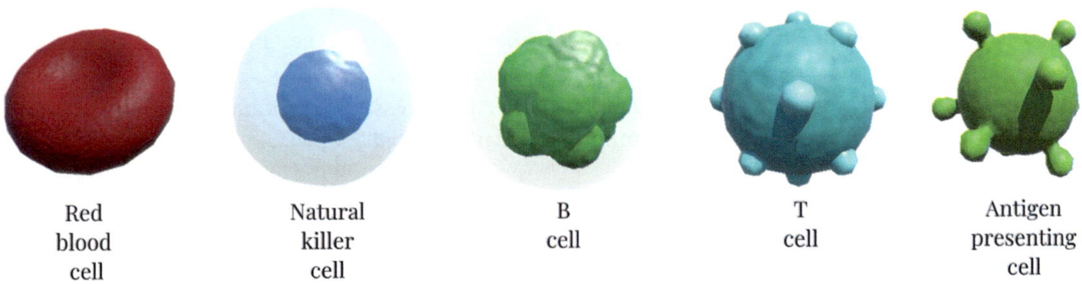

Fig. 9.10 Cells involved in the game

3 seconds simulating secreting interfering signals to make disorder in immune cells. The second type is the 'Flame Bullet', which inflicts damage on immune cells until they are killed simulating the hazardous substances the parasite generated in life activity which would impair the human immune system. The last one is collecting human-derived antigens to cover surface molecular patterns. Immune cells would check the human leukocyte antigen (HLA) to identify whether the cell they check is autologous or allogeneic. The schistosome would intake the fragment of human-owned surface antigen and produce similar ones on their body surface to avoid being marked. The three methods mentioned above are the core mechanism of its immune evasion and are reflected well in the game presentation.

9.2.2.5 Non-playing Characters: 'Enemy' Cells

In the game, five types of cells are represented, four of which are immune system cells (see Fig. 9.10).

Red blood cells (RBC) are used as food for the schistosome; therefore in the game, intaking them increases the player's hit points (HPs).

Natural killer cells (NK) and T cells are two types of cells that directly attack the schistosome, but the value is different. NK cells are an important part of innate immunity, but due to lack of specificity, their damage to schistosomes is very limited. T cells are produced by acquired immunity, so they are more targeted and cause more damage to players in the game.

On the other hand, B cells secrete antibodies to enhance the damage dealt by other cells; this phenomenon is called antibody-dependent cell-mediated cytotoxicity (ADCC). ADCC is a core mechanism of the human immune system for schistosome infection. Antibodies produced by B cells do not have a protective effect on the first-infected adult worms, but they are lethal to the re-infected worms, which is why the antibodies do not cause direct damage to the player in the game because it was the first-time infection.

Antigen-presenting cells (APCs) are responsible for identifying pathogenic microorganisms. Since APCs largely only recognise schistosomiasis infections, they are also not given the ability to harm players in the game. However, when touched by APCs, the player will be prompted, and the number of times the touch is recorded and presented. Being marked by APCs activates the host's acquired immunity; therefore, players who avoid being marked by APCs face fewer enemy-acquired immune cells in later levels.

As for their behaviours, APCs and T cells actively pursue the enemy (the player) when they detect the enemy invading their domain, while the rest of the cells either remain stationary or move along predefined paths. This is true for these cells' habits physiologically.

Therefore, it can be seen that all game behaviours and mechanics either overtly or more subtly inform the player about accurate real-life behaviours of this parasite and our immune system response.

9.3 Results

9.3.1 Menu Scene

The menu scene is in accordance with the game's poster (see Fig. 9.11). Three different stages of schistosome involved in the game take the visual centre of the menu scene. The title is a little lower than the schistosome. Players press the round button to start the game.

After pressing, the main elements disappear, but the global map background remains. Three stains would mark the three locations in the world

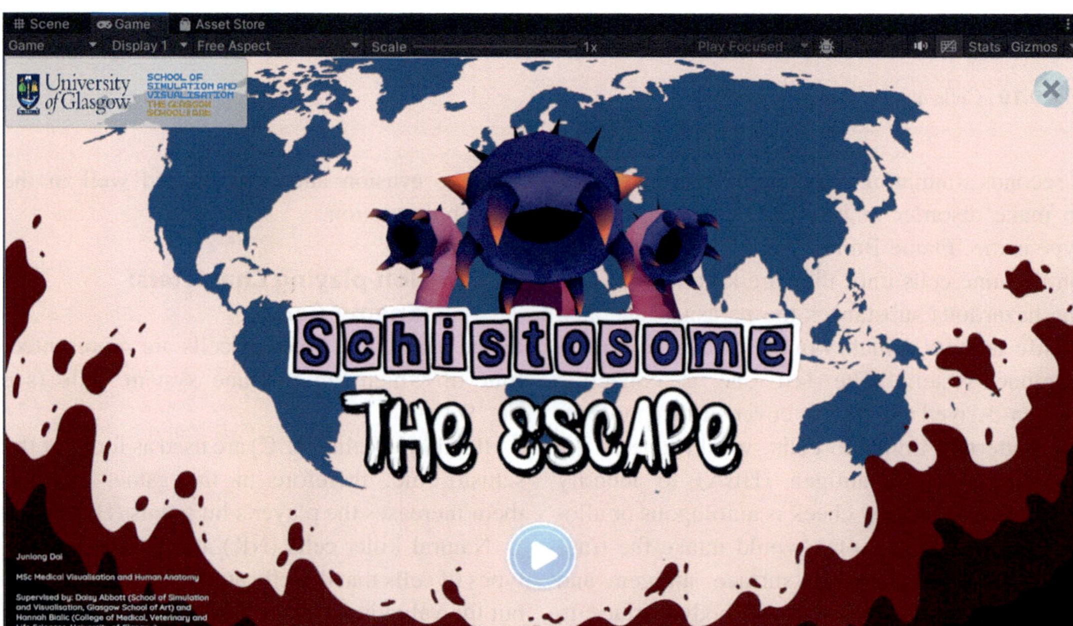

Fig. 9.11 Menu scene

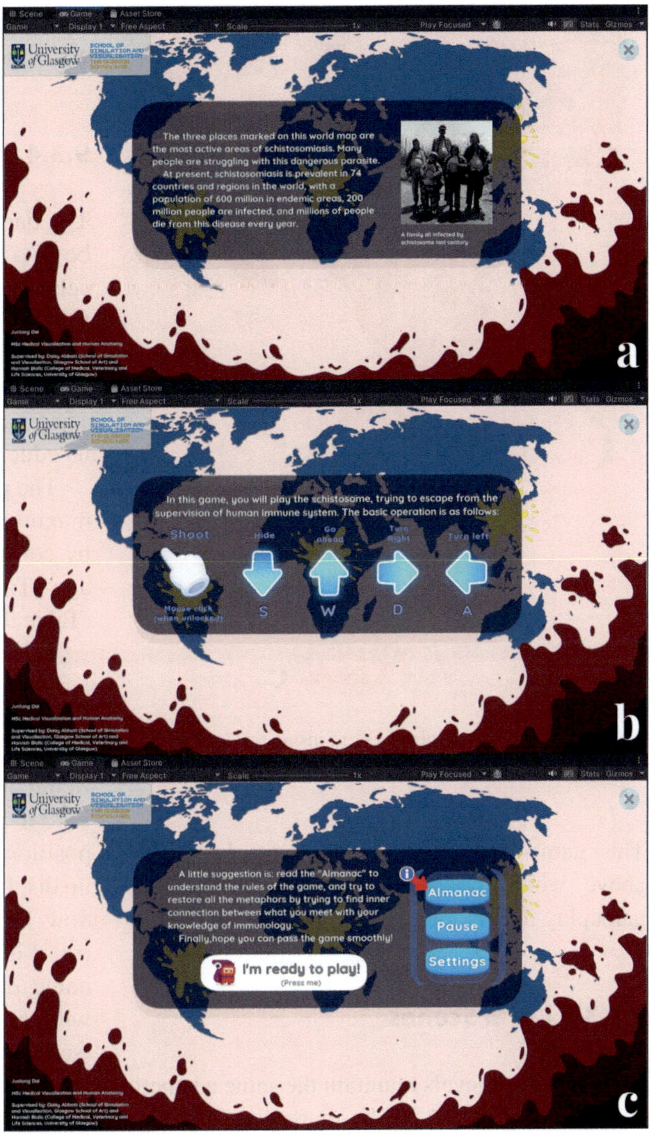

Fig. 9.12 Instructions following menu scene. (**a**) Epidemiology; (**b**) manipulation; c almanack system

which have the highest schistosomiasis morbidity. Then, three pop-up instructions introduce schistosomiasis epidemiology, teach players how to manipulate and highlight the importance of using the almanack system (see Fig. 9.12).

9.3.2 Head-Up Display System

This is a first-person game, so the head-up display (HUD) system was designed to show essential information. When the players get hurt, the specific value number appears over the schistosome (see Fig. 9.13a). When players come in contact with antibodies and are in ADCC status, a label appears reminding players that they should be careful at the middle bottom of the screen (see Fig. 9.13b). Another example is that a label appears to show that their game progress has been saved automatically after passing the save point (see Fig. 9.13c).

The HUD system is a potent tool for information supplements. It requires guide accuracy and a well-planned area to avoid any overlapping.

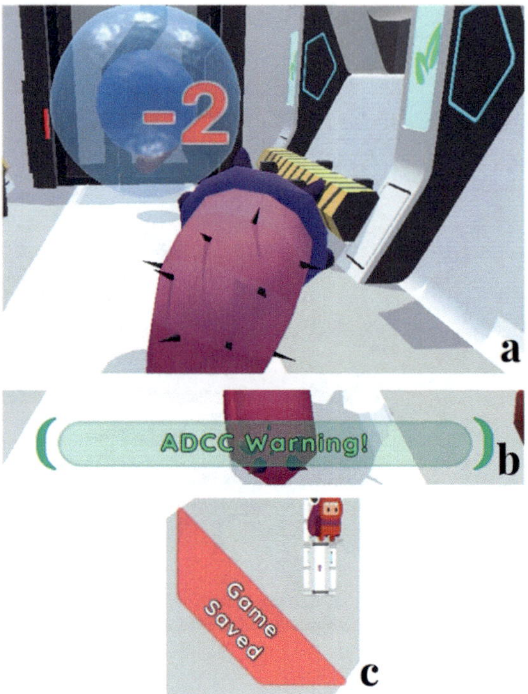

Fig. 9.13 Head-up display system instances. (**a**) Damage value; (**b**) ADCC status label; (**c**) game saved label

This game has many similar examples to the above which present important learning and gameplay information.

9.3.3 Level Scenes

All three game levels maintain the same aesthetic style (see Fig. 9.14). To be more detailed, Sect. 2.2.3 provides a more specific depiction of environment building.

At the beginning of each level, quotes about learning from some famous persons are added to the transitional scenes (see Fig. 9.15). The purpose of designing these transitional scenes is not only to relieve the players' stress but also to exert subtle influences to reinvigorate their study attitude.

In practical terms, these scenes' details were adjusted during the testing period according to comments from players. But the changes were minor; these adjustments aimed at solving game running problems and fixing bugs to ensure players' satisfactory whole game experience.

9.3.4 Damage Detection System

The damage which leads to HP reduction could be divided into two sorts. One is the immune cells factor, and the other is the environmental factor. When setting the damage values and mechanisms, we took great inspiration from actual immune response principles while considering gameplay elements and striving to achieve its educational purpose.

The player starts with five HPs and can have a maximum of 10 HPs, which can be replenished by consuming red blood cells after taking damage. The specific damage logic is as follows (Table 9.3).

9.3.5 Navigation System

In the original game version, three methods were used to ensure players clearly knew their current position and next steps. The first method is a pop-up display: when players enter a new zone, a window will appear to provide hints or information (see Fig. 9.16a). The second method is location name display: when each door opens, players will trigger the appearance of the location name (see Fig. 9.16b). The third method involves environmental cues like electric wires and railings, which are non-verbal (see Fig. 9.16c, d). This method is set to mitigate the text-reading burden of the game.

But through preliminary testing, the feedback pointed out that these methods could not make a precise and efficient guide for players. Especially for level 3, most players were confused about where to go for the next game step. Considering their suggestions, a real-time navigation system was added to the game's final version (see Fig. 9.17 arrow a). Players can use a toggle to show or hide the map when playing (see Fig. 9.17 arrow b). In follow-up testing, participants highly commended this navigation system.

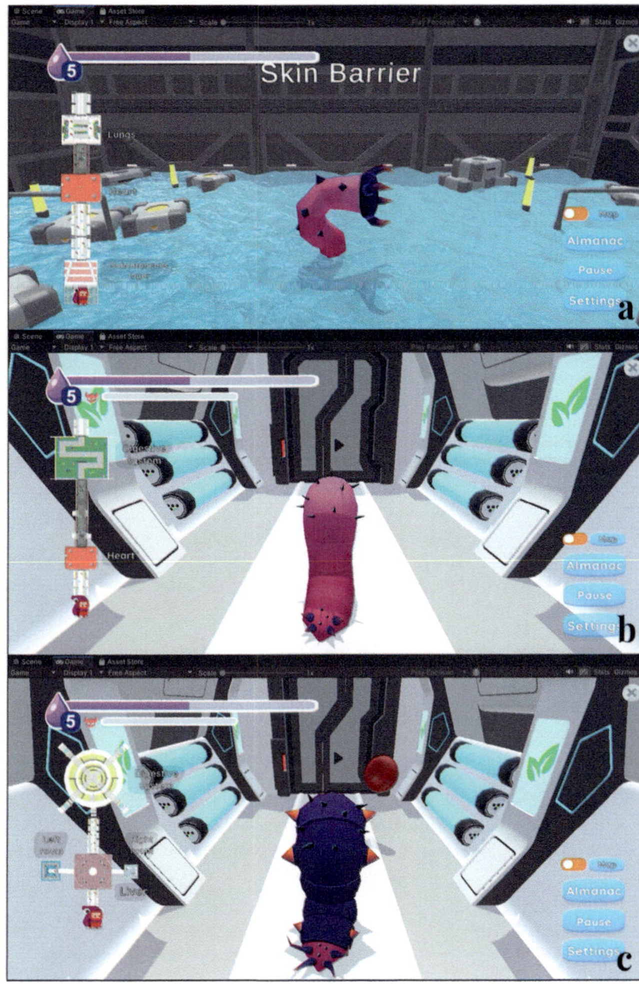

Fig. 9.14 Game scene screenshots. (**a**) Level 1 screenshot; (**b**) level 2 screenshot; (**c**) level 3 screenshot

9.3.6 User Interface System

9.3.6.1 Basic UI

First, players are informed of their HP by viewing their health bars in the top left-hand corner (see Fig. 9.18 arrow a). The specific number is shown there as well (see arrow b). When the protagonist is in ADCC status, the countdown bar is activated to inform players how long it will take to recover (see arrow c).

In the bottom left-hand corner, the real-time navigation system and game-saving label play a game-process driving role (see arrow d). And the navigation system can be hidden by a map toggle on the other side for a better game visual field (see arrow e).

A quit button is in the top right-hand corner (see arrow f). When players want to read the almanack, pause the game, or adjust sound settings, they can press buttons in the bottom right-hand corner (see arrows g, h, i).

Last, when entering the final battleground, a small starboard which has four slots appears under the ADCC countdown bar (see arrow j).

9.3.6.2 Outcome UI

A special UI appears as a guide when players trigger different game outcomes. After the unsuccessful completion of the game objectives, the Death UI stresses the importance of the almanack system, suggesting players read it to find game tricks (see Fig. 9.19). After passing one level or

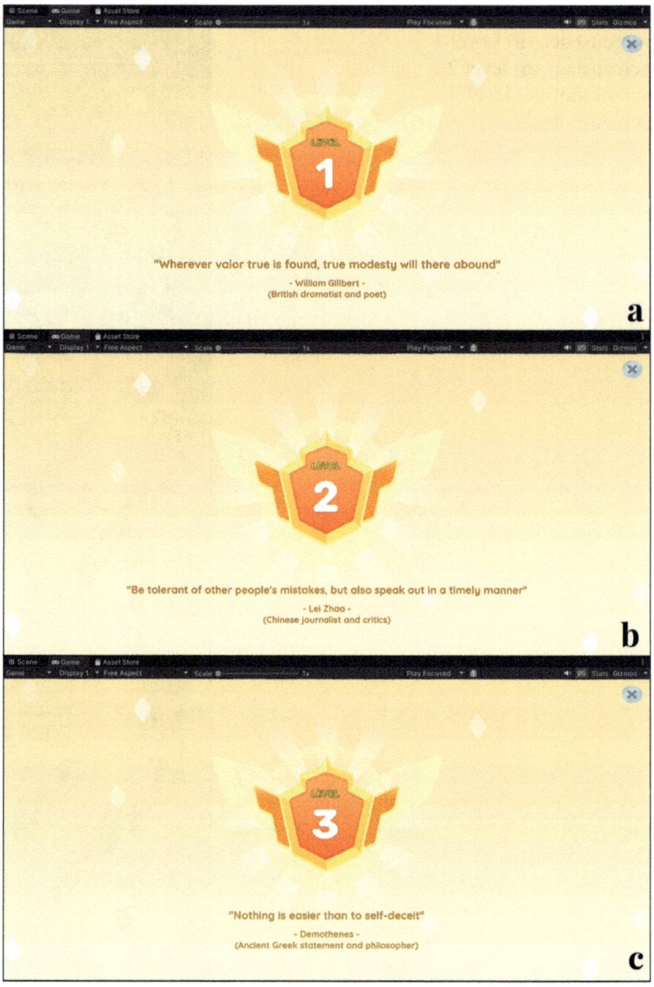

Fig. 9.15 Transitional scenes

winning the game, celebrating UIs send congratulatory messages to the player (see Figs. 9.20 and 9.21). When pausing the game, the timescale is frozen, and the pause UI does not disappear until players press the pause button again (see Fig. 9.22).

9.3.7 Almanack System

The almanack system is the key for players to find the relationship between their game experience and scientific knowledge. In fact, players can better understand the game rules and strategies by reading the almanack system (see Fig. 9.23), namely, the inner logic of the game is the parasite knowledge itself. On the one hand, by playing such a kind of game, players could develop a strong interest in exploring the almanack system. On the other hand, by reading the almanack system, players could transform their text memory into graphic memory. This transformation could mitigate the learning burden of students and establish a stronger long-term learning effect.

Table 9.3 Damage detection system

Picture	Name	HP change	Special effect
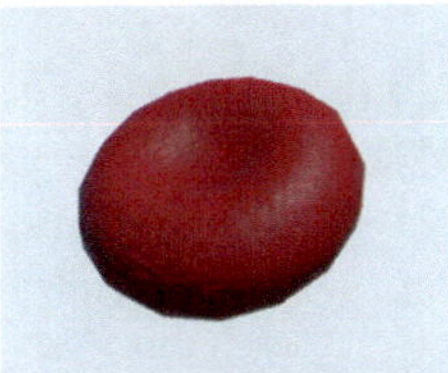	Red blood cells	+1	
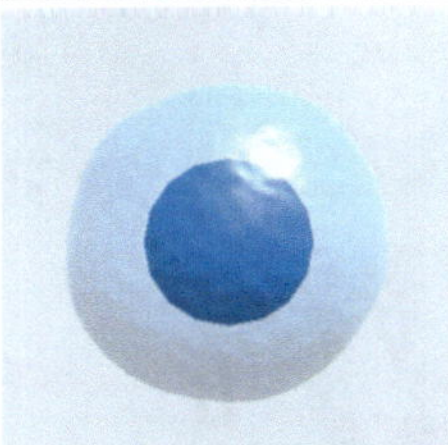	Natural killer cells	−1/−2	When the schistosome is tagged by antibodies launched by B cells, the damage caused by NK cells is doubled.
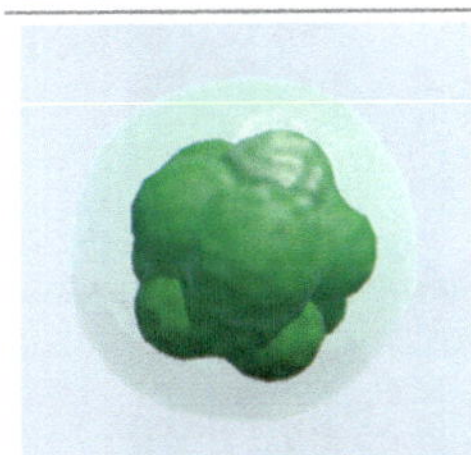	B cells	0	
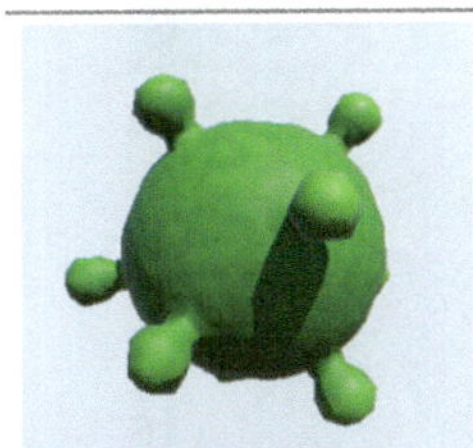	Antigen-presenting cells	0	
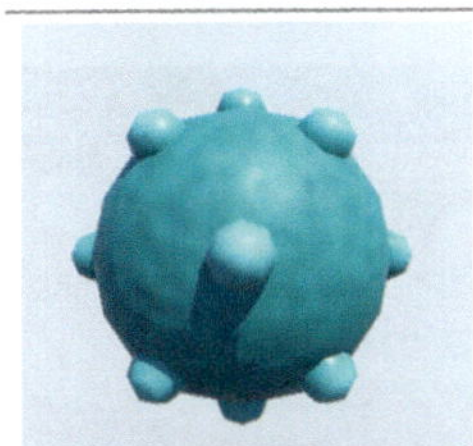	T cells	−2/−3	In the final battleground, the T cells generated there would cause more damage to the player than the liver.
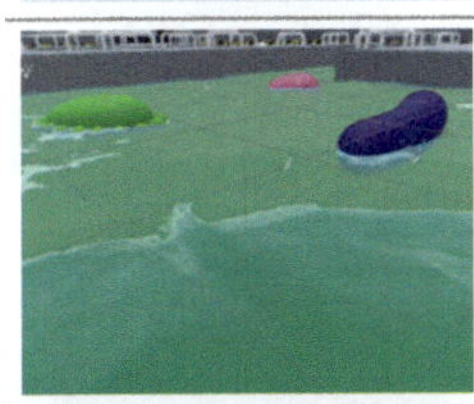	Acid pool	Death	Falling into the acid pool or getting hit by acid splashes instantly clears the HP.
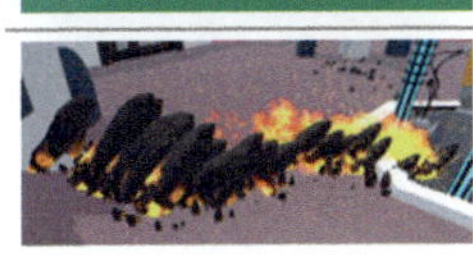	Fire	−1	

Fig. 9.16 Game navigation guide

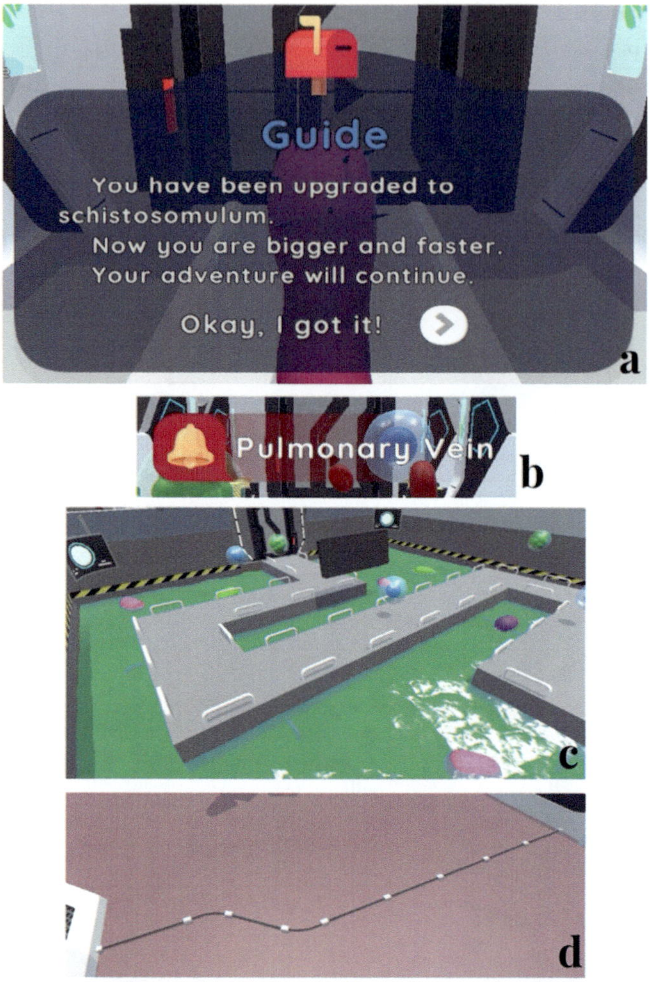

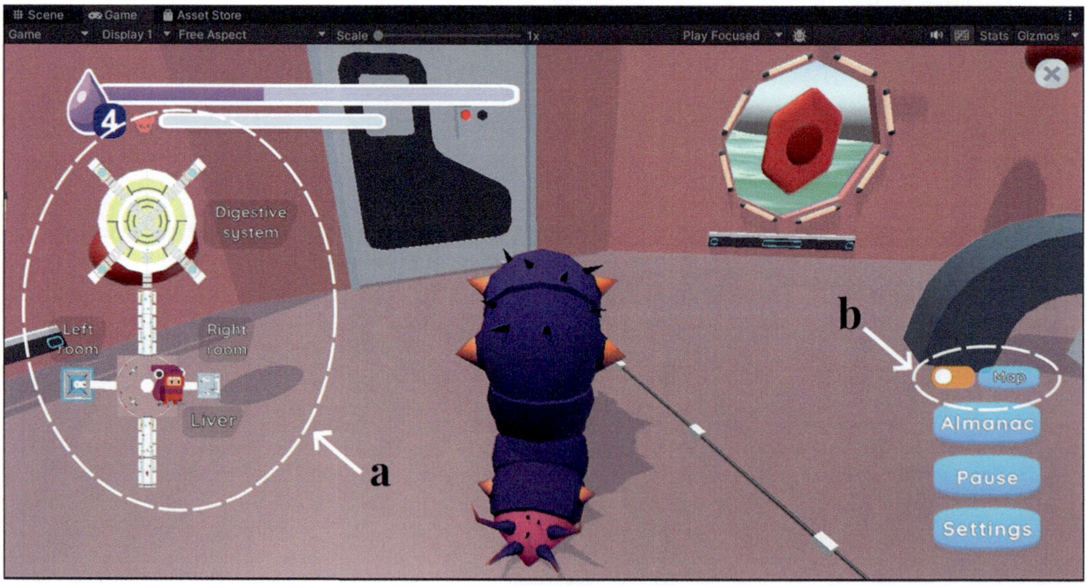

Fig. 9.17 Game real-time navigation system

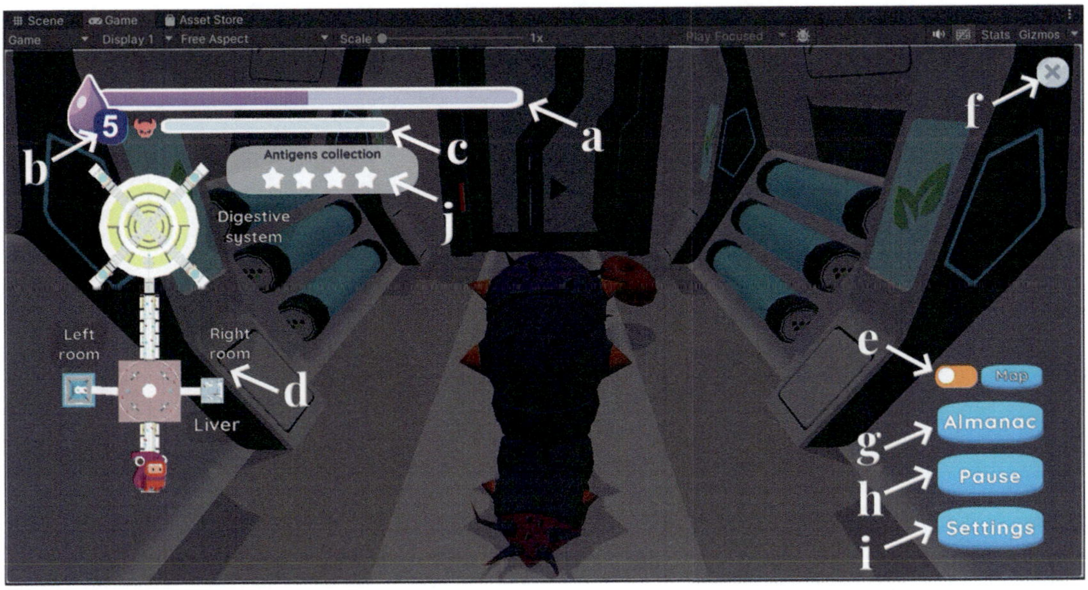

Fig. 9.18 Basic UI system

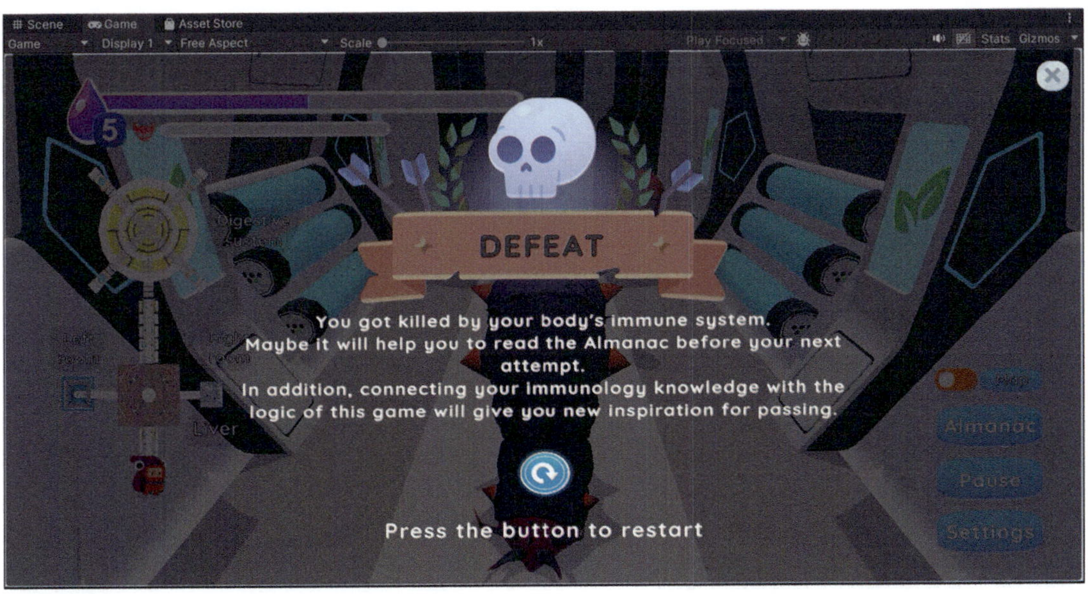

Fig. 9.19 Death UI

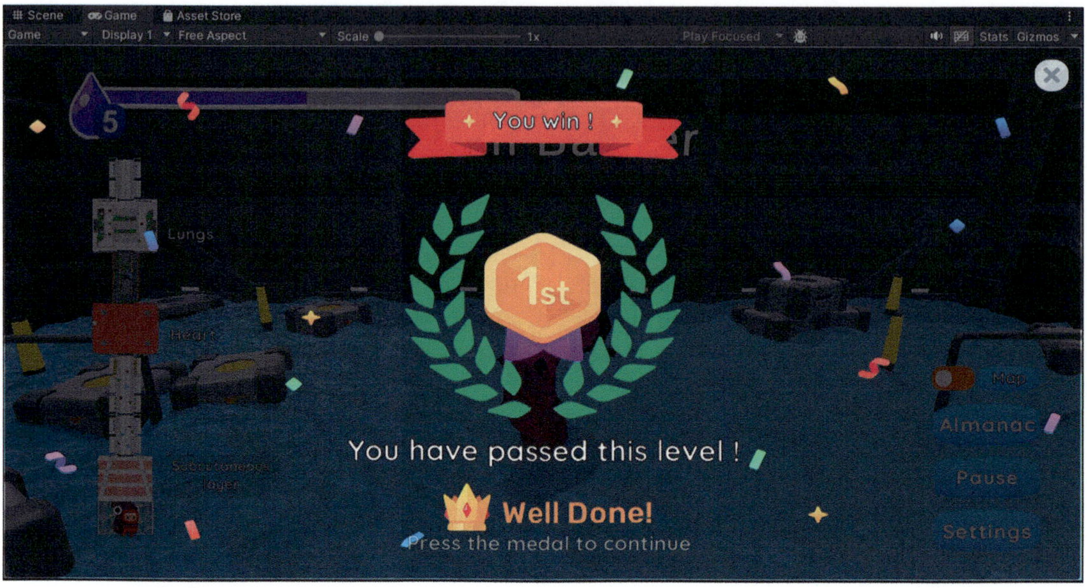

Fig. 9.20 Level pass UI

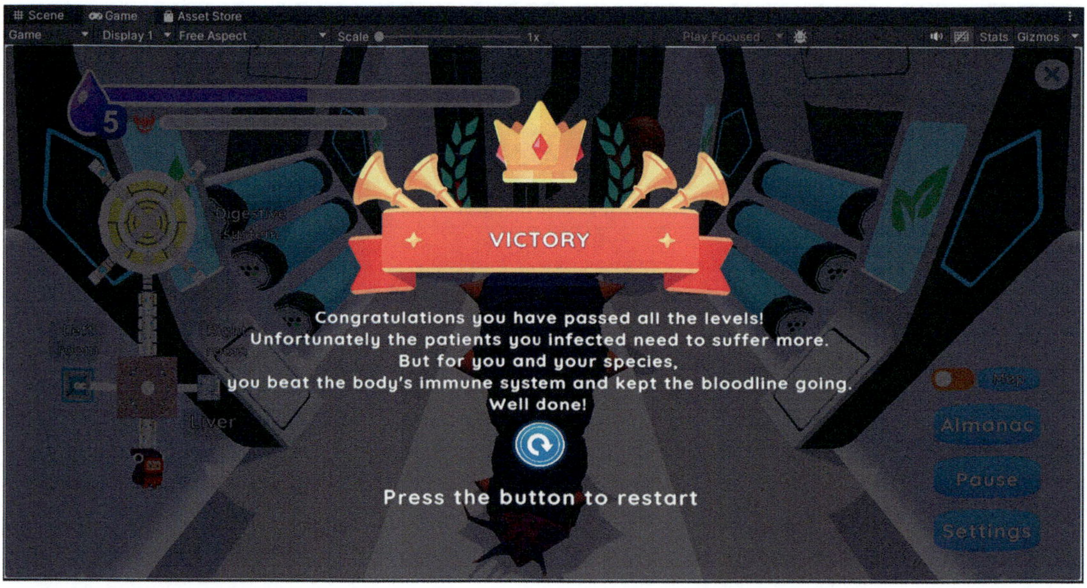

Fig. 9.21 Game win UI

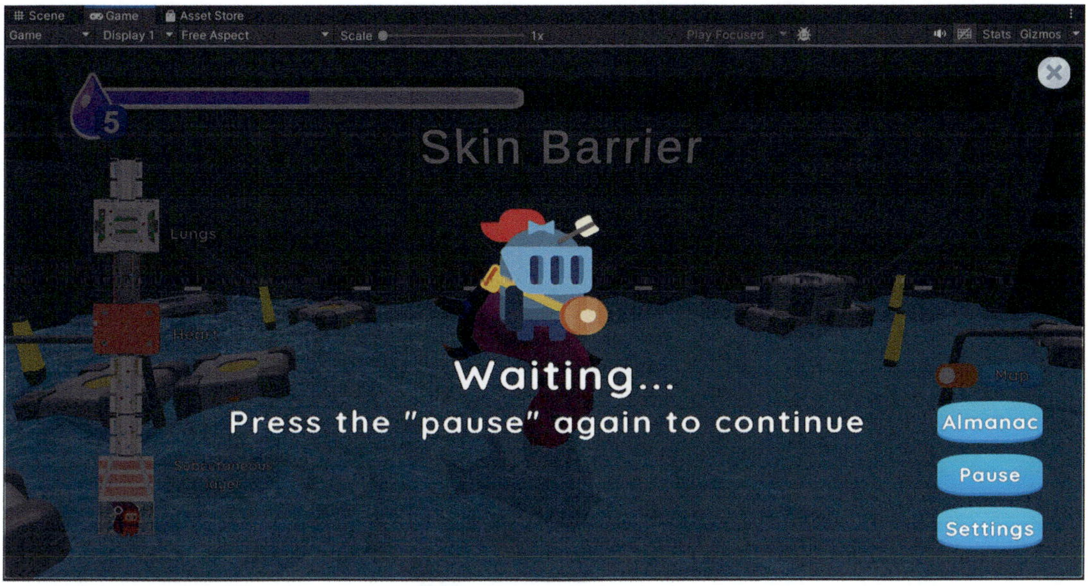

Fig. 9.22 Game pause UI

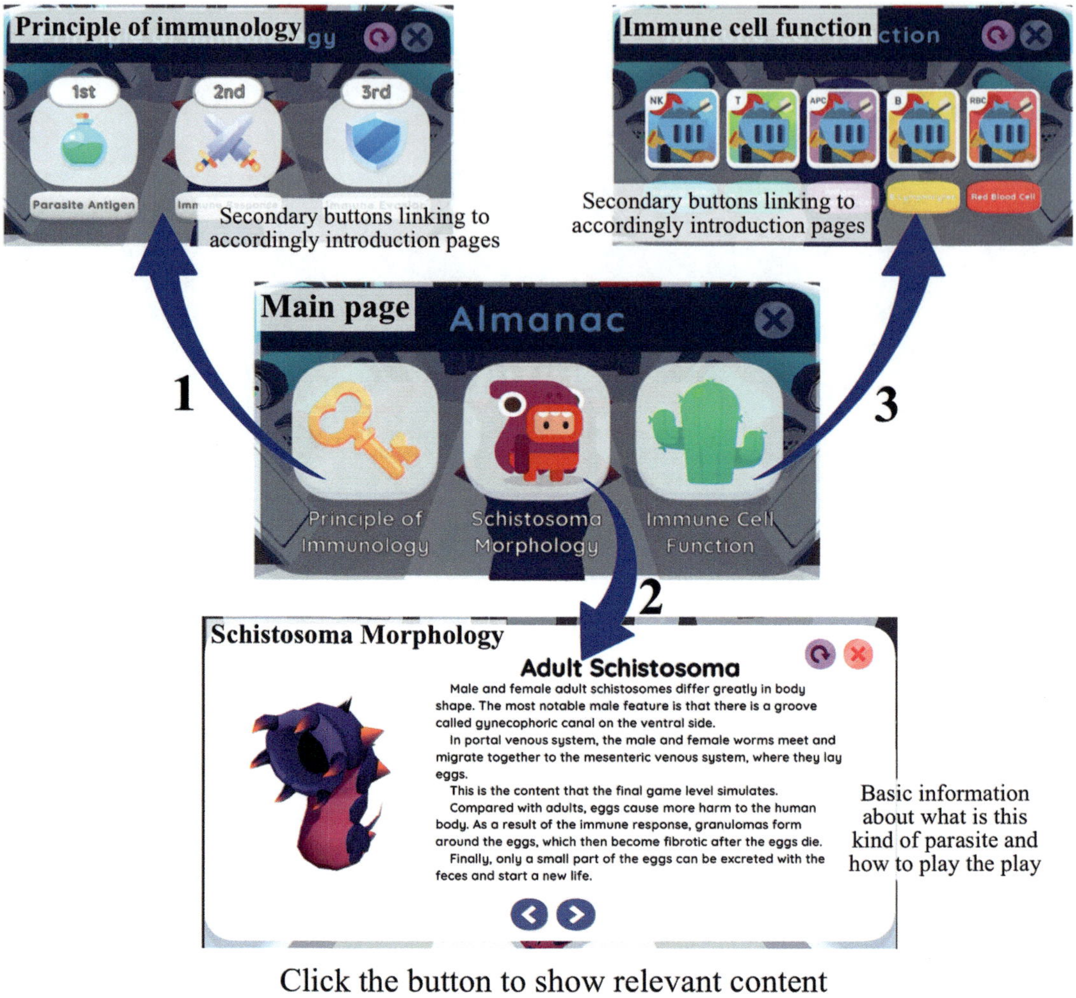

Fig. 9.23 Almanack system frame

9.3.8 Hidden Achievement System

Long-term memory is the result of repetitions (Plater et al. 2023). So the design of giving players a constant sense of fulfilment is crucial for an educational game. In order to encourage players to replay, a hidden achievement system was developed. This system is shown in settings along with the sound volume control slides (see Fig. 9.24). Players could infer the condition by the achievements' name (see Table 9.4).

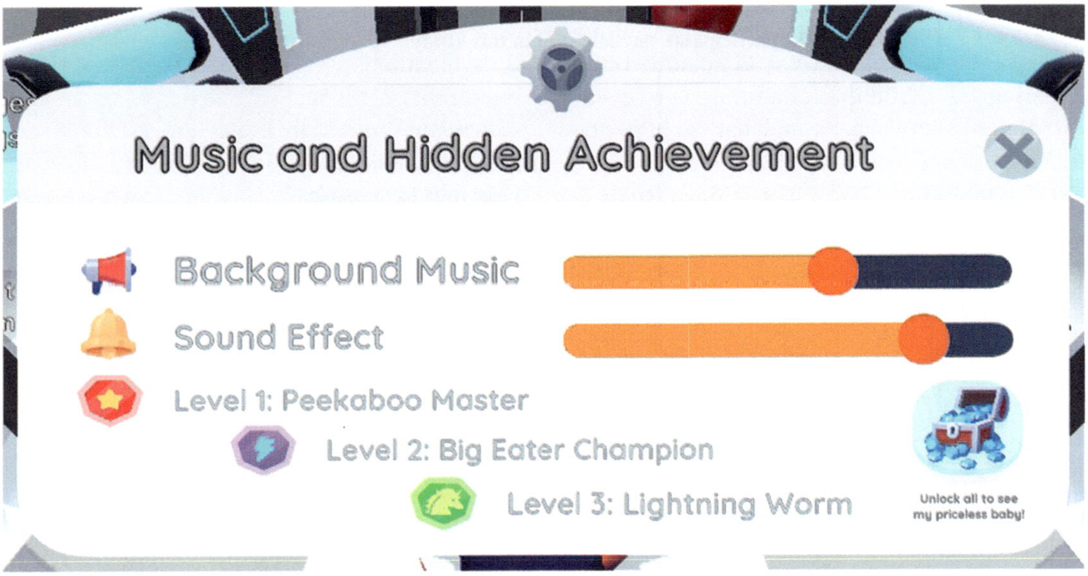

Fig. 9.24 Hidden achievement system

Table 9.4 Hidden achievement names and unlock conditions

Logo	Name	Unlock Condition
	*Peekaboo Master*	Pass the first level without being marked by any APC
	*Big Eater Champion*	Pass the second level with HP of 10/10
	*Lightning Worm*	Finish the final mission (collect antigens) of the third level in a limited time

9.4 Evaluation Design

The game's effectiveness was evaluated by comparison with the cohort study.

9.4.1 Participants

A total of 27 participants were included in this study. The inclusion criteria were as follows: (1) age over 18 years old, (2) the educational level is higher than high school and (3) have enough time and energy to finish the whole process and be willing to be followed up. And the exclusion criteria is found in Fig. 9.25.

Overall, 12 of the 27 people were assigned to the game-based group. There were fewer males in the game-based group (66.7% vs. 73.3%), and the average age of participants in the game-based group was higher ($M = 25.1 \pm 3.5$ vs. $M = 22.8 \pm 5.3$). However, these differences are

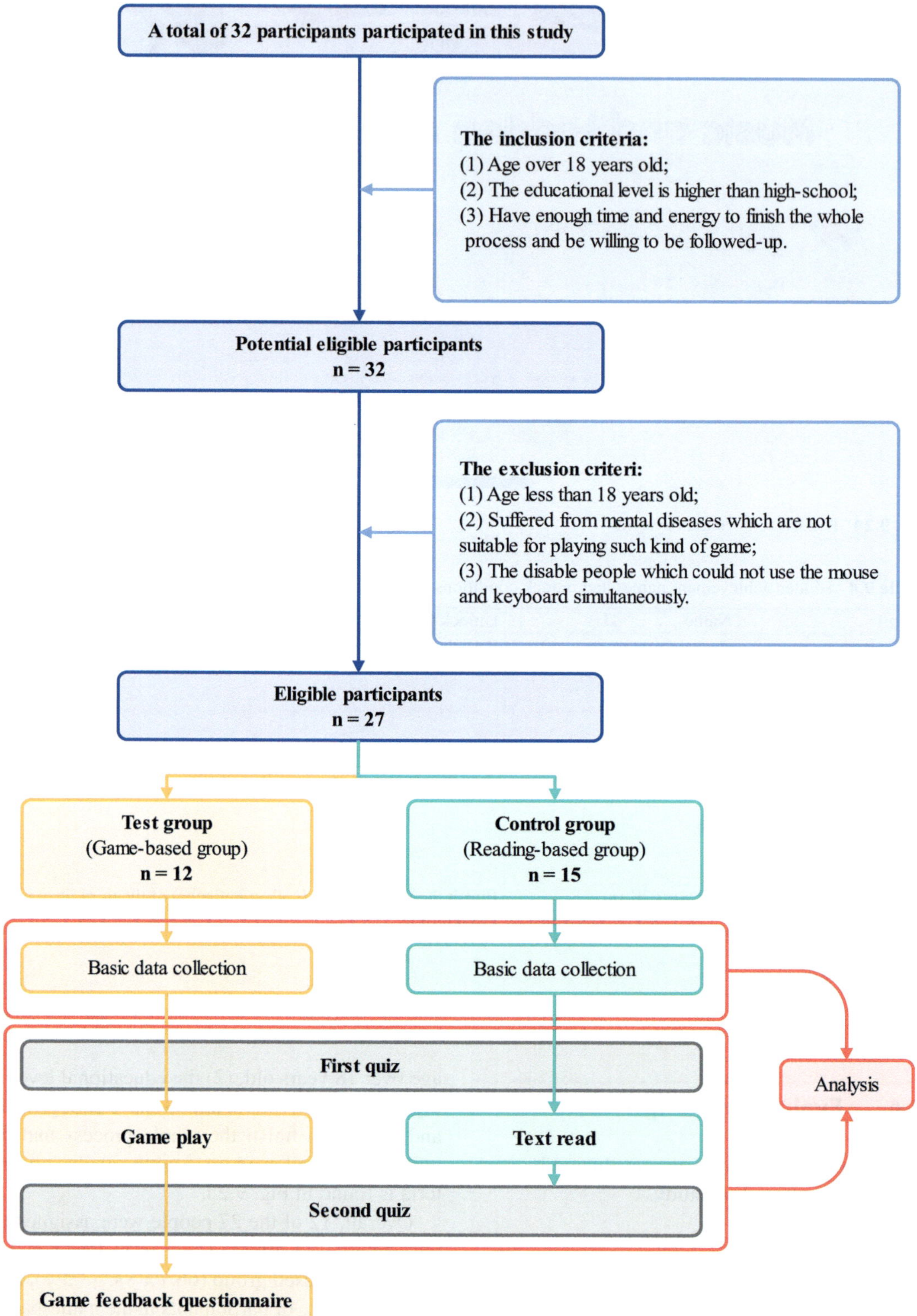

Fig. 9.25 Inclusion and exclusion criteria and research design

Table 9.5 Demographic characteristics

Items		Game-based learning group	Reading-based learning group	p-value
Men		8 (66.7%)	11 (73.3%)	0.706
Age		25.1 ± 3.5	22.8 ± 5.3	0.361
Educational level	High school	1 (8.3%)	3 (20.0%)	0.184
	Undergraduate	8 (66.7%)	4 (26.7%)	
	Postgraduate	2 (16.7%)	7 (46.7%)	
	Doctor	1 (8.3%)	1 (6.7%)	
Student		10 (83.3%)	12 (80%)	0.825
Medical student		2 (16.7%)	4 (26.7%)	0.535
Game habit		10 (83.3%)	8 (53.3%)	0.100
Know SGs before		3 (25.0%)	1 (6.7%)	0.183
Have parasitic basis		7 (58.3%)	8 (53.3%)	0.795

not expected to influence the results. The educational level composition was similar for each group. Student rates among both groups were close as well. Notably, most participants had not heard of SGs in the past (25.0% vs. 6.7%). In addition, a potentially influential factor, the basic knowledge of schistosome before testing, was almost equal (58.3% vs. 53.3%, $p = 0.795$). By and large, the baseline information shows good comparability (see Table 9.5).

9.4.2 Experimental Procedure

After entering the testing period, the participants were assigned to a test group (game-based learning group) and a control group (reading-based learning group) by lottery. Detailed background information was collected. Before reading the learning material or playing the game, participants were asked to complete a small quiz about the parasite to get a baseline of their initial knowledge.

Then, the test group was asked to play the game, while the control group was asked to read a parasite-related article. The intervention lasted up to 15 minutes, stopping prior to that if participants reported that they were finished. The same quiz with no change to the question order was used to test their new understanding of schistosome parasites. A separate questionnaire about their feedback and preferences was attached to the quiz for the gameplay group. The testing process was performed in a quiet, bright and independent space, preventing being bothered by any environmental factors (see Fig. 9.26). When the participants asked to discontinue, or something happened accidentally that may lead to a false result, the testing stopped immediately, and the data was discarded.

By comparing knowledge gained between groups, the effect difference between both experimental conditions could be discerned (see Fig. 9.25).

9.4.3 Data Analysis

First, the Shapiro-Wilk and Anderson-Darling tests were used to check whether the data followed a normal distribution. Continuous variables were presented as the means ± standard deviations ($M \pm SD$). If the variable follows a normal distribution and the sample size is small ($n < 30$), use the t-test; however, if the variable does not, use the Wilcoxon rank-sum test (also known as the Mann-Whitney U). Categorical data were shown as frequencies and were compared using the χ^2 test or Fisher's exact test. All statistical tests were performed using *SPSS* version 27 (International Business Machines Corporation, New York, America). A two-sided p-value < 0.05 was considered statistically significant.

Finally, heuristic feedback was also collected. Playability Heuristic Evaluation for Educational Computer Games (PHEG) has been developed to evaluate educational computer games (Mohamed

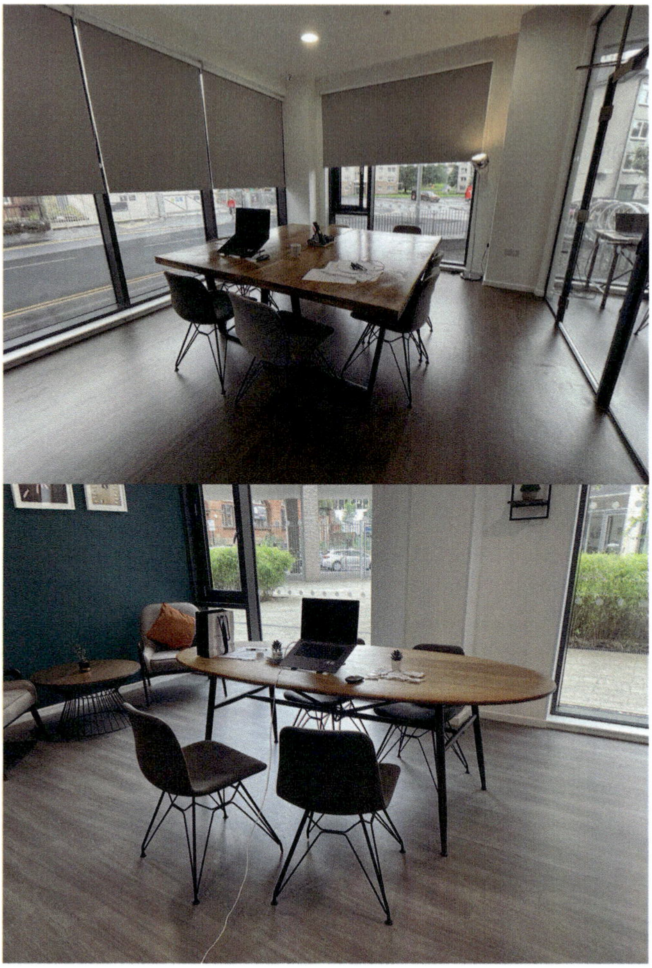

Fig. 9.26 Testing environment

and Jaafar 2013). At first, PHEG was designed as a guideline for educational game development. Later, it was generalised to SG evaluation because of its prominent evaluating function. All participants in the game-based learning group were asked to fill in this questionnaire.

9.4.4 Ethics

This study conformed to the ethical guidelines of the 1975 Declaration of Helsinki, and the ethical approach was approved by the Glasgow School of Art. All the participants were required to sign an informed consent form, and the data collection was undertaken under the supervision of the main researcher.

9.4.5 Experimental Outcomes

9.4.5.1 Learning Mode Comparison

Before the intervention, the knowledge basis of schistosome was similar between the game-based learning group (test group) and reading-based learning group (control group) ($M = 46.7 \pm 3.8$ vs. $M = 58.5 \pm 5.6$). After game playing, the test group made significant progress in knowledge acquisition ($M = 46.7 \pm 3.8$ vs. $M = 72.5 \pm 3.5$), a score increase of 25.8 on average between the pre-test and the post-test. A similar phenomenon could also be observed in the control group ($M = 58.5 \pm 5.6$ vs. $M = 69.3 \pm 4.4$) and the score increase of 10.8. The result illustrates that both methods are effective ways for people to learn parasite knowledge.

There is no statistical difference in results in the second quiz after the intervention ($M = 72.5 \pm 3.5$ vs. $M = 69.3 \pm 4.4$), which shows that playing SGs can achieve the same learning effect as text reading (see Tables 9.6 and 9.7 and Fig. 9.27). Though both groups' score increases are significant, it is notable that the specific increasing score after gameplay shows a much higher average knowledge acquisition than the text-reading group (25.8 vs. 10.8), which reflects a higher efficiency in using the game as a parasite knowledge-imparting medium.

Table 9.6 Specific quiz result

	Correct rate			
	Game-based learning group		Reading-based learning group	
Participant number	First time (%)	Second time (%)	First time (%)	Second time (%)
1	40.0	50.0	40.0	60.0
2	60.0	80.0	40.0	80.0
3	30.0	60.0	40.0	70.0
4	50.0	70.0	30.0	60.0
5	20.0	60.0	30.0	60.0
6	40.0	90.0	30.0	50.0
7	60.0	70.0	20.0	50.0
8	50.0	80.0	10.0	40.0
9	40.0	80.0	40.0	70.0
10	60.0	70.0	40.0	60.0
11	60.0	90.0	40.0	90.0
12	50.0	70.0	90.0	100.0
13	–	–	50.0	80.0
14	–	–	80.0	90.0
15	–	–	70.0	80.0
Average	46.7	72.5	58.5	69.3

9.4.5.2 Heuristic Feedback

Playability Heuristic Evaluation for Educational Computer Games (PHEG) was developed to evaluate educational computer games (Mohamed and Jaafar 2013). At first, PHEG was designed as a guideline for educational game development. Later, it was generalized to SGs evaluation because of its prominent evaluating function. All participants in the game-based learning group were asked to fill in this questionnaire. The result shows that users were generally satisfied with the game. All of them (100.0%) said they would choose SGs as a learning tool in the future and believe that SGs could be constructive for acquiring relevant parasite knowledge. Most (91.7%) would recommend this game to their friends.

The below data shows the player-reported problems from the PHEG questionnaire. Players give a score about problems they met when playing the game according to specific items. The

Table 9.7 Learning mode comparison result

Correct rate	Game-based learning group (%)	Reading-based learning group (%)	*P*-value
First time	46.7	58.5	0.281
Second time	72.5	69.3	0.170
p-value	<0.001	<0.001	——

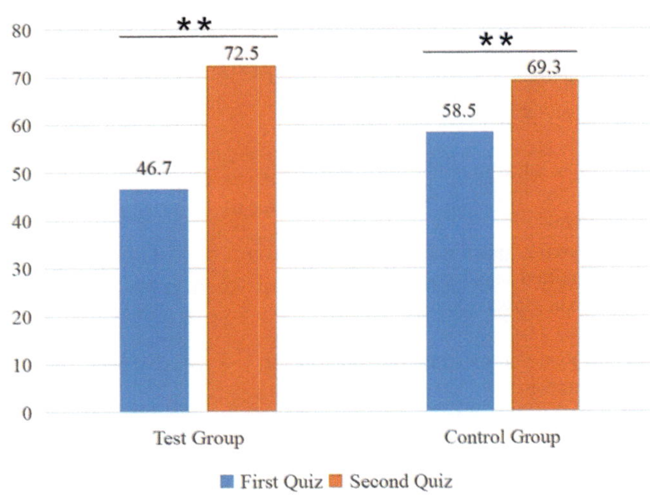

Fig. 9.27 Visual result for comparison result

lower the mark the better. A high mark means the problem is urgent or impairs quality (see Table 9.8). What needs special explanation is that, in the final version, all game problems with higher marks were improved or corrected according to the test result.

9.4.5.2.1 User Interface

Problems were mainly reflected in operational flexibility and learner-level adaptation. Overall, based on user feedback, the UI design was suitable for purpose (Table 9.9).

Table 9.8 Scoring criteria

Level	Descriptive standard
0	A problem that does not necessarily impair the use/no problem
1	An aesthetic problem that does not necessarily require correction/cosmetic problem
2	Low-priority problem/minor problem
3	High-priority problem/major problem
4	Urgent priority problem/usability catastrophe

9.4.5.2.2 Education

Most people recognised the educational features of the game. However, in terms of individual differences and game difficulty settings, some users expressed the need for improvement (Table 9.10).

9.4.5.2.3 Content

The lack of a real-time navigation system affected the user experience, which was made up for in the subsequent development. The content of the game is generally appropriate (Table 9.11).

9.4.5.2.4 Playability

There was a flaw in the visibility of the game's progress. But it was solved by the development of a real-time navigation system. Besides, it is worth noting that some players report they believed they did not perform best at the first game attempt (Table 9.12).

Table 9.9 General percentage of problems for UI

	Total problems/total users				
Heuristic—UI	Level 0 (%)	Level 1 (%)	Level 2 (%)	Level 3 (%)	Level 4 (%)
UI1—Uses aesthetic and minimalist design	11 (91.7)	1 (8.3)	0	0	0
UI2—Maximises consistency and matches standards	10 (83.3)	2 (16.7)	0	0	0
UI3—The uses of space, colour and text are according to the principles of screen design	10 (83.3)	1 (8.3)	1 (8.3)	0	0
UI4—The uses of text, colour and font follow the principles of readability	9 (75.0)	2 (16.7)	1 (8.3)	0	0
UI5—Ensure appropriate use of standard and propriety control	6 (50.0)	6 (50.0)	0	0	0
UI6—The interactivity of the game is suitable for learner level	7 (58.3)	3 (25.0)	2 (16.7)	0	0
UI7—The integration of presentation means is well coordinated	8 (66.6)	4 (33.3)	0	0	0
UI8—Provide specific and self-identified keys for specific tasks (exit, glossary, main, objective)	11 (91.7)	0	1 (8.3)	0	0
UI9—Quality of user interface is acceptable	9 (75.0)	2 (16.7)	0	1 (8.3)	0
UI10—Overall interface of the game is appealing	9 (75.0)	3 (25.0)	0	0	0

Table 9.10 General percentage of problems for education

	Total problems/total users				
Heuristic—ED	Level 0 (%)	Level 1 (%)	Level 2 (%)	Level 3 (%)	Level 4 (%)
ED1—Clear goal and learning objectives	9 (75.0)	3 (25.0)	0	0	0
ED2—The activities are interesting and engaging	9 (75.0)	3 (25.0)	0	0	0
ED3—The design and the contents are reliable and proven	12 (100.0)	0	0	0	0
ED4—Can be used as self-directed learning tools	8 (66.6)	4 (33.3)	0	0	0
ED5—Support for self-learning skills	10 (83.3)	2 (16.7)	0	0	0
ED6—Medium for learning by doing	9 (75.0)	2 (16.7)	1 (8.3)	0	0
ED7—Considers the individual differences	7 (58.3)	4 (33.3)	1 (8.3)	0	0
ED8—Performance should be an outcome-based	10 (83.3)	1 (8.3)	0	1 (8.3)	0
ED9—Offers the ability to select the level of difficulty in games/game difficulty should be progressive	7 (58.3)	3 (25.0)	2 (16.7)	0	0
ED10—Ability to work at their own pace	8 (66.6)	4 (33.3)	0	0	0

Table 9.11 General percentage of problems for content

	Total problems/total users				
Heuristic—CO	Level 0 (%)	Level 1 (%)	Level 2 (%)	Level 3 (%)	Level 4 (%)
CO1—Reliable content with correct flow	12 (100.0)	0	0	0	0
CO2—Clear and understandable structure of contents	10 (83.3)	2 (16.7)	0	0	0
CO3—Navigation of content is easy and accurate	6 (50.0)	3 (25.0)	3 (25.0)	0	0
CO4—Supporting materials are sufficient and relevant (quiz)	10 (83.3)	2 (16.7)	0	0	0
CO5—Materials are interesting and engaging	10 (83.3)	2 (16.7)	0	0	0
CO6—Players able to understand the learning goal	9 (75.0)	2 (16.7)	1 (8.3)	0	0
CO7—The content is chunk based on topic and subtopic	10 (83.3)	2 (16.7)	0	0	0
CO8—Major and minor topic is clearly differentiated	8 (66.6)	3 (25.0)	1 (8.3)	0	0

Table 9.12 General percentage of problems for playability

	Total problems/total users				
Heuristic—PL	Level 0 (%)	Level 1 (%)	Level 2 (%)	Level 3 (%)	Level 4 (%)
PL1—Challenge provided is up to the user's standard/level	12 (100.0)	0	0	0	0
PL2—Users able to strategies	10 (83.3)	1 (8.3)	1 (8.3)	0	0
PL3—The pace of the game is in balance	9 (75.0)	2 (16.7)	1 (8.3)	0	0
PL4—Players able to control the game	10 (83.3)	1 (8.3)	0	1 (8.3)	0
PL5—Progress of the game can be seen at anytime	4 (33.3)	4 (33.3)	4 (33.3)	0	0
PL6—Players able to perform to their best ability	7 (58.3)	4 (33.3)	1 (8.3)	0	0
PL7—Challenge is adequate—not too easy and not too difficult	12 (100.0)	0	0	0	0

Table 9.13 General percentage of problems for multimedia

Heuristic—MM	Total problems/total users				
	Level 0 (%)	Level 1 (%)	Level 2 (%)	Level 3 (%)	Level 4 (%)
MM1—Usage of multimedia elements is acceptable	12 (100.0)	0	0	0	0
MM2—Combination of multimedia elements is adequate	10 (83.3)	1 (8.3)	1 (8.3)	0	0
MM3—The presentation of multimedia elements is well managed	11 (91.7)	1 (8.3)	0	0	0
MM4—Suitability of multimedia elements for specific use	9 (75.0)	3 (25.0)	0	0	0
MM5—Not too many multimedia elements in one screen	10 (83.3)	2 (16.7)	0	0	0
MM6—The use of multimedia elements supports meaningfully the text provided	11 (91.7)	1 (8.3)	0	0	0
MM7—The quality of multimedia elements (text, image, animation, video and sound) used is acceptable	11 (91.7)	1 (8.3)	0	0	0
MM8—The uses of multimedia elements enhances the presentation of information	11 (91.7)	0	1 (8.3)	0	0

9.4.5.2.5 Multimedia

Overall, the multimedia settings received good feedback from players. All background music and sound effects can well match the game plot and scene switching. In interviews after the questionnaire, the testers said that the exciting music also gave them a stronger sense of accomplishment when passing levels and upgrading the protagonist (Table 9.13).

9.5 Discussion

9.5.1 Achievement

This study presents a rigorously designed serious game for learning about the schistosome parasite and a comparison of the effectiveness between game-based learning and text-based learning. This is not commonly seen in related game development projects (Olszewski and Wolbrink 2017). Many studies tend to focus on user feedback as the primary goal without genuinely testing the game's educational/learning effects. A game that effectively combines knowledge acquisition and playability is the true embodiment of the standards for educational serious games (Graafland et al. 2014). The between-group comparison suggested that the game-based approach could achieve a similar score increase as with the text-reading approach in the quiz. Both conditions have enriched people's understanding of the schistosome parasite, although the game-based learning mode shows greater potential for knowledge acquisition. Users strongly recognise the game's educational value. During the initial data collection, the majority of testers were unfamiliar with the concept of serious games. This indicates that the promotion of serious games is still insufficient, especially for games like this project that are not developed exclusively for professionals, requiring more societal attention (Graafland et al. 2014). In terms of UI design, many participants appreciated the aesthetic style and layout. The game mechanics were considered to portray immunological principles effectively. Although a small portion of players found professional terminology challenging to comprehend, in the final testing phase, all users were able to translate their gaming experience into short-term learning outcomes, as evidenced by the increased quiz scores. The multimedia aspects received high praise, which is crucial for catering to user preferences and creating immersion. While there is room for further refinement in the game content, imperfections were minimal. Despite significant differences in participants' opinions, overall, they effectively utilised the game for learning, successfully completing the game. This indicates that the game's difficulty level was appropriately set, and the gameplay was smooth.

The development technology utilised in this game allowed us to test a unique example of a 3D game within the realm of serious medical gaming. Moreover, the expanded inclusion criteria have endowed this game with a larger audience base. The outcome also demonstrates that a game-based learning approach serves as a valuable complement to, and innovation upon, existing conventional learning methods.

9.5.2 Limitation

Despite attempting to balance the representativeness of the research population during the recruitment of participants, the vast majority included in this study are students due to objective constraints. Moreover, the average age is relatively young. This demographic possesses a quick adaptability to new things and high efficiency. However, whether similar experimental outcomes can be observed within even younger or less educated demographics requires further investigation through more extensive sub-group studies with expanded sample sizes.

Additionally, due to workload constraints, no differentiation was made between medical students and regular students, which requires improvement. Because of their distinct knowledge foundations, there are significant differences in their abilities to acquire relevant knowledge. This discrepancy is also evident in knowledge assessments. Although, in the initial plan, conducting univariate and multivariate analysis that could influence game-based knowledge acquisition was deemed important, this aspect was not ultimately executed considering the various limitations mentioned. This could serve as a part of future efforts to enhance the project and be addressed in the upcoming phases of work.

For the game, the optimization of keyboard and mouse controls needs further enhancement to align with user habits. The game's difficulty also requires adjustments; testers generally indicated that the final acid pool challenge in the second level was quite challenging. In the subsequent development, the number of NK cells in that part has been reduced, and the speed of acid spray pipelines has been slowed down. However, further feedback is needed to confirm the effectiveness of these difficulty reductions.

Another issue that received complaints was the lack of game progression and the excessive volume of the hint system text. These aspects significantly affected user ratings in both the 'Content' and 'Playability' categories. These concerns were addressed by implementing a real-time navigation system in the secondary develop ment phase. However, this solution has yet to undergo user testing due to time constraints. These shortcomings are also anticipated to be improved in the subsequent phases of research.

9.5.3 Considerations for Future Work

Based on the current development status of SGs used in medical education and this project's developing experience, the following suggestions are proposed:

1. Emphasise the optimization design of SGs in medical education.

   For the design of SGs, it is important to focus on how to enhance the learning of medical knowledge and skills. Additionally, the content and complexity of the game should be optimised to cater to learners with different proficiency levels. It is recommended to integrate the content of SGs with medical curricula or professional training materials. Moreover, the primary designers of SGs should possess qualifications as medical professionals or educators and follow a formal educational theory framework or set of guidelines for game design.
2. Avoid rigidly separating the entertainment value of games from their serious purposes.

   The use of SGs in medical education does not solely emphasise the educational value of the games. An important aspect is that the games must be engaging and enjoyable. Therefore, high levels of both content accuracy and accessibility are required alongside reinforcing and motivating game mechanics. This is often described in serious game literature as a 'balance' between fun and learning; however, it is possible to achieve highly in both the entertainment and the purposeful aspects of a well-designed serious game. Nevertheless, this is a challenge requiring significant multidisciplinary and interdisciplinary expertise.

3. Rigorously evaluate the effectiveness of SGs in improving medical education.

   With the development of SGs and their application in medical education, it is necessary to rigorously evaluate the effectiveness of SGs in improving medical education. After all, as serious games, their main purpose is education. If they fail to achieve educational effectiveness, it can lead to student distraction or excessive engagement in entertainment activities, thereby losing the original intent of SGs.

4. Encourage more experimentation and exploration from developers and medical students as game users.

   Various new technologies are emerging, bringing about numerous transformations in SGs. Game developers must keep up with the times and develop new games by incorporating the latest technologies or concepts. Additionally, medical institutions should encourage medical students to explore SGs and discover how they can be utilised for learning. This ideal state is achieved through dynamic feedback and iteration, overcoming biases against SGs, managing fruitful collaborations between subject specialists and serious game designers and ensuring developers stay connected with the users.

9.6 Conclusion

This project created a game for learning schistosomiasis-related immune knowledge and validated its effectiveness. Through a questionnaire-based survey, participants highly rated this game's entertainment, educational value and comprehensiveness. Regarding specific educational outcomes, the game achieved knowledge gains similar to text-based reading results.

These findings indicate that the game has achieved the intended effects of the study and has undertaken a forward-looking attempt to promote parasitic immunity through SGs. Despite various imperfections in the game itself, the result of this study still provides evidence for the further application of serious games in parasitic immune education.

References

Buijs-Spanjers KR, Hegge HHM, Cnossen F, Hoogendoorn E, Jaarsma D, de Rooij SE (2019) Dark play of serious games: effectiveness and features (G4HE2018). Games Health J 8:301–306

Costain AH, Macdonald AS, Smits HH (2018) Schistosome egg migration: mechanisms, pathogenesis and host immune responses. Front Immunol 9:3042

García-Redondo P, García T, Areces D, Núñez JC, Rodríguez C (2019) Serious games and their effect improving attention in students with learning disabilities. Int J Environ Res Public Health 16:2480

Graafland M, Dankbaar M, Mert A, Lagro J, de Wit-Zuurendonk L, Schuit S, Schaafstal A, Schijven M (2014) How to systematically assess serious games applied to health care. Jmir Serious Games 2:73–80

Gryseels B, Polman K, Clerinx J, Kestens L (2006) Human schistosomiasis. Lancet (London, England) 368:1106–1118

Hu GH, Hu J, Song KY, Lin DD, Zhang J, Cao CL, Xu J, Li D, Jiang WS (2005) The role of health education and health promotion in the control of schistosomiasis: experiences from a 12-year intervention study in the Poyang Lake area. Acta Trop 96:232–241

Leitao TM, Navarro LLL, Cameira RF, Silva ER (2021) Serious games in business process management: a systematic literature review. Bus Process Manag J 27:685–721

Lima IDD, de Leon C, Ribeiro LM, da Silva ICR, Vilela DM, Fonseca LMM et al (2022) A serious game (immunitates) about immunization: development and validation study. JMIR Serious Games 10(1). https://doi.org/10.2196/30738

Mcmanus DP, Dunne DW, Sacko M, Utzinger J, Vennervald BJ, Zhou X-N (2018) Schistosomiasis. Nat Rev Dis Primers 4:13

Mohamed H, Jaafar A (2013) Playability assessment for educational computer games: pilot study for model development. In: Zaman HB, Robinson P, Olivier P, Shih TK, Velastin S (eds) Advances in visual informatics. Springer, Cham

Nation CS, Da'dara AA, Marchant JK, Skelly PJ (2020) Schistosome migration in the definitive host. PLoS Negl Trop Dis 14:e0007951

Olgers TJ, de Weg AAB, Ter Maaten JC (2021) Serious games for improving technical skills in medicine: scoping review. JMIR Serious Games 9:e24093

Olszewski AE, Wolbrink TA (2017) Serious gaming in medical education a proposed structured framework for game development. Simul Healthc J Soc Simul Healthc 12:240–253

Plater L, Nyman S, Joubran S, Al-Aidroos N (2023) Repetition enhances the effects of activated long-term memory. Q J Exp Psychol 76:621–631

Suppan M, Stuby L, Harbarth S, Fehlmann CA, Achab S, Abbas M, Suppan L (2021) Nationwide deployment of a serious game designed to improve covid-19 infection prevention practices in Switzerland: prospective web-based study. JMIR Serious Games 9(4):e33003. https://doi.org/10.2196/33003

Tori AA, Tori R, Nunes FDD (2022) Serious game Design in Health Education: a systematic review. IEEE Trans Learn Technol 15:827–846

Tsopra R, Courtine M, Sedki K, Eap D, Cabal M, Cohen S, Bouchaud O, Mechai F, Lamy JB (2020) AntibioGame (R): a serious game for teaching medical students about antibiotic use. Int J Med Inform 136:104074

Wilkinson P (2016) A brief history of serious games. In: Dörner R, Göbel S, Kickmeier-Rust M, Masuch M, Zweig K (eds) Entertainment computing and serious games. Springer, Cham

MindMap: Developing and Evaluating a Novel Digital Revision Tool for Cranial Nerve Nuclei and Their Resulting Pathways

10

Ryan McGonagle, Emma Bailey, and Fraser Dougan

Abstract

The cranial nerves are 12 pairs of nerves which emerge from the base of the brain brainstem and are responsible for a myriad of sensory and motor functions across the head and neck. Learning the anatomy of these nerves is difficult, requiring strong spatial skills, mental visualisation of abstract anatomy and an understanding of the internal brainstem histology (Lack et al. 2022). Despite this, most teaching resources available to students rely solely on 2D histology. This research therefore aims to design and develop a novel cranial nerve revision resource which embeds 2D histology within a digital 3D model. Developed as an online application, 'MindMap' targets this gap in the current literature, and its effectiveness was evaluated through a variety of feedback acquired from life science student and staff cohorts within the University of Glasgow. This feedback provided a mixture of quantitative and qualitative data which highlight the application's impact on student comprehension, usability and motivation. Open-feedback responses provided further insight into the student and staff user experience. Unexpectedly, the results obtained contradicted the hypothesised response—with student and staff participants in disagreement. Staff responded more positively to the application than students. Although mixed responses were collected, the findings suggest participants were receptive to the concept of an integrated resource which highlights histology and gross anatomy features of the cranial nerves within a single 3D model. With development, 'MindMap' has the potential to improve student comprehension of the cranial nerve pathways and act as a supplementary revision resource. Further research is required to determine whether the feedback from the student participant reflects that of a wider student population or if this response is a potential outlier.

R. McGonagle (✉)
School of Innovation and Technology, The Glasgow School of Art, Glasgow, UK

School of Medicine, Dentistry and Nursing, College of Medical, Veterinary and Life Sciences, University of Glasgow, Glasgow, UK

E. Bailey
School of Medicine, Dentistry and Nursing, College of Medical, Veterinary and Life Sciences, University of Glasgow, Glasgow, UK
e-mail: emma.bailey@glasgow.ac.uk

F. Dougan
School of Innovation and Technology, The Glasgow School of Art, Glasgow, UK
e-mail: F.dougan@gsa.ac.uk

J. Clancy, M. Poyade (eds.), *Medical Visualization and Applications of Technology – Volume 2*, Biomedical Visualization 5, https://doi.org/10.1007/978-3-031-63463-5_10

Keywords

Cranial nerve pathways · Internal brainstem anatomy · Histology · Digital 3D visualisation · Online interactive application

be to review and improve upon their current pedagogical resources. Further research is vital to determine the potential impacts of 3D visualisation in the improvement of student spatial awareness and comprehension of neuroanatomy.

10.1 Introduction

10.1.1 Introduction to Neurophobia

Neuroanatomy is an extremely complex discipline of life science which focusses on learning the structure of the brain and spinal cord and—to determine their effects on the human body. Studying this field requires strong skills in mental 3D visualisation and spatial awareness. Despite the three-dimensional nature of this discipline, resources provided to students throughout higher education institutions are predominantly 2D. From the current literature, it can be determined that neuroanatomy is an area of common difficulty for both students and professionals alike (Pakpoor et al. 2014; Hall et al. 2018; Javaid et al. 2018; Geoghegan et al. 2019 & Venter et al. 2022), and it is likely that the combination of difficulty and lack of effective 3D resources has contributed to 'neurophobia'. This is an informal term used throughout the literature to address the fear of neuroanatomy which is prevalent among students and professionals of the life sciences (Pakpoor et al. 2014; Javaid et al. 2018 & Venter et al. 2022). Not only does this fear impact the academic performance of students throughout their neuroscience-related modules, but it is often carried into their future careers. As frivolous as this may seem, it has led to a reduction in neuroanatomy specialists and clinicians, as well as a noticeable rise in referrals from GPs, as they feel unequipped to tackle neurology-related consultations effectively and with confidence (Chhetri 2017; Javaid et al. 2018; Hernando-Requejo 2020; Edwards-Bailey et al. 2022). If not addressed, neurophobia will continue to stunt the progression of the neurosciences and impact the medical care of those who require it. It is concluded that an effective way to reduce neurophobia within student cohorts may

10.1.2 Neuroanatomy Education

Neuroanatomy is most commonly taught through the use of didactic lectures across higher education institutions in the UK (Edwards-Bailey et al. 2022). Although these are undoubtedly effective, it should be noted that lectures are only able to provide information and diagrams in a two-dimensional format. Despite this limitation, lectures are usually available to students online, providing means for revision of the complex topics taught. Peculiarly, the same study found the second most common teaching method to be self-directed study, with e-learning and prosections following closely behind (Edwards-Bailey et al. 2022). Since this research was conducted in 2022, the increase in self-directed study may be closely correlated to the impacts of the COVID-19 pandemic. As well as this, many higher education institutions have reduced their allocated laboratory time across life science undergraduate courses, causing many students to search elsewhere for supplementary revision resources (Hall et al. 2018; Venter et al. 2022). With reduced laboratory experience, the student's exposure to prosection and cadaveric models is also impacted. These are crucial tools used throughout higher education institutions and are especially effective at improving student comprehension of the complicated spatial relationships between structures in an exclusively three-dimensional format (McLachlan et al. 2004; Mathiowetz et al. 2016). Despite their effectiveness, prosection models are often aged, fragile and, in some cases, damaged. Alongside prosections, cadaveric materials assist in student comprehension of 3D neuroanatomy and are often coined as the pinnacle of anatomical teaching resources (Krähenbühl et al. 2017; Iwanaga et al. 2021). As well as spatial awareness, cadaveric models also provide insight into the relationships between differing tissues as well as haptic feedback when dissecting—which is difficult to digitally recreate (Mathiowetz et al. 2016). Although effective, cadavers are scarce and highly regulated and, most importantly, may only be dissected once. It is important that students are provided the resources that they may access beyond their university campus, which represent accurate 3D anatomy, and may be revisited by students as required.

10.1.3 Histology in Neuroanatomy

Histology is a 2D teaching resource used throughout higher education institutions to provide insight into the microscopic composition of anatomy. Within cranial nerve education, histology often represents the landmarks of the internal brainstem, in relation to each nerve's origin and site of emergence. Histology and gross anatomy models remain separate resources which are often used by students in unison in order to comprehend the cranial nerve anatomy. Unfortunately, this method is often ineffective and leads to unmotivated, disheartened students. Additionally, histology sections are often difficult to decipher and are dependent on clear slicing of the specimen. Due to this, comprehension of brainstem histology depends on each individual's ability to distinguish between minute variations in hue and tone. Recognising this issue within current teaching methodologies, a group of research has emerged in recent years which aims to target these issues through the integration of histology within digital 3D models, redefining the current methodology for cranial nerve pedagogy (Henssen et al. 2020).

10.1.4 Current Research

Inspired by the current literature which highlights neurophobia as a prominent barrier for higher education students, many researchers have ventured into the design and development of digital 3D resources. There are many different ways these resources may be formatted including, but not limited to, online anatomical atlases, interactive 3D applications and extended reality software (including both augmented and virtual reality) (Nowinski et al. 2012, Richardson-Hatcher et al. 2014, Wimsatt et al. 2017, Henssen et al. 2020). The development of these resources targets two main regions of the students' neuroanatomical learning experience. Firstly, they expand upon traditional 2D resources such as lectures and textbooks—which in turn aims to improve student motivation and engagement with their learning. Secondly, they provide 3D representations of their chosen anatomy, which are available off-campus and provide the means to strengthen the vital spatial awareness skills required for the study of neuroanatomy. Interesting research conducted by Nowinski et al. (2012) documents the creation of an online neuroanatomy atlas (Nowinski et al. 2012). Although this atlas is no doubt impressive and has great potential, its efficacy was not tested on a student population. Despite the quantity and usefulness of the provided information, the user interface of this particular resource is cluttered and difficult to navigate. This considered, the atlas may be overwhelming to a user at the level of higher education and may even invoke neurophobia. Instead, this atlas may be better suited for neuroscience professionals and practicing clinicians.

A more appropriate student resource may be found in the atlas developed by Wimsatt and colleagues in 2017, titled '3D Brain' (available at https://www.brainfacts.org/3d-brain). This atlas is openly available online and, so, can be accessed from anywhere and across multiple devices, as long as the student has Internet access (Wimsatt et al. 2017). Not only is the user interface of this atlas simplified for ease of use, but it implements a tab system which improves information provision. This allows users to be more deliberate with their learning as they may select a specific region of neuroanatomy and remove anything unnecessary. The colour palette consists of muted greys and pinks. Although aesthetically pleasing, this palette leads to low-contrast regions throughout its user interface. This is a vital factor to consider within application design, especially when applying these principles to pedagogical resources. The text should be clear and visible to all students, including those with visual impairments or any category of colour blindness (Sawyer et al. 2020). Accessibility of this atlas may have been improved through a revision of the current palette or an alternate colour setting which allows users to adjust the settings to suit their personal requirements.

Despite hosting a wealth of neuroanatomy information and 3D models, this style of resource fails to directly address the recurrent issue of weak spatial awareness of the cranial nerves within student populations. The cranial nerves are most frequently taught through cross-sectional histology and plastinated or cadaveric specimens. Although students are able to view these specimens within their allocated laboratory time, this is limited and requires strict access. Due to this, many students are not able to access 3D models of the cranial nerves outside their university campus laboratories. Current revision resources available to students are predominantly 2D, further reducing their exposure to 3D models when revising.

'The Cranial Nerve Skywalk', developed by Richardson-Hatcher et al. (2014), is an online learning platform dedicated to the physical pathways of the cranial nerves. This online application included a selection of the 12 cranial nerves (III, V, VII and IX), each aided by information panels, labelled diagrams and 3D models. By combining the 3D models and 2D diagrams within one virtual space, it was hoped that users may begin to build correlations between the 2D and 3D data, strengthening their spatial awareness of the cranial nerves and how their 3D form may link to each nerve's function. As well as providing 3D visualisation, this application was developed for use within 'Second Life', a digital space which allows for student collaboration, by providing the ability to communicate through voice and text-chat systems (Richardson-Hatcher et al. 2014). In spite of this innovative feature, the application's interface may be perceived as difficult to read and navigate. Although further information is provided, this is difficult to decipher, and the font is unclear and small. As well as this, the nerves are difficult to distinguish as they are differentiated merely by the type of dotted line and minor tonal differences. With cognitive load being a focal theme of this research, adapting the colour scheme used (e.g. enhancing the contrast between nerves to improve accessibility for those with colour blindness) or improving the UI components may have improved the student experience.

Earlier research conducted by Yeung et al. (2011) described the design and development of a neuroanatomical visualisation aimed at improving student spatial awareness of the cranial nerves, as well as their physiological relation to their sites of emergence from the brainstem. This application utilised a multimedia approach to test the potential impact on student comprehension when 2D and 3D data are combined within a single resource (Yeung et al. 2011). In a later study, Yeung et al. (2012) conducted an evaluation to determine the effectiveness of their novel neuroanatomy application against the traditional 2D text–based learning methodologies, with a specific focus on student spatial awareness of the trigeminal nerve (V). Fascinatingly, this research found no significant differences in spatial awareness between their student cohorts when comparing 2D methods with their novel 3D resource; however, students exposed to 3D visualisation reported stronger feelings of engagement and motivation (Yeung et al. 2012). Interestingly, this is a recurrent theme which presents itself throughout similar literature (Bye et al. 2009; Drapkin et al. 2015; Stepan et al. 2017). Despite this, researchers are determined to refine this theory and continue to produce applications which combine 2D and 3D information to improve the student learning experience.

Alternatively, some research utilise different mediums to tackle these issues. For instance, Henssen et al. (2020) developed an augmented reality (AR) application, due to their inherent 3D nature, to target student comprehension of another subtopic within neuroanatomy education: the limbic system. Even with the use of AR, this research found no significant difference in student comprehension between 2D or 3D methodologies when quizzed on 3D gross anatomy. In fact, they found that when questioned on aspects of the 2D anatomy (e.g. histology), those within the 2D methods cohort scored higher. This therefore highlights the potential idea that perhaps these findings are not a direct result of the specific technology used to present 2D and 3D visualisations to students, but the ways in which this information is combined within these resources. Within Henssen and colleagues' work, there is a distinction between the histological and gross anatomy information throughout their AR application, potentially leading to a lack of correlation between both sets of information. This may ultimately limit its potential impact on student spatial awareness and, so, the effectiveness of this application. Instead, it may be more appropriate to combine histology and gross anatomy within a single 3D visualisation rather than presenting this information to students independently. The use of AR within this research also led to no significant student-reported improvement in their motivation when compared to traditional 2D methods (Henssen et al. 2020). This contradicts other research in that despite a lack of improved neuroanatomy knowledge, students often report a positive correlation between 3D digital visualisation and their levels of motivation and enjoyment (Bye et al. 2009; Drapkin et al. 2015; Stepan et al. 2017). Based on this, it was decided that AR would not be utilised in the context of this research to reduce its potential influence over participant's engagement.

Although rare, the concept of integrating 2D and 3D data within neuroanatomy revision resources has been explored. With the cranial nerves emerging from specific brainstem nuclei, comprehension of these nerves relies heavily on a combination of gross anatomy and histology knowledge (Pedersen et al. 2013). Nowinski, as previously mentioned for their work in the development of a neuroanatomical atlas, has developed a novel resource which overlays 3D models onto medical scan data. These are presented side-by-side in two forms: one being the scan alone and the other containing the 3D model representation of different structures (e.g. intracranial arteries or cranial nerves) (Nowinski 2023). This concept allows for easy comparison between each data type and is accessible to students due to its online format—allowing for supplementary use outside university laboratories. Even though the trigeminal nerve pathway is physically represented with accuracy, there are key details missing from the visualisation which are expected knowledge for those studying within higher education institutions such as origin nuclei, exit foramen within the skull or sites of action. Additionally, the visualisation is limited to planar views, by incorporating a 360-degree range of motion, and spatial awareness skills may be targeted more directly. Furthermore, it may be more appropriate to combine 3D models with histological information in the context of cranial nerve anatomy education, rather than radiology, as this is the predominant source of 2D data used throughout higher education institutions.

One example utilised the combination of 2D cross-sectional anatomy within the brainstem and digital 3D models to highlight potential safe entry zones and internal landmarks for neurosurgery (Guberinic et al. 2022). As a result, neurosurgeons were found to have an improved understanding of the internal structure of the brainstem; however, it is uncertain whether these findings are directly correlated to the combination of 2D and 3D data within the model. Further research is required to determine this impact. Although targeted at neurosurgeons, a similar methodology could be used in the context of cranial nerve anatomy and applied to the different nuclei present at various levels of the internal brainstem.

To summarise, there are many ways in which neuroanatomy may be visualised digitally through the use of 3D models. As there is a recurrent issue within student populations with spatial awareness skills, this area should be targeted directly and may benefit from the incorporation of these novel visualisation techniques. Despite the creation of 3D digital visualisation applications, there are only a select few attempts to embed 2D data (e.g. histology) with 3D structure—and these are often overbearing to the user, reducing their potential impact. This research attempts to address these main issues in the creation of 'MindMap': A Cranial Nerve Crash Course.

10.2 Materials and Methods

10.2.1 Materials

A range of materials (both software and hardware) were used throughout this research to aid in the design and development of the 'MindMap' application (Tables 10.1 and 10.2). Additionally, existing assets were utilised throughout its development for user interface design and 3D model creation (Table 10.3).

10.2.2 Methods

10.2.2.1 Design and Development

The main aim of this research was to develop an online 3D interactive application to assist higher education students with their revision of the cranial nerve nuclei and resulting pathways—by highlighting the relationship between their gross anatomy and histology. The content of this application was carefully selected to align with the information taught to Anatomy and Neuroscience

Table 10.1 Software used during application design and development

Software	Publisher	Use
3D Slicer	Slicer3D	Used to create the skull model within the application
Autodesk 3DSMax	Autodesk, Inc.	Used for model creation and editing for the application
ZBrush	Pixologic, Inc.	Used to refine, add details and retopologise models for application
Unity	Unity Technologies	Used to create and build the application
Visual Studio (Code)	Microsoft	Used to add C# code to the application
Free Form	Apple	Used to design the storyboard and user interface button images
Adobe Color	Adobe, Inc.	Used to test the accessibility of the colour scheme within the application
Microsoft Excel	Microsoft	Used to visualise data acquired through participant feedback
Microsoft Forms	Microsoft	Used to acquire participant feedback online
Canva	Canva	Used to create project workflow diagram

Table 10.2 Hardware used for application design and development

Hardware	Publisher	Use
HP Probook 640 G5 Laptop	Hewlett-Packard Inc.	Used to run all software and create the application in Unity
Apple iPad Air (4th generation)	Apple	Used to draw storyboards and create user interface buttons in Canva

Table 10.3 Data used during application design and development

Software	Publisher	Use
'The Visible Human' Female CT Head Data	The National Library of Medicine	Used to create the skull model within 3D Slicer
Satoshi Font Family	Fontshare: designed by Indian Type Foundry	Used as font throughout entire application. This is an open-source font family downloaded from 'Fontshare', an online font database (*https://www.fontshare.com/*)
Eyeball Material Image	By creator named 'BienenFisch' on 3DXO	Material to make the eyeball look more realistic
Brainstem Reference Image	Image downloaded from Radiology Key	Brainstem reference image used within 3DS Max during the model creation period
Histology	Provided by Dr. Emma Bailey	Histology images used within the application to represent the internal brainstem anatomy

BSc junior students at the University of Glasgow. It is hypothesised that this resource will improve student comprehension of the cranial nerve pathways and their relation to internal brainstem anatomy by combining 3D gross anatomical models with 2D histological data in a single resource. A storyboard was first created to provide a visual representation of the application. By providing a clear and concise workflow, the development process was more efficient. Each scene would highlight required models, interactive components and the user interface organisation within each scene. It was determined that 13 scenes would be required including an introduction, main scene and individual scenes dedicated to each cranial nerve which emerges at the level of the brainstem (CNIII–CNXII), as well as one final scene which combines gross anatomy with histology within one model. Unfortunately, due to time constraints, the final application contained fewer scenes than initially intended. The final application omitted cranial nerves V, VII, X, XI and XII.

Each scene required a range of models including a section of the human skull, the brainstem, an eyeball and each cranial nerve pathway (dependent on the scene selected). The use of a cropped skull model resulted in a lower final polygon count, reducing the burden of the final application to a user's computer. This also provided greater visualisation of the accompanying models within each scene, as well as providing a means of comparison. The introductory scene of the application, although not interactive, presented rotating models to attract the user's attention and encourage their curiosity.

10.2.2.2 Development of 3D Models

10.2.2.2.1 The Skull

The skull model for this application was created from a stack of DICOM images downloaded from the open-source 'Visible Human Project' (specifically, the Female CT Dataset titled 'VHFCT1mm—Head'). These were imported into a 3D Slicer, unedited, and a 3D visualisation was generated using the pre-installed 'Grayscale Modelmaker' module available within the programme. The bone in this case was segmented at a threshold value of 105. Creating the skull model directly from this dataset allowed for improved anatomical accuracy—this was vital as the scale and position of all remaining models would be determined by the skull. To further reduce the polygon count of this model, the spinal vertebrae and mandible also selected throughout the segmentation process were discarded as they were deemed unnecessary in this case. The final cropped skull model was saved and exported as a .obj (object) file and imported into 3DS Max for 'smoothing' and then ZBrush for further refinements. This allowed for further retopology and smoothing of the skull model through a combination of modifiers including: 'DynaMesh' and 'ZRemesher'—closing unwanted holes while maintaining the foramen at the base of the skull. By allowing the foramen at the base of the skull to remain identifiable, the appropriate cranial nerve pathways could be more accurately mapped during their modelling process. Once satisfied, the skull was then re-imported into 3DS Max where it would be sliced along the mid-sagittal plane. Finally, the cranium of the skull was sliced along the transverse plane to provide the potential for a top-down view into the model as well as a final reduction to the number of polygons. In total, the polygon count for this model was 20,970.

10.2.2.2.2 The Eyeball

The eyeball model within this application was used as a landmark for the cranial nerves due to the relation between the extrinsic eye muscles and multiple cranial nerves. This may also improve student spatial awareness of the pathways and their points of termination of the oculomotor, trochlear and abducens nerves. A YouTube tutorial titled 'Modelling an Eyeball', published by 'Clint DiClementi' (2014) (available at https://youtu.be/eb6sS6YXpc0?si=HsKsP5FSvGlUyHGJ), was followed to create this model. The tapered cone shape of the pupil allowed for a more realistic response to light and avoided a potentially unsettling flat appearance. The original model contained a cornea, of a semi-transparent nature; however, due to difficulties with the transparent texture, this was removed. The final model contained 576 polygons.

10.2.2.2.3 The Brainstem

The brainstem model is of the utmost importance within this application due to its relation to the cranial nerves through surface-level and internal anatomy. With the achievement of accurate points of emergence for each cranial nerve being reliant on the brainstem model, its development required the utmost care and attention to detail. Ideally, the same Visible Human Dataset would have been utilised within 3D Slicer to generate a brainstem segmentation. Unfortunately, this proved difficult due to the quality of these DICOM images. The isodensity values within the dataset were not distinguishable enough to accurately determine regions of brainstem anatomy for manual segmentation. As a result, it was decided that the model should be created manually within 3DS Max and ZBrush alongside reference photos to generate an anatomically accurate mesh. A reference containing the anterior, lateral and posterior views of the brainstem was acquired through 'RadiologyKey'. From these reference images, the brainstem was divided into its three main components (midbrain, pons and medulla oblongata) and box modelled. Box modelling is a technique often used in the organic modelling process as it allows for complex geometries to be broken down into simpler forms. These can then be altered using a variety of modifiers to adjust from angular to smooth meshes. This technique was used to divide the complex brainstem structure into the three aforementioned regions—making this task more manageable.

NURMS (non-uniform rational mesh smooth) is a modifier available within 3DS Max and was used to smooth these box models, altering each component into a high-polygon mesh. This therefore created an organically shaped base to import into ZBrush for further refinement. ZRemesher was used to re-topologize the models, in turn increasing the number of polygons. When adding finer detail to a model, it is important to work from a high polygon count as this allows for more accurate modelling while minimising the potential disruption to an area's surrounding mesh. Consequently, this provided a greater degree of control when adjusting external landmarks of the brainstem such as the superior and inferior colliculi. With detail added, the final brainstem model was re-topologized to reduce the final polygon count.

To assist the modelling process of the cerebellar peduncles which required a bit more insight, access was provided by the anatomy department of the University of Glasgow to inspect a brainstem from available cadaveric material. Photographs were taken of the brainstem specimen to aid the development of the brainstem model. These images were subject to strict adherence to the 'Code of Conduct for Image Handling in Anatomy' as outlined by the university. By providing greater insight into the 3D form of the brainstem, the brainstem model was adapted to more appropriately represent the region of the cerebellar peduncles, improving the model's overall anatomical accuracy. The final polygon count for the brainstem was 9414.

10.2.2.2.4 The Internal Brainstem

In order to provide a view of the internal histology, the brainstem model was duplicated and divided into segments. Each of these sections was deliberately sliced at levels of importance throughout the three main regions of the brainstem. Each cross-section was 'detached' from the model within 3DS Max and created as clones of the original model. Considering the 'hollow' nature of this model—as it was merely represented by a surface mesh with no internal structure—the superior and inferior surfaces remained open. 'Cap Holes' (modifier within 3DS Max) was used to recognise the gaps within the models and bridge them. This process was repeated for each segment, with a final sum of nine models, representing motor decussation, sensory decussation, level of lower olives, upper olives, inferior, middle and superior pons and, finally, the inferior and superior colliculi. Each region was selected due to the relationships between each level of the brainstem and histology materials provided to higher education students.

10.2.2.2.5 The Cranial Nerves

The final models to be developed were the cranial nerves. Unfortunately, due to time constraints, some nerves were omitted from this application. The final resource contained oculomotor (III), trochlear (IV), abducens (VI), vestibulocochlear (VIII) and glossopharyngeal (IX). To begin, the pathway of each nerve was researched and planned out in terms of its relation to the brainstem, skull and, in relevant cases, the eyeball. 'Splines' (3D line models) allowed for freeform lines to be created, representing each cranial nerve pathway—producing organic and low poly adjustable nerves. As this technique is limited to a 2D format, the 3DS Max viewport was locked to the left, ensuring models would only be present on the *x*-axis. Finally, the 3D form of each nerve pathway was further adjusted using the *y*- and *z*-axis viewports. Several cranial nerve pathways required the creation of multiple line models which were later grouped together to form the complex nerve model. A similar methodology was adopted and repeated for the creation of each of the remaining nerves. With all nerve models created and adjusted, a symmetry modifier was applied to each nerve group to provide a visual representation of the models on both sides of the skull.

10.2.2.3 User Interface Design

Accessibility was a major guiding factor throughout the entire design and development process for the User Interface components used throughout this application. Due to its intended use as a revision resource, it is crucial that it is designed with accessibility at the forefront to ensure accessibility to a broad range of students. The Web Content Accessibility Guidelines (WCAG) influenced design decisions throughout this process, and adherence to this allowed for optimised accessibility (available at https://www.w3.org/WAI/standards-guidelines/wcag/).

10.2.2.3.1 Style

A simple and professional design style was adopted to encourage users to perceive the application as appropriate to their academic level of study. Font and colour choices further emphasised the theme of this application. The buttons, however, contradict the serious tone through their stylised and gamified aesthetic. Introducing this contrast aimed to emphasise the playful nature of the application.

10.2.2.3.2 Colour

The contrast was heavily considered throughout the creation of this application's colour scheme. Across anatomical resources, yellow is often associated with nerves and nervous tissue within diagrams and anatomical imagery. Implementing this within the application should encourage immediate recognition of nerve pathways within student users. With yellow selected, it was decided that contrast would be most effectively achieved through the use of purple (yellow's complementary colour). The final palette remained simple consisting of four colours: dark purple (#301E2C), light purple (#5D3754), yellow (#F0CF60) and white (#FFFFFF) (see Fig. 10.1). Contrast was tested using Adobe Color, specifically, its colour contrast analyser tool. Each of the four colours were compared to determine the most and least effective colour pairings.

Each colour combination was found to be of high contrast, with the exception of yellow and white. These colours were used within the buttons of the application. To combat their potential impact, each button was placed on an area of purple—creating greater contrast. If to be repeated, button colours may be adjusted for improved accessibility.

As well as contrast, common categories of colour blindness were also considered throughout the design process. Adobe Color allows for testing of the palette by adjusting each hue with regard to deuteranopia, protanopia and tritanopia. The results identified no issues for any of these conditions (see Fig. 10.2).

10.2.2.3.3 Buttons

Apple 'Freeform' was used to create buttons for the application. A general background was created and duplicated for the use of all buttons to encourage coherence throughout each scene of the application. Open-source iconography, avail-

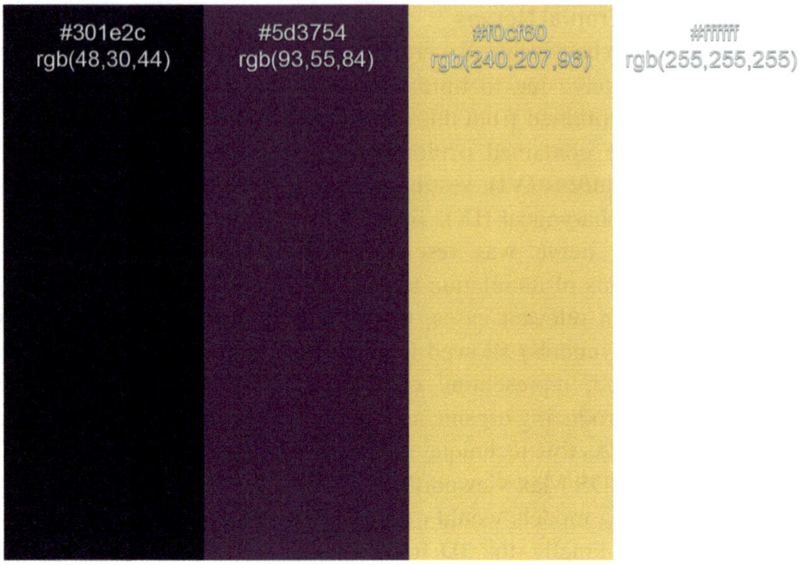

Fig. 10.1 Representation of the final colour scheme used within the application

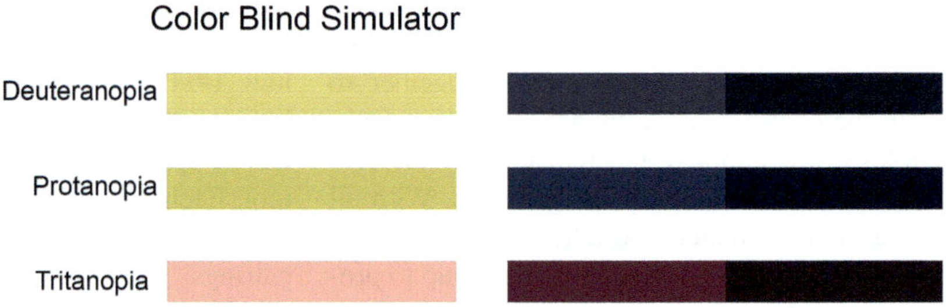

Fig. 10.2 Colour blindness simulator within Adobe Color with relation to deuteranopia, protanopia and tritanopia

able within freeform, was searched, choosing appropriate symbols for each button which would correlate to its intended purpose. The stylised icons emphasise the playful theme of the UI, and the use of graphics reduced the volume of unrequired text within each scene. Each UI button was imported into Unity and converted to sprites. Adjustment of the filter mode and compression of each sprite resulted in high-definition and appropriately scaled files which may be attached to the UI button elements within the Unity application. Placement of buttons also remained identical throughout the application, through the implementation of a vertical layout group, improving user flow and creating a sense of familiarity.

10.2.2.3.4 Font

The Satoshi font family is utilised throughout the application as it is simple, clear and bold, improving its readability. This is important as this font was used for paragraphs of informative text within each scene.

10.2.2.4 Application Development

The platform Unity 3D (version 2021.4f1) allowed for the development of this application. An initial version was constructed based on the originally proposed plan for each scene, and all main user interface components were appropriately oriented and anchored within each scene. All required models were imported, and functionalities were added to each individual component, as appropriate. Each interactive functionality appointed to objects within the scene may arise from pre-existing functions within Unity 3D or through the implementation of the script. The Microsoft coding language C# was adopted throughout the application development process, alongside the source code editor 'Visual Studio Code'. Table 10.4 presents an overview of all C# scripts included within the application. The final application was built as an executable file compatible with Windows operating systems and also published on 'itch.io', an independent game host site. This ensures easy distribution to users for access throughout the participant testing portion of this research.

10.3 Results

Three main scene styles were created for this application: firstly, the introductory scene which is presented to a user upon opening the application (see Fig. 10.3); secondly, the main scene style contained the majority of interactive components and information about the cranial nerves, as well as the required 3D models for each scene (see Fig. 10.4); and lastly, the histology scene, which provided a 3D digital reference with embedded internal brainstem anatomy in the form of 2D histology sections at each appropriate level of the brainstem—each segment triggering an animation when selected (see Figs. 10.5 and 10.6).

Table 10.4 List of C# scripts created for the MindMap application—and their functions

C# script name	Function
UIManager	Control scene load and application quit
SliderToRotate	Allows models to rotate on the y-axis
ViewModel	Allows the visibility of models to be easily toggled on/off
AnimationOnClick	When left mouse button is clicked over a brainstem segment's box collider, animation will play
CameraRotator	Rotates camera around model centre of rotation at a steady pace
InfoPanelController	Controls info panel activity when object is clicked to ensure only one panel is visible at any given time

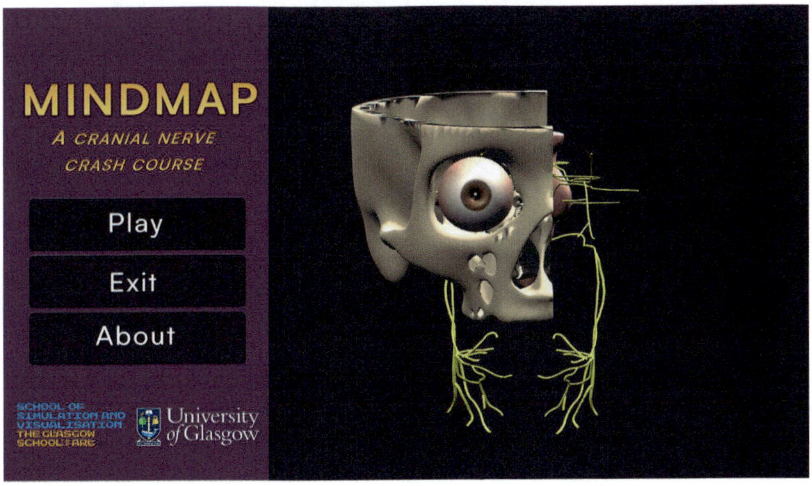

Fig. 10.3 Screenshot of the introductory scene for the MindMap application

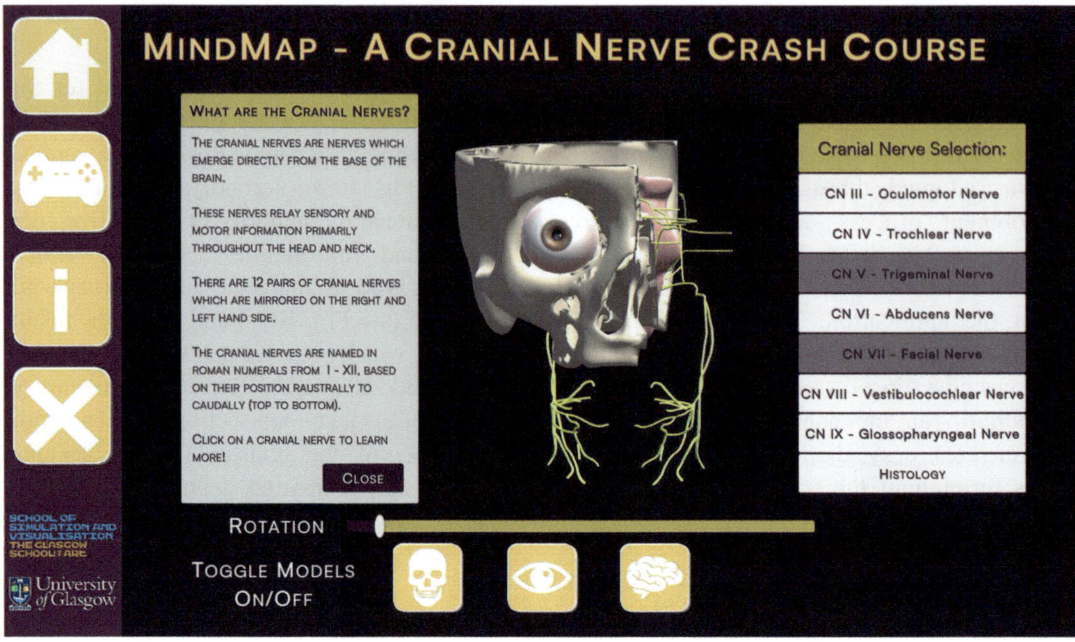

Fig. 10.4 Screenshot of the main scene from the MindMap application

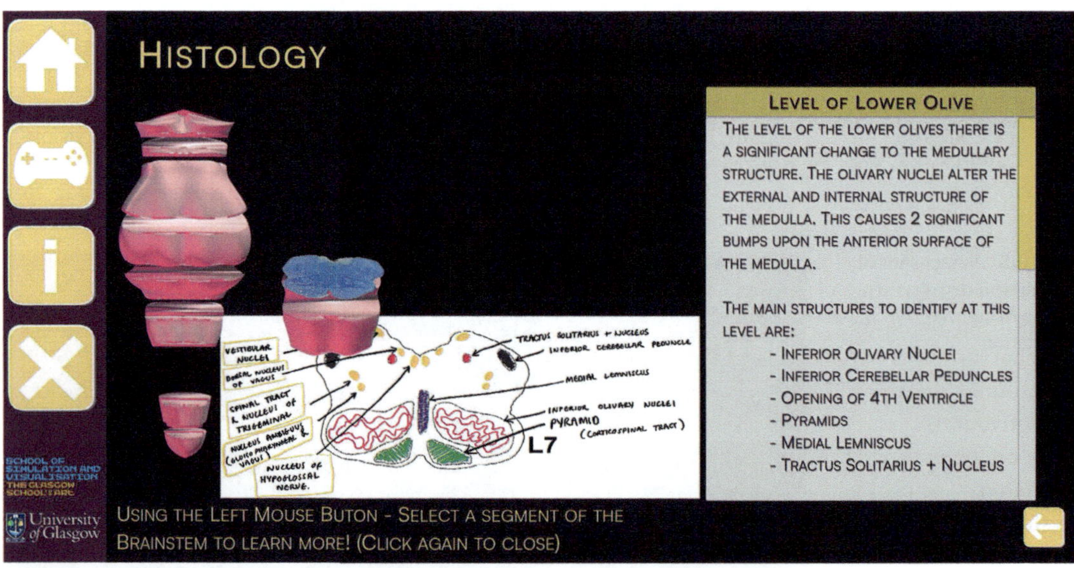

Fig. 10.5 A screenshot of the animation process for the selection of an individual brainstem segment (in this example, the lower olive). The arrows represent the direction of movement in the animation

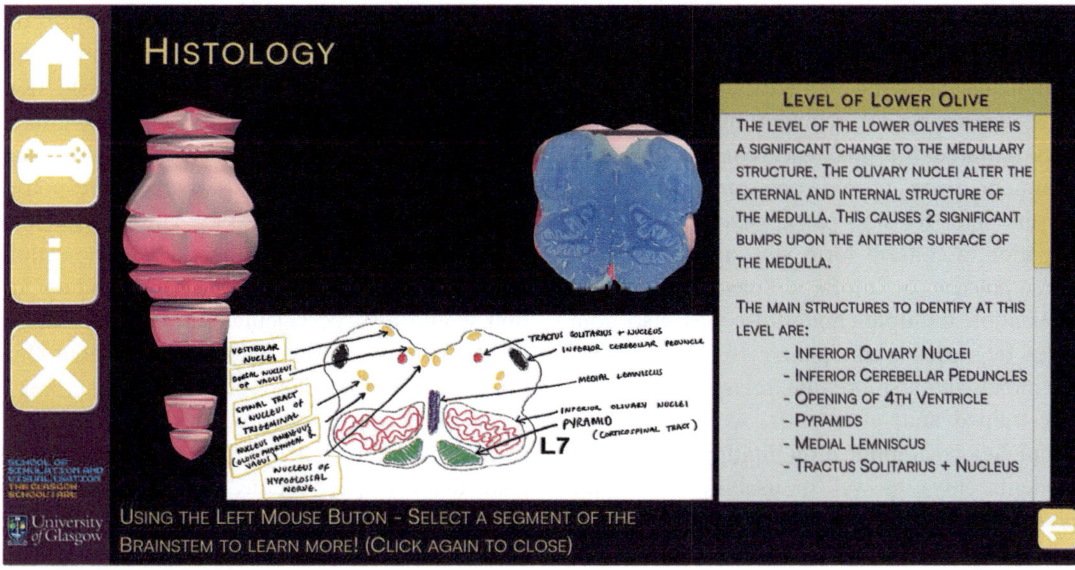

Fig. 10.6 The final positioning of the segment after animation, as well as the information panels and brainstem model within the scene

10.4 Evaluation

An experimental approach was used to determine user opinions about this resource. There were three main research questions which directed the evaluation of this application:

- How does 'MindMap' impact student comprehension of the cranial nerve nuclei and resulting pathways?
- What are the user's opinions of the novel resource (with a focus on usability and motivation)?
- Does the combination of histology and gross anatomy improve the user's spatial understanding of the cranial nerves?

10.4.1 Participants

There were two groups of targeted participant cohorts within this research: staff (professionals, $n = 3$) and higher education students (at level 3, $n = 1$). All contacted members of staff worked within the School of Medicine, Veterinary and Life Science at the University of Glasgow. Student participants of Anatomy and Neuroscience undergraduate degrees were contacted. The National Undergraduate Neuroanatomy Competition (NUNC) team were also contacted for potential participation in this research. Participant information remained anonymous throughout the entire testing process as no identifiable personal data was collected.

10.4.2 Apparatus

The final application was built to run on PCs or laptops supported by Windows operating systems. Emails containing guidelines for participation as well as links to the application were distributed to the required student and staff populations by a member of the Life Science team at the university and the supervisor of this project, Dr. Emma Bailey. 'MindMap', available to download through itch.io, could be retrieved by anyone with access to the Internet and the application's link (https://ryanmcgonagle1.itch.io/mindmap). Microsoft Forms provided a means for anonymous user feedback and were attached along with the user information documents provided to participants.

10.4.3 Procedure

Participants were first emailed a user information form containing all relevant instructions and links required for this research. Two alternate documents were created: one aimed at students and the other for staff participants. Prior to participation, a consent form was signed to ensure the acquisition of informed consent, and a pre-application multiple-choice test was also completed by student participants. Users were able to download and explore the created application unrestrained and, afterwards, were required to complete a post-application multiple-choice quiz (students only), as well as usability (SUS) and motivation questionnaires (RIMMS).

10.4.4 Data Analysis

Pre- and post-application multiple-choice quizzes contained 15 identical questions, in a randomised order, and were divided equally into three main sub-topics: structure, function and histology. Average grades were calculated for both pre- and post-application quiz scores and converted into percentage values within Microsoft Forms. Exporting results to Microsoft Excel allowed for the generation of a visual comparison between the data, in the form of a bar graph.

The System Usability Scale (SUS) (Brooke 1996) determined the usability of the final 'MindMap' application. This scale provides pre-determined questions, answered using a Likert scale ranging from 'strongly agree' to 'strongly disagree'. Responses to this questionnaire provide a final value grade for the application usability for each participant. The higher this value (0–100), the more usable the application is deemed to be. Ideally, confidence intervals for average SUS scores would be calculated to predict how these results may be reflected across a larger cohort—unfortunately, with one student participant, this was not an option.

To determine the impact of the resource on motivation, the Reduced Instructional Materials Motivation Survey (RIMMS), a reduced and validated format of the original IMMS survey (Loorbach et al. 2015), was used. This focuses on four contributing factors to user motivation: attention, relevance, confidence and satisfaction (ARCS). This further provides quantitative data through a Likert scale response system ranging from 'not true' to 'very true'—with each response representing a value from 1–5. The mean of the recorded data is then calculated for each section of the questionnaire. Usually, the standard deviation would also be calculated; however, due to the limited responses acquired throughout this research, this was not possible.

Open-response style feedback opportunities were provided to both staff and student participants to allow space for any general comments or critiques relating to any aspect of their participation in this research and/or their experience with the application. The question asked 'Is there any extra feedback you wish to add? If so, please use the text box below'. All responses were recorded on Microsoft Forms to ensure the participant's anonymity. Responses were read and categorised based on their relation to either visual aspects of the application or the educational content. Feedback responses provided greater insight into the user's unique perspective and would allow the author to address key points of concern which may arise across both participant groups.

10.4.5 Ethics

Ethical approval to conduct this research was granted by the School of Simulation and Visualisation at the Glasgow School of Art.

10.4.6 Evaluation Results

10.4.6.1 Student Comprehension

The single student participant was found to improve their quiz result after exposure to the novel application, increasing from 73 to 93% (see Fig. 10.7).

10.4.6.2 Usability

The responses from the SUS survey of both staff and student participants were combined within a single bar graph to allow comparison. From the SUS student feedback, the application was rated at SUS = 57.50 (represented in purple); contrarily, of the three staff responses acquired, the SUS value averaged at a rating of SUS = 82.5 (yellow) (see Fig. 10.8). The individual results were recorded as 85, 80 and 82.5 from participants 1, 2 and 3, respectively.

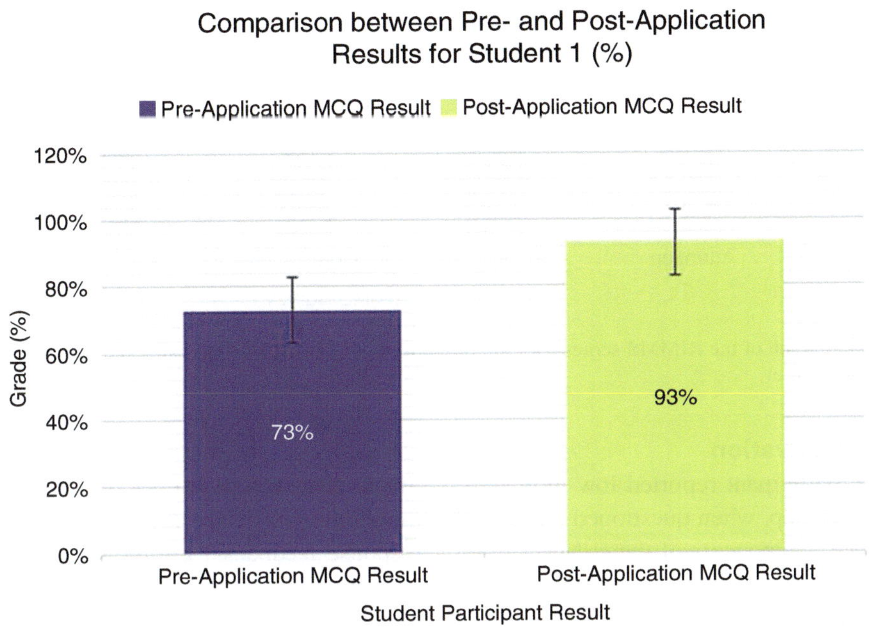

Fig. 10.7 A bar graph which represents the student participant's pre- and post-application MCQ results, in percentages (%). Created using Microsoft Excel. Standard Error bars added within Excel

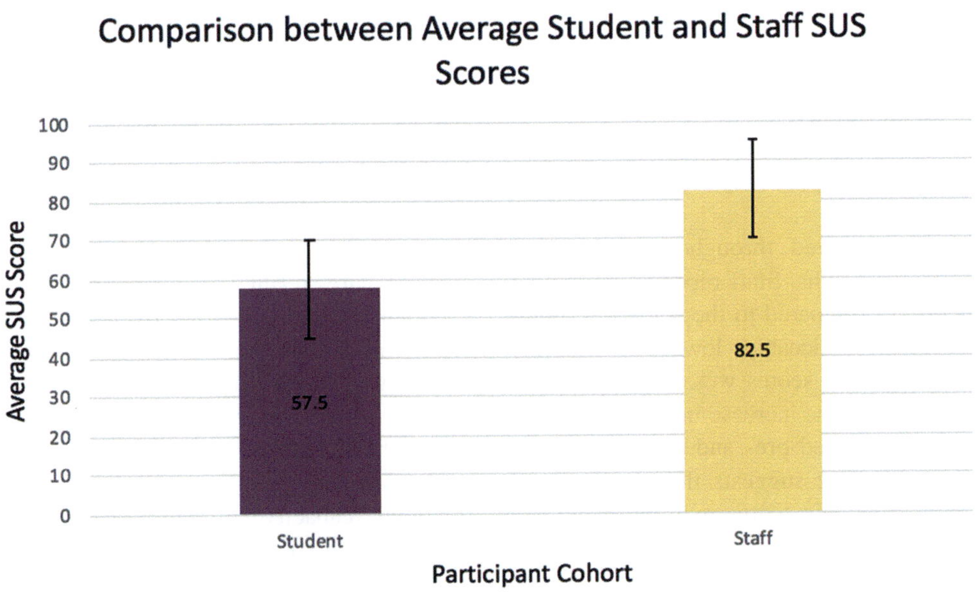

Fig. 10.8 Bar graph which represents a comparison between the student SUS score (purple) and the average of the staff SUS scores (yellow) calculated from the SUS questionnaire. Created using Microsoft Excel. Standard error bars added within Excel

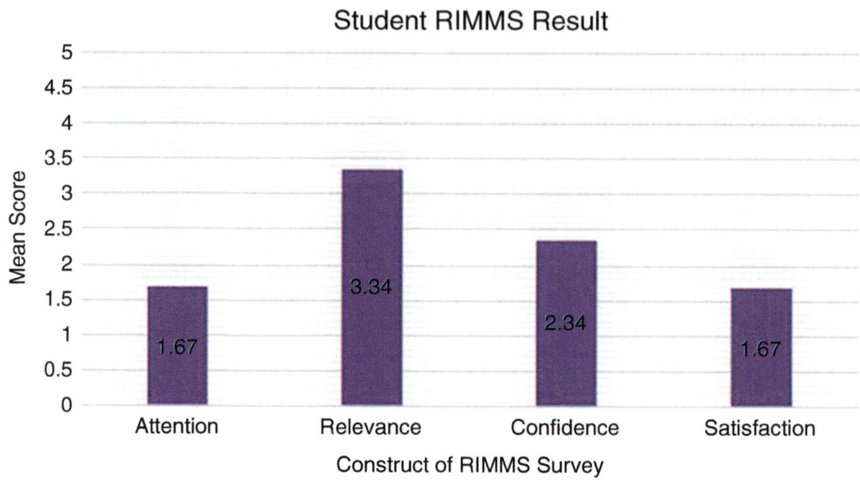

Fig. 10.9 A bar graph of the RIMMS scores for each of the four constructs assessed using the ARCS model. Created within Microsoft Excel

10.4.6.3 Motivation

The student participant reported low motivation when using the app, when questioned on each of the four main components of the RIMMS questionnaire for attention, relevance, confidence and satisfaction (ARCS). Each comprised of three questions (12 in total). The average values across each category were 1.67, 3.34, 2.34 and 1.67, respectively. Relevance was the highest-rated category at 3.34 out of 5 (see Fig. 10.9).

10.5 Discussion

10.5.1 Summary of Key Findings

The results acquired throughout user testing yielded mixed results. Staff reported more positive feedback, compared to the student response which scored noticeably lower in usability. Student motivation scores were also lower than expected, despite the increase in multiple-choice quiz results acquired pre- and post-application. This data therefore suggests that the improvement in student quiz scores may be linked to a factor other than student motivation and usability in this instance. These findings contradict most similar research (Bye et al. 2009; Yeung et al. 2011, 2012; Drapkin et al. 2015; Stepan et al. 2017); despite having no increase in student performance, usability and motivation are rated positively. This research does, however, align with the findings of Henssen et al. (2020). Open-response feedback from the student participants also highlighted that despite appreciating the integration of gross anatomy and histology, the chosen technique for this integration was not to their preference. In the future, it may be beneficial to correct the presentation of histological data within the application through the use of multi-sub-object materials within 3DS Max, allowing for the presentation of 2D data on the surface of the model as opposed to a 2D sprite overlay.

Conversely, staff participants in this research responded positively, producing higher usability scores, when compared to the students. Staff questionnaire results also implied a positive experience overall, relating to the application's style, content, appropriateness and engagement. Throughout user testing, a few similar responses were acquired across participants' open feedback. The readability of certain text within the application was reported to be difficult, and the rotational capacity of the models within the application restricted their view of the anatomy. Utilising their feedback, the informative text within the application was adjusted, improving its readability and consistency throughout the app. Unfortunately, after some difficulty, it was determined that it would not be possible under the time constraints of this research to adjust the rotation of the models within the application. Future research is needed to determine the potential reasons for the distinct contrast in student and staff feedback and to gauge whether this trend continues within a larger participant cohort.

10.5.2 'MindMap' Critical Analysis

Many challenges presented themselves throughout the development of this application. When creating the skull model from the Visible Human Dataset, the resulting mesh contained multiple unintentional holes. To resolve this, a variety of techniques were used in an attempt to bridge the gaps across 3DS Max and ZBrush; unfortunately, none were successful. Upon reflection, these holes may have been best targeted during the segmentation process in 3D Slicer. Improving the precision of the threshold value used or applying a filter to the data such as the 'Laplacian Sharpening Image Filter' may have improved the resulting skull model. Alternatively, a histogram equalisation may have been used to further improve the contrast between structures.

The nerves also proved challenging to model, due to their meandering and complex forms. Initially, it was thought that ZBrush may be used to generate organic models of the nerves; however, in practice, this proved beyond the authors' acquired skill level. The resulting methodology, as previously described, allowed for the creation of splines, although their accuracy was diminished. As this method proved time-consuming, the trigeminal and facial nerves were revoked from the application in the interest of progress.

The histology scene of this application was found to contain the only identified 'bug'. Despite the authors' awareness, the code for this interactive component remained unresolved within the final application due to the limited timeframe. Although minor, the issue was identified by participants throughout their user testing. When a single segment of the brainstem model was selected, it would trigger an animation. This animation would adjust the component's transform to a pre-determined location on the screen. Unfortunately, the component could not return automatically and would therefore require a further mouse click to trigger its reverse animation sequence—re-adjusting the segment's transformation matrix to its original position. Interestingly, despite being a flaw, some participants praised this feature as they believed, if adjusted correctly, the ability to overlap segments may be beneficial to their comprehension of internal brainstem anatomy. Future development of this application should consider the potential refinement of this feature.

10.5.3 Limitations

Firstly, it is important to address the limitation of the low participant numbers within this research ($N = 4$). From this, it is difficult to derive accurate conclusions from the data acquired. Fascinatingly, from the limited responses obtained, it was concluded that staff and student experiences differed. This result was unexpected, and its cause remains unidentified. It is difficult to determine the reliability of the concluding results; further testing is required to assess whether the student response obtained would be echoed by a larger group of students or if these results are a potential outlier. Due to the date at which this research was conducted (non-term time), student participation may improve if conducted on term time (September–May), despite its online format.

Secondly, the user testing process was restricted by an unforeseen issue. The limited access to Windows PCs or student preference for devices running Apple operating systems had not been considered. The reason for this accessibility issue remains unknown; however, improvements to the student information documentation or the use of a physical testing environment may have reduced this risk.

Next, with the online nature of this research, it was impossible to control each participant's testing conditions—resulting in a plethora of external variables which may have impacted these findings. Providing a space for participants to conduct this research may have yielded more accurate and dependable results.

Finally, as the post-application quiz results are revealed to participants after the test's completion, there runs the risk that students may potentially use these results to forge their initial test result if completed in an incorrect sequence. This risk is mitigated by the provision of the instructional document available to all student participants. From the results obtained, it is also assumed that this is unlikely, due to the alignment with the results obtained, and the expected results.

10.5.4 Future Development

Future development of this application should prioritise the creation of models for the omitted cranial nerve pathways (trigeminal and facial). Animations may also improve the engagement with this application as well as provide an extra medium from which students may utilise for their consolidation of the information presented. To improve accessibility, a toggle could be integrated into the menu panel which manages the application's colour scheme. Selection of this toggle would customise the colour scheme as required, according to each user's personal needs (for example, the use of soft and light colours may be preferred for users on the autistic spectrum). This feature would be a focal point in the future development of this application. Lastly, the inclusion of an internal quizzing system may improve student motivation as well as provide an aspect of gamification, encouraging users to return to 'MindMap' repeatedly.

10.6 Conclusion

This research aimed to develop and evaluate a novel teaching resource for cranial nerve nuclei and their pathways, in the format of an interactive online application. The main results of this research are conflicting, with staff perceiving the application more positively than the student participant. This suggests that the application did not improve student motivation to learn the cranial nerve pathways, and its format was not easy to use, which was an unexpected response. Further research is required to determine the accuracy and reliability of these results within a larger student cohort. Despite this, both groups responded positively to the idea of integration between 2D histology within 3D gross anatomy. Future research is required to gain a more complete understanding of the impacts of combined histology and gross anatomy in cranial nerve and neuroanatomical education.

References

Brooke J (1996) SUS: a "quick and dirty" usability scale. In: Jordan PW, Thomas B, McClelland IL, Weerdmeester B (eds) Usability evaluation in industry. Taylor and Francis, Boca Raton, FL, pp 189–194

Bye AM, Connolly AM, Farrar M, Lawson JA, Lonergan A (2009) Teaching paediatric epilepsy to medical students: a randomised crossover trial. J Paediatr Child Health 45(12):727–730. https://doi.org/10.1111/j.1440-1754.2009.01602.x

Chhetri SK (2017) E-learning in neurology education: principles, opportunities and challenges in combating neurophobia. J Clin Neurosci 44:80–83. https://doi.org/10.1016/j.jocn.2017.06.049

Drapkin ZA, Lindgren KA, Lopez MJ, Stabio ME (2015) Development and assessment of a new 3D neuroanatomy teaching tool for MRI training. Anat Sci Educ 8(6):502–509. https://doi.org/10.1002/ase.1509

Edwards-Bailey A, Ktayen H, Solomou G, Bligh E, Boyle A, Gharooni A-A, Lim GHT, Varma A, Standring S, Santarius T, Fountain D (2022) A survey of teaching undergraduate neuroanatomy in the United Kingdom and Ireland. Br J Neurosurg 36(1):52–57. https://doi.org/10.1080/02688697.2021.1902942

Geoghegan K, Payne DR, Myers MA, Hall S, Elmansouri A, Parton WJC, Harrison CH, Stephens J, Parker R, Rae S, Merzougui W, Nagy E, Venkatesh P, Parrott R, Border S (2019) The National Undergraduate Neuroanatomy Competition: lessons learned from partnering with students to innovate undergraduate neuroanatomy education. Neuroscientist 25(3):271–280. https://doi.org/10.1177/1073858418788000

Guberinic A, van den Elshout R, Kozicz T, ter Laan M, Henssen D (2022) Overview of the microanatomy of the human brainstem in relation to the safe entry zones. J Neurosurg 137(5):1524–1534. https://doi.org/10.3171/2022.2.JNS211997

Hall S, Stephens J, Parton W, Myers M, Harrison C, Elmansouri A, Lowry A, Border S (2018) Identifying medical student perceptions on the difficulty of learning different topics of the undergraduate anatomy curriculum. Med Sci Educ 28(3):469–472. https://doi.org/10.1007/s40670-018-0572-z

Henssen DJHA, van den Heuvel L, De Jong G, Vorstenbosch MATM, van Walsum AMC, Van den Hurk MM, Kooloos JGM, Bartels RHMA (2020) Neuroanatomy learning: augmented reality vs. cross-sections. Anat Sci Educ 13(3):353–365. https://doi.org/10.1002/ase.1912

Hernando-Requejo V (2020) Neurophobia: why, how much, consequences and solutions. MedEdPublish 9:3. https://doi.org/10.15694/mep.2020.000003.1

Iwanaga J, Loukas M, Dumont AS, Tubbs RS (2021) A review of anatomy education during and after the COVID-19 pandemic: revisiting traditional and modern methods to achieve future innovation. Clin Anat 34(1):108–114. https://doi.org/10.1002/ca.23655

Javaid MA, Chakraborty S, Cryan JF, Schellekens H, Toulouse A (2018) Understanding neurophobia: reasons behind impaired understanding and learning of neuroanatomy in cross-disciplinary healthcare students. Anat Sci Educ 11(1):81–93. https://doi.org/10.1002/ase.1711

Krähenbühl SM, Čvančara P, Stieglitz T, Bonvin R, Michetti M, Flahaut M, Durand S, Deghayli L, Applegate LA, Raffoul W (2017) Return of the cadaver. Medicine 96(29):e7528. https://doi.org/10.1097/MD.0000000000007528

Lack CM, Pena J, Grubb EXL, Shen E, Hiatt KD, Benayoun MD, Jones FS, West TG (2022) Cranial nerve anatomy using a modular and multimodal radiologic approach. MedEdPORTAL 18:11261. https://doi.org/10.15766/mep_2374-8265.11261

Loorbach N, Peters O, Karreman J, Steehouder M (2015) Validation of the instructional materials motivation survey (IMMS) in a self-directed instructional setting aimed at working with technology. Br J Educ Technol 46(1):204–218. https://doi.org/10.1111/bjet.12138

Mathiowetz V, Yu C-H, Quake-Rapp C (2016) Comparison of a gross anatomy laboratory to online anatomy software for teaching anatomy. Anat Sci Educ 9(1):52–59. https://doi.org/10.1002/ase.1528

McLachlan JC, Bligh J, Bradley P, Searle J (2004) Teaching anatomy without cadavers. Med Educ 38(4):418–424. https://doi.org/10.1046/j.1365-2923.2004.01795.x

Nowinski WL (2023) Bridging neuroradiology and neuroanatomy: NOW in BRAIN—a repository with sequences of correlated and labeled planar-surface neuroimages. Neuroradiol J 36(1):94–103. https://doi.org/10.1177/19714009221108674

Nowinski WL, Johnson A, Chua BC, Nowinska NG (2012) Three-dimensional interactive and stereotactic atlas of the cranial nerves and their nuclei correlated with surface neuroanatomy, vasculature and magnetic resonance imaging. J Neurosci Methods 206(2):205–216. https://doi.org/10.1016/j.jneumeth.2012.02.026

Pakpoor J, Handel AE, Disanto G, Davenport RJ, Giovannoni G, Ramagopalan SV (2014) National survey of UK medical students on the perception of neurology. BMC Med Educ 14(1):225. https://doi.org/10.1186/1472-6920-14-225

Pedersen K, Wilson TD, De Ribaupierre S (2013) An interactive program to conceptualize the anatomy of the internal brainstem in 3D. Stud Health Technol Inform 184:319–323

Richardson-Hatcher A, Hazzard M, Ramirez-Yanez G (2014) The cranial nerve skywalk: A 3D tutorial of cranial nerves in a virtual platform. Anat Sci Educ 7(6):469–478. https://doi.org/10.1002/ase.1445

Sawyer B, Dobres J, Chahine N, Reimer B (2020) The great typography bake-off: comparing legibility at-a-glance. Ergonomics 63(4):391–398. https://doi.org/10.1080/00140139.2020.1714748

Stepan K, Zeiger J, Hanchuk S, Del Signore A, Shrivastava R, Govindaraj S, Iloreta A (2017) Immersive virtual reality as a teaching tool for neuroanatomy. Int Forum of Allergy Rhinol 7(10):1006–1013. https://doi.org/10.1002/alr.21986

Venter G, Lubbe JC, Bosman MC (2022) Neurophobia: A side effect of neuroanatomy education? J Med Syst 46(12):99. https://doi.org/10.1007/s10916-022-01885-1

Wimsatt M, Simpson J, Morrison J, Hof P, Lein E, Gadye L, Wnuk A, Roskams J (2017) 3D-brain. Available at 3D brain (brainfacts.org) Accessed 05 Oct 2022

Yeung JC, Fung K, Wilson TD (2011) Development of a computer-assisted cranial nerve simulation from the visible human dataset. Anat Sci Educ 4(2):92–97. https://doi.org/10.1002/ase.190

Yeung JC, Fung K, Wilson TD (2012) Prospective evaluation of a web-based three-dimensional cranial nerve simulation. J Otolaryngol - Head Neck Surg = Le Journal d'oto-Rhino-Laryngologie et de Chirurgie Cervico-Faciale 41(6):426–436

GPSR Compliance

The European Union's (EU) General Product Safety Regulation (GPSR) is a set of rules that requires consumer products to be safe and our obligations to ensure this.

If you have any concerns about our products, you can contact us on ProductSafety@springernature.com

In case Publisher is established outside the EU, the EU authorized representative is:

Springer Nature Customer Service Center GmbH
Europaplatz 3
69115 Heidelberg, Germany

Batch number: 10615152

Printed by Printforce, the Netherlands